PHYSICAL THERAPY
of the LOW BACK

CLINICS IN PHYSICAL THERAPY
VOLUME 13

PHYSICAL THERAPY
of the LOW BACK

Edited by
Lance T. Twomey, PhD

Professor and Head
School of Physiotherapy
Curtin University of Technology
Shenton Park, Western Australia
Australia

James R. Taylor, MD, PhD

Senior Lecturer in Anatomy and Human Biology
University of Western Australia
Nedlands, Western Australia
Australia

CHURCHILL LIVINGSTONE
NEW YORK, EDINBURGH, LONDON, MELBOURNE
1987

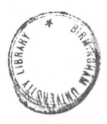

Library of Congress Cataloging-in-Publication Data

Physical therapy of the low back.

(Clinics in physical therapy ; vol. 13)
Includes bibliographies and index.

1. Backache.   2. Backache—Treatment.   3. Physical
therapy.   I. Twomey, Lance T.   II. Taylor, James R.,
Ph.D.   III. Series: Clinics in physical therapy ; v. 13.
[DNLM: 1. Backache—rehabilitation.   2. Physical
Therapy.   W1 CL831CN v.13 / WE 755 P578]
RD768.P49   1987   617'.56062   87-11654
ISBN 0-443-08493-9

1820148 2

© **Churchill Livingstone Inc. 1987**

Distributed in the United Kingdom by Churchill Livingstone,
Robert Stevenson House, 1-3 Baxter's Place, Leith Walk, Edinburgh
EH1 3AF, and by associated companies, branches, and representatives
throughout the world.

Accurate indications, adverse reactions, and dosage schedules
for drugs are provided in this book, but it is possible that they
may change. The reader is urged to review the package information
data of the manufacturers of the medications mentioned.

Acquisitions Editor: *Kim Loretucci*
Copy Editor: *Ann Ruzycka*
Production Designer: *Gloria Milner*
Production Supervisor: *Jocelyn Eckstein*

Printed in the United States of America

First published in 1987
Second printing in 1990

*To our respective wives,
Meg and Mamie*

Contributors

Nikolai Bogduk, MD, PhD
Reader in Anatomy, University of Queensland; Visiting Medical Officer to the Pain Clinic, Princess Alexandra Hospital, St. Lucia, Queensland, Australia

Brian C. Edwards, BAppSc, BSc, GradDipManTher
Specialist Manipulative Physiotherapist, Honorary Fellow, Curtin University of Technology, Shenton Park, Western Australia, Australia

Ruth Grant, MAppSc, GradDipAdvManTher
Head, School of Physiotherapy, South Australian Institute of Technology, Adelaide, South Australia, Australia

Vladimir Janda, MD, DSc
Professor of Rehabilitation Medicine, Postgraduate Medical Institute; Director, Department of Rehabilitation Medicine, Charles University Hospital, Prague, Czechoslovakia

Gwendolen A. Jull, MPThy, GradDipManTher
Senior Lecturer in Physiotherapy, University of Queensland, St. Lucia, Queensland, Australia

Colleen B. Liston, AUA
Senior Lecturer in Physiotherapy, Curtin University of Technology, Shenton Park, Western Australia, Australia

James W. Lynn, BSc(PT), GradDipManTher
Private Practitioner; Faculty, McKenzie Institute, Perth, Western Australia, Australia

Jennifer M. Lynn, PT
Private Practitioner; Faculty, McKenzie Institute, Perth, Western Australia, Australia

Janet E. Macintosh, BSc(Hons)
Department of Anatomy, University of Queensland, St. Lucia, Queensland, Australia

Geoffrey D. Maitland, MBE, MAppSc, AUA
Specialist Manipulative Physiotherapist, School of Physiotherapy, South Australian Institute of Technology, Adelaide, South Australia, Australia

Robin A. McKenzie, DipMT
Consultant in Spinal Therapy, The End Farm, Waikanae, New Zealand

Mark J. Oliver, DipPhys(NZ), DipMT(NZ)
Research Fellow, Curtin University of Technology, Shenton Park; Private Practitioner, Perth, Western Australia, Australia

James R. Taylor, MD, PhD
Senior Lecturer in Anatomy and Human Biology, University of Western Australia, Nedlands, Western Australia, Australia

Patricia H. Trott, MSc, GradDipAdvManTher
Specialist Manipulative Physiotherapist, Principal Lecturer, South Australian Institute of Technology, Adelaide, South Australia, Australia

Lance T. Twomey, PhD
Professor and Head, School of Physiotherapy, Curtin University of Technology, Shenton Park, Western Australia, Australia

Preface

Back pain is as common as headache in Western society; it is estimated that 30 to 35 percent of any large group, at any point in time, will have some degree of backache, and that 80 percent of us will suffer at least one disabling bout of back pain during our lives.[1] It is the most costly musculoskeletal disorder in Western society, both in terms of cost to the community in working days lost, and in terms of treatment costs.[2] Many occupational groups, including physical therapists, make an excellent living by treating back pain.

Physical therapy of the low back has, historically, been largely empirical in its choice of treatments. A wide variety of treatment methods and techniques have been vigorously recommended and defended by their different advocates as providing the "answer" to this very complex problem. The multiplicity of empirical treatments and the persistent and recurrent nature of the problem of back pain are both testimony to our lack of definitive success in solving this problem.

In spite of all this, the area of back pain and dysfunction has been largely neglected by biological and clinical scientists; there is still widespread ignorance of the structure and function of the vertebral column among health professionals and many of the problems of etiology and pathogenesis of back pain have been left in the "too hard basket." It is only in comparatively recent times that much of the detailed knowledge of anatomy, function, and biomechanics of the spine has been gathered to provide a much better understanding of the region than has been generally available in the past.

Against this background, this book brings together a number of largely empirical, but successful, physical therapy procedures. These procedures are successful, in our view, because of the innovative response of their proponents to the experience gained by close attention to physical diagnosis and careful clinical assessment of patients' response to treatment. We have also endeavored to bring to the attention of our readers recent advances in knowledge of the development, structure, function, and biomechanics of the low back and to apply this knowledge to the clinical techniques described, in an attempt to provide more soundly based rationales for these different approaches. Finally, we have highlighted the importance of prevention of low back pain by education, changes in lifestyle, and a more intelligent approach to work and sporting activities.

Lance T. Twomey, PhD
James R. Taylor, MD, PhD

REFERENCES

1. Nachemson A: The lumbar spine: An orthopaedic challenge. Spine 1:59, 1976
2. Kelsey J, White AA: Epidemiology and impact of low back pain. Spine 5:133, 1980

Acknowledgments

The authors wish to acknowledge the valuable assistance of Jenny Cook and Joan Reyland (secretarial), David Watkins (photography and artwork), Martin Thompson (artwork), and John Owens (technical assistance).

Contents

1 | The Lumbar Spine from Infancy to Old Age

James R. Taylor
Lance T. Twomey

Anatomy is commonly misconceived to be about knowledge that does not change from year to year gained only from the study of aged cadavers. On the contrary, there are many important "dynamic" elements in the study of anatomy, including the relation of structure to function, and the continuing changes in structure during life due to the processes of development, growth, and aging. In studies of developmental variation and aging, it is often difficult to define boundaries between normal anatomy and pathology. In addition, those anatomists with clinical and research interests cannot study variations in structure without attempting to relate them to clinical conditions although these relationships are difficult to establish. With these "dynamic" concepts in mind, this chapter has the following three sections: Functional Anatomy of the Adult Lumbar Spine; Development and Growth of the Spine and Related Pathology; and Age Changes in the Lumbar Spine.

FUNCTIONAL ANATOMY OF THE ADULT LUMBAR SPINE

The spine is the principal, central part of the axial skeleton. However, this is altogether too static a description for such a dynamic structure!

1

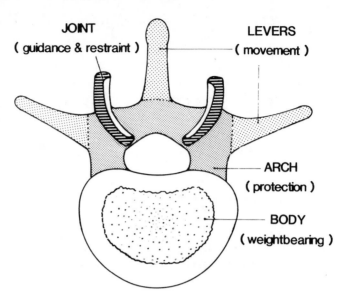

Fig. 1-1.   Diagram relating the structures of vertebral parts to their functions.

A spine made up of many parts ensures a full mobility,
Strong discs and facet joints together give a good stability.
To bend down low, the discs must have a full and free compliance,
To stand erect, good posture needs a muscle–joint alliance.

The vertebral column forms the stable but mobile axis of the human skeleton. Considering the lumbosacral spine in particular, its strength, resilience, and mobility are essential to normal human posture and activity. Its position affects the posture of the whole spine and head. Stiffness in the lumbosacral spine restricts mobility in locomotion, bending, and lifting, and many other normal, everyday activities. Lumbar spinal osteoporosis and shortening with aging allow the rib cage to abut on the pelvis, further restricting movement and respiration. A thorough knowledge of normal anatomy is essential to a study of the effects of age changes.

The functional anatomy of the human vertebral column can be conveniently summarized (Fig. 1-1) under the general headings, Anterior Elements and Posterior Elements (Table 1-1).

The functional anatomy of the lumbar spine will be described in the following sequence: *vertebrae, vertebral and intervertebral canals*, and *ligaments*, followed by the *joints–intervertebral discs and zygaphophyseal (facet) joints.*

Vertebral Bodies and Weight Bearing

In the adult male, lumbar-vertebral bodies are about 2.5 cm tall and are separated by discs about 1 cm thick. They have anteroposterior dimensions of 3 to 3.5 cm and transverse dimensions increasing from about 4 cm at L1 to

Table 1-1. A Summary of the Relation between Structure and Function

	Structure	Function
Anterior elements	Vertebral bodies	Weight bearing
	Intervertebral discs	Shock-absorbing load-bearing joints, combining strength with limited mobility
Posterior elements	Vertebral arches and associated ligaments	Protection of the spinal cord, cauda equina, meninges, and vessels
	Transverse and spinous processes	Levers for muscles
	Articular processes	Guidance and restraint of movements

about 5 cm at L5. Female dimensions are on average about 15 percent smaller than those in males. There are sex differences in vertebral body shape that will be described later. Vertebral bodies are generally said to increase in end-surface area from L1 to S1, as weight-bearing stress increases as one progresses down the column. But according to Davis,[2] end-surface area is maximal at L4. The large increase in the dimensions of the pedicles and transverse processes of L5 compensates for the reduction in its end-surface area.

A cartilage plate covers each upper and lower vertebral-body surface (cp. Fig. 1-2). This cartilage plate is surrounded at the vertebral margin by a compact rim of bone formed by the ring apophysis. A thin shell of compact bone forms the anterolateral and posterior surfaces of each kidney-shaped vertebral body. Within this shell, thin irregular beams, or *trabeculae*, of bone crisscross to form a network of cancellous bone. Vertical weight-bearing trabeculae predominate in this network (Fig. 1-2). These vertical beams are supported at regular intervals by cross-ties formed by horizontal trabeculae. Without this support, the vertical beams would buckle and fracture under loading. The fine horizontal trabeculae make the lightly built vertical beams more rigid and give the whole structure the considerable strength it needs to bear large axial loads. Red marrow fills the "honeycomb" spaces between the trabeculae in the cancellous or "spongy" bone. This composite architecture strikes a good compromise between rigidity and resilience appropriate to the intermittent increases and decreases in loading associated with many normal human activities.[3]

Vertebral Arches and "Protection"

Two *pedicles* project backward from each vertebral body, lateral to the spinal canal. They are oval in cross-section and attach to the upper lateral margins of the posterior aspect of each vertebral body. The pedicles are continuous medially around the posterior aspect of the vertebral canal with flat plates of bone called *laminae*. The pedicles and laminae form the vertebral arch, and together with the posterior surfaces of the vertebral bodies, encircle

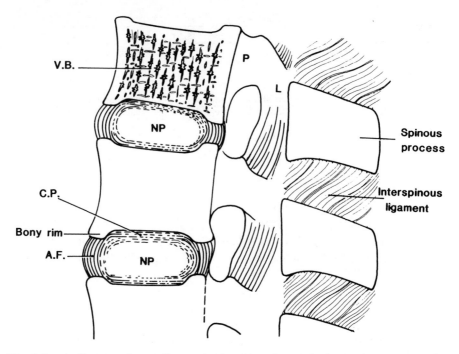

Fig. 1-2.   A diagram of a median sagittal section shows the internal structure or "architecture" of a vertebral body and an intervertebral disc. The vertebral body has vertically oriented weight-bearing, trabeculae and cross ties formed by transverse trabeculae. The intervertebral disc has a lamellar outer anulus fibrosus (AF). The inner lamellae of the anulus are continous with the lamellar structure of the cartilage plates (CP) as revealed by polarized light. The anulus and cartilage plates form an envelope enclosing the nucleus pulposus (NP). Fusion of the ring apophysis with the centrum forms the bony rim. P = pedicle; L = lamina; the interlaminar ligaments are the ligamenta flava.

the vertebral canal, protecting the lower end of the spinal cord, the *cauda equina*, and their membranes and vessels. It is possible to enter the spinal canal with a needle passed through an interlaminar space, e.g., between the laminae of L3 and L4, piercing the *ligamentum flavum* and the *dura mater* and arachnoid membranes, to enter the fluid-filled subarachnoid space.

Two transverse, one spinous and four articular processes project from each vertebral arch. In the column as a whole, the ligaments flava bridge the gaps between adjacent laminae and interspinous and supraspinous ligaments join the spinous processes. The articular processes project upward and downward from the laminae near their junction with the pedicles to form synovial zygapophyseal joints with neighboring vertebrae. Each joint is enclosed by a capsule, which is fibrous above, below, and behind and formed by the yellow, elastic ligamentum flavum in front (Fig. 1-3).

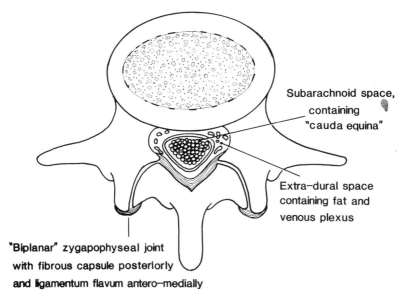

Subarachnoid space, containing "cauda equina"

Extra-dural space containing fat and venous plexus

"Biplanar" zygapophyseal joint with fibrous capsule posteriorly and ligamentum flavum antero-medially

Fig. 1-3. The appearance of the zygapophyseal (facet) joints is shown in horizontal section. The cancellous bone of the vertebral body can be seen within the compact bony ring. The contents of the vertebral canal in the lower lumbar region include the cauda equina within the dural sac. The extradural veins form a valveless venous plexus that connects regional veins outside the vertebral column with basivertebral veins at the center of each vertebral body.

The Vertebral Canal and the Intervertebral Foramen

The lumbar vertebral canal contains the lower end, or conus of the spinal cord, which terminates at the level of the L1–2 interspace, and the nerve roots or cauda equina descending to their respective intervertebral foramina. These are contained within the dural sac, which is lined internally by the arachnoid membrane. The dural sac, the arachnoid, and the subarachnoid space containing the cerebrospinal fluid extend down to the level of S2. This level may be conveniently located visually by finding the two dimples that overlie the palpable posterior superior iliac spines (Fig. 1-4). Lumbar spinous processes can be easily identified by counting up from L5 above the angular depression marking the posterior lumbosacral angle ("sacral shelf").

The spinal canal varies in size and shape according to spinal level and age. Average dimensions at the L1 level are 20 mm in the sagittal plane and 25 mm in the coronal plane.[4] The upper lumbar canal is usually oval in transverse section at L1 and triangular below this level in young people, becoming trefoil in outline in old people, especially at lower lumbar levels.[5,6] The change to a trefoil shape is due to the osteophytic overgrowth at the anterior margins of the zygapophyseal joint facets, which push the ligaments flava forwards, narrowing the lateral recesses of the canal.

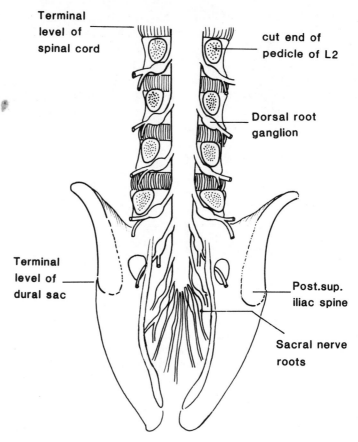

Terminal
level of
spinal cord

cut end of
pedicle of L2

Dorsal root
ganglion

Terminal
level of
dural sac

Post.sup.
iliac spine

Sacral nerve
roots

Fig. 1-4. A dorsal view of the lumbosacral spine from which the vertebral arches have been removed shows the spinal canal containing the dural sac, which terminates opposite the posterior superior iliac spines. The dura fuses with the outer fibrous covering (epineurium) of each spinal nerve as it exits the dural sac.

The regularly-spaced lateral openings from the vertebral canal, called the *intervertebral foramina*, are better described as intervertebral canals, as they range from 9 mm long at L1–2 to 2 cm long at the lumbosacral level.[1] They transmit the lumbar spinal nerves and accompanying vessels. The remainder of the space is fat-filled. The spinal nerves are formed medially within the canal by the union of multiple anterior and posterior rootlets; they pass obliquely in a downward and lateral direction through the canal. The somatic motor and sympathetic preganglionic axons pass out from the spinal cord through the anterior roots. The sensory fibers have their cell bodies in the dorsal-root ganglia and generally enter the spinal cord through the dorsal roots. Small arteries and somewhat larger veins accompany the nerves. The veins connect segmental lumbar and sacral veins to the large venous plexuses in the extradural space of the spinal canal. The tiny arteries supply the bones, meninges, and nerves and occasionally supply "feeders" to reinforce the arteries of the spinal cord.

As the nerve roots exit from the spinal canal, they are followed into the medial end of the intervertebral canal by lateral projections of the arachnoid membrane and the subarachnoid space, which end in the canal where the arachnoid is pierced by the spinal nerve and the dura fuses with its outer connective tissue covering or epineurium.[7] The lateral recesses of the subarachnoid space are closely related to the posterolateral surfaces of the intervertebral discs. Here, extruded nucleus pulposus tissue from a ruptured disc may impinge upon and deform the subarachnoid space. This would be visible on a myelogram as a "filling defect." The dorsal-root ganglion, containing the cell bodies of the sensory neurons, forms an enlargement on the posterior root just as it joins the anterior root to form the mixed spinal nerve. There is plenty of room in the normal intervertebral canal for all these structures, which descend obliquely from medial to lateral through the wider upper part of the canal, surrounded extradurally by fat, but extrusion of part of the nucleus through a ruptured anulus may entrap a spinal nerve in the canal.

The lumbar spinal nerves, containing mixed sensory and motor axons, divide into ventral and dorsal rami as soon as they pass out of the intervertebral canal. Ventral rami participate with sacral nerves in the lumbosacral plexus, forming femoral, obturator, gluteal, and sciatic nerves to supply distant lower-limb structures. The dorsal rami supply local dorsal structures including the zygapophyseal joints, postvertebral muscles, and the skin of the low back and gluteal region (Fig. 1-5). The ventral, and dorsal rami of sacral nerves exit separately through the anterior and posterior sacral foramina. The ventral rami of S1–3 groove the anterior aspect of the lateral mass of the sacrum as they pass to join the lumbosacral trunk (L4–5), which descends over the ala of the sacrum. These five spinal nerves are stretched fairly taut over the ala and anterior surface of the sacrum as they form the sciatic nerve. The sciatic nerve passes out of the pelvis through the greater sciatic notch, then over the back of the ischial spine, and behind the hip joint. When a lower-lumbar or upper-sacral nerve is entrapped by a ruptured disc, the combined hip flexion and knee extension of the straight leg raising test stretches the sciatic nerve. This pulls on the entrapped root of the sciatic nerve, eliciting pain and reflex spasm of hip extensors.

Vessels

The small artery entering each intervertebral canal from a lumbar or lateral sacral artery, divides into three branches.[8] The anterior branch supplies the vertebral bodies and discs, anastomosing with adjacent vessels above and below in a ladder pattern. The posterior branch supplies the posterior elements, and the middle radicular branch travels along and supplies the nerve roots. In the case of the upper lumbar vessels, the radicular vessels may reinforce the anterior and posterior arteries of the spinal cord. The great spinal artery (of Adamkiewicz), which supplies the lumbosacral part of the spinal cord, usually

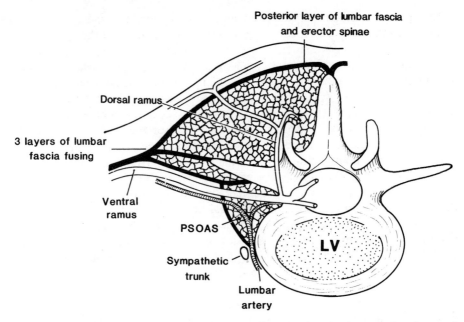

Fig. 1-5. Diagram illustrating the three layers of the lumbar fascia enclosing the quadratus lumborum in a lateral compartment and the dorsal spinal muscles in a posterior compartment (showing erector spinae and multifidus as one muscle mass). The psoas is enclosed by its own psoas fascia. The division of the spinal nerve into dorsal and ventral rami and of the dorsal ramus into medial and lateral branches is shown. (Modified from Last S: Anatomy: Regional and Applied. 2nd Ed. Churchill Livingstone, Edinburgh, 1959.)

arises from a lower posterior intercostal artery, most often T10 on the left side.[9,10]

The extradural internal vertebral venous plexus and the veins connecting the segmental lumbar and sacral veins to the internal vertebral venous plexus (see Fig. 1-3) are valveless. This system of valveless veins connects the basivertebral vein at the center of each vertebral body through the extradural internal vertebral venous plexus, and the veins passing out of the intervertebral foramina to the external vertebral venous plexus around the vertebral column. This in turn connects with body-wall veins and visceral veins in the pelvis (e.g., prostatic and vesical plexuses). These venous pathways permit transmission of any rise in intraabdominal pressure to the internal vertebral venous plexus, and they are also notoriously common routes for spread of cancer cells (e.g., from prostatic carcinoma to lumbar vertebrae), leading to pathologic fractures and vertebral collapse.

Transverse and Spinous Processes: Levers

The lumbar transverse processes project laterally from the junction of the pedicle and lamina. They tend to be long and flat (L3 is longest) with anterior and posterior surfaces. Their anterior surfaces serve as attachments to psoas and quadratus lumborum muscles. Posteriorly, the superficial, longitudinally running erector spinae and the deeper, obliquely oriented transversospinalis muscles are attached.

The transverse processes of L5 are exceptionally thick and strong because of their response to the particular stresses at the lumbosacral joint. The tendency to forward slippage of the lumbar column off the sacrum is resisted in part by the attachment of the L5 transverse processes to the iliac crests by the iliolumbar ligaments. The principal stabilizing structures at this joint are the lumbosacral zygapophyseal-joint facets and the lumbosacral intervertebral disc itself.[2]

The lumbar transverse processes are homologous with the ribs, and the small accessory tubercles behind the base of each lumbar transverse process are homologous with the thoracic transverse processes. The mamilloaccessory ligament bridges over the groove between this accessory process and the mamillary tubercle on the back of the superior articular process. This forms a little tunnel through which the medial branch of the dorsal ramus passes downward to supply the lower part of the adjacent zygapophyseal joint and descends to supply the upper part of the zygapophyseal joint below (see Ch. 3).

The lumbar spinous processes are large and hatchet-shaped, projecting straight backward in the midline from the junction of the two laminae at a level about 1 cm below the corresponding vertebral bodies. In the articulated column, there is a large squared-off hollow on each side between the transverse and spinous processes, into the angle of which the zygapophyseal joints project.

Muscles and Fasciae

The lumbar postvertebral muscle masses (erector spinae and multifidus) are larger than the space between the spinous and transverse processes. Thus the tips of the spinous processes are palpated in a longitudinal midline groove between the two muscle masses and the tips of the transverse processes lie deep to the lateral parts of the muscles. The middle layer of the lumbar fascia passes laterally from the tips of the transverse processes, separating quadratus lumborum from erector spinae, and the posterior layer of the lumbar fascia extends laterally from the tips of the spinous processes, the two layers enclosing the erector spinae and multifidus muscles (see Fig. 1-5). The term *erector spinae* is reserved for the superficial, longitudinally running fibers that span many segments. The muscle erector spinae forms a compact mass in the lumbar region and splits into three columns, the spinalis, longissimus, and iliocostalis, as it ascends into the thoracic region. Multifidus lies deep and medial to erector spinae. The fascicles of multifidus run in an oblique direction and only span two or three segments as they ascend or descend. The deeply placed zygapophyseal joints are covered by the fascicles of multifidus, which are in turn covered by the erector spinae and the posterior, aponeurotic lumbar fascia. The deeper parts of multifidus may play an important role in stabilizing the zygapophyseal joints (see Zygapophyseal (Facet) Joints). Detailed descriptions of spinal musculature appear in Chapter 4.

Ligaments

The anterior and posterior longitudinal ligaments line the anterior and posterior surfaces of the vertebral bodies and intervertebral discs. They contrast with one another in their shape and attachments. The anterior ligament is a broad, flat ribbon, attached with equal strength to both the vertebral periosteum and the anterior anulus of the disc. The posterior ligament is wide where it is strongly attached to the disc, but narrow where it is separated from the back of the vertebral body by a space containing blood vessels.

The ligaments of the posterior elements are functionally more important than those of the anterior elements. The posterior elements are "discontinuous", with spaces between the laminae and spaces between the spinous processes. The ligaments bridging these spaces provide continuity between these parts of the posterior elements. These ligaments and the good fit of the zygapophyseal joint facets, guide and restrain intervertebral movements.

Ligamenta Flava

These elastic ligaments, which are thickest in the lumbar region and about 2 mm thick at lumbosacral levels in adults, pass vertically between adjacent laminae. With the laminae, they form the posterior boundary of the vertebral canal. Each ligament also forms the anteromedial capsule of a zygapophyseal joint (see Figs. 1-2 and 1-3), and extends laterally around the anterior margin of each superior articular facet to form part of the posterior boundary of the intervertebral foramen. Where the ligamenta flava form part of the posterior boundary of the vertebral canal, their elasticity maintains the smooth regular outline of the dural sac during movement and in all postures of the vertebral column. With the other posterior ligaments, which are more obliquely oriented (see Fig. 1-2), the ligamenta flava are "put on the stretch" by flexion. The ligaments therefore provide some protection to the mobile segment. Since the ligamenta flava are the strongest of the posterior ligaments, their protective effect would be greatest. However, the ligaments collectively are less important than the zygapophyseal joints in restraining or limiting lumbar-spinal flexion.[11] The lumbar ligamenta flava are said to thicken with age and lose some of their elasticity.[12,13] Part of the apparent thickening is due to bony hypertrophy of the anterior margins of the zygapophyseal joint facets beneath the ligaments.

Supraspinous and Interspinous Ligaments

The supraspinous ligaments and most of the interspinous ligaments are collagenous, reinforced by the most medial fibers of insertion of the erector spinae. The supraspinous ligaments do not extend below L5 except as fibrous muscle insertions. The interspinous ligaments run obliquely upward and backward from one spinous process to the one above as a double layer with a narrow

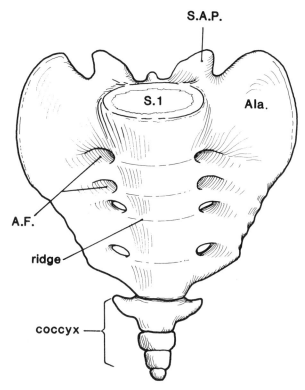

Fig. 1-6.   Anterior and superior surfaces of a female sacrum. The superior articular process (SAP) of S1 and the anterior sacral foramina (AF) which transmit the ventral rami of sacral spinal nerves are designated. The ridges mark the positions of fusion between the five centra forming the central part of the sacrum. The ala, or upper end of the sacral lateral mass, is crossed by the lumbosacral trunk as it descends to form the sciatic nerve with S1, S2, and S3.

space in between. Their anterior parts are continous with the ligamenta flava and contain elastic fibers. All appear designed to limit flexion,[14] but posterior release experiments[11] suggest that their capacity to do so is limited.

Sacrum and Sacroiliac Joints

Five centra fuse to form the central part of the sacrum, which contains remnants of intervertebral discs enclosed by bone. The transverse elements fuse to form the alae and lateral masses. The sacrum is triangular with its base above and anterior and its apex below and posterior. The anterior surface is relatively smooth, with transverse ridges at the positions where the discs would have been, and anterior sacral foramina lateral to these ridges, between the fused bodies and the lateral masses (Fig. 1-6). On the rough posterior surface, spinous processes form a midline spinous crest, and articular processes are

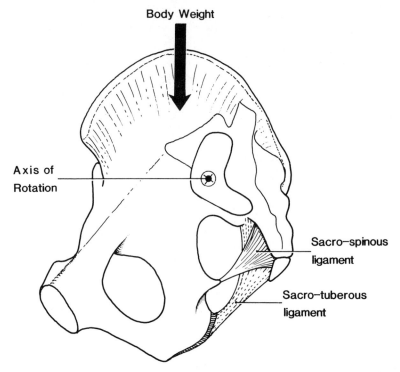

Fig. 1-7. Diagram illustrating how body weight, acting through the lumbar vertebral column, would tend to rotate the sacrum forwards if its lower end were not "anchored" by the sacrospinous and sacrotuberous ligaments. The ligaments resist the anterior rotational effect of body weight.

represented by articular crests. The posterior foramina lie lateral to the articular crests and medial to the crest marking the lateral extremity of the posterior surface.

On each lateral sacral surface, two areas can be distinguished. The rough posterior area is for the attachment of the enormously strong sacroiliac ligaments, which suspend the sacrum between the two ilia. The smooth anterior area is the articular surface of the sacroiliac joint. The superior surface of the S1 vertebral body of the sacrum bears the weight of the head, trunk, and upper limbs, transmitted through the lumbar vertebral column. This axial force would tend to rotate the sacrum forward, but this tendency is resisted by the sacrotuberous and sacrospinous accessory ligaments (Fig. 1-7), which bind the lower parts of the sacrum and coccyx down to the lower parts of the hip bones. Equally important in preventing or reducing sacroiliac movement, are the reciprocal irregularities of the adult joint surfaces together with the great strength of the posterior and interosseous sacroiliac ligaments (Fig. 1-8). These ear-shaped or C-shaped articular surfaces are smooth and flat in the child, where some "nutation" or rotary movement in the sagittal plane is possible. They

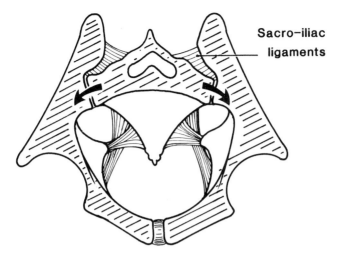

Fig. 1-8. The sacrum is "suspended" between the two ilia by very strong posterior sacroiliac ligaments. Body weight tends to compress the ilia against the sacrum at the sacroiliac joints.

become irregular in the mature adult due to the growth of a ridge or ridges on the iliac surfaces. This makes movement almost impossible in most adults.[15,16] In young females, 8 degrees of movement is said to be possible[17], and in some females, particularly during pregnancy, there is a degree of ligamentous laxity, probably due to the effect of the hormone relaxin on fibrous tissues.

Bilateral differences in sacroiliac joint posture are sometimes seen on radiographs of adolescents who have a leg length discrepancy. Pelvic torsion occurs when one sacroiliac joint is rotated more than the other and a "step" is apparent between the right and left pubic bones on the anteroposterior radiograph.[18,19]

Joints: Mobility with Stability

The multisegmental construction of the spine combines strength with stability. The lumbar vertebral column is required to provide stability in load bearing and a wide range of mobility. Mobility and stability are usually in inverse proportion to each other, but these two apparently contradictory requirements are achieved in the lumbar vertebral column by virtue of its multisegmental construction. Each mobile segment, consisting of one intervertebral disc and two zygapophyseal joints, has only a limited range of movement and therefore remains stable. However, five mobile segments together provide large ranges of sagittal and coronal plane movement, plus some axial rotation.

Articular Triad

The intervertebral disc and its two associated synovial joints combine in a unique way to enhance the strength of the mobile segment, but at the same time provide it with adequate mobility.

The Intervertebral Disc. The disc provides enough strength and stiffness for stability, but by its thickness gives enough compliance for a useful movement range. It is a structure of unique simplicity in concept, but with a complexity of fine structure in its parts. Though generally described as formed by the *anulus fibrosus* and the *nucleus pulposus*, it should be regarded functionally as including the *cartilage plates*, which bind and unite it to the vertebral bodies above and below. It is not generally realized that the cartilage plates and the anulus fibrosus form a continuous envelope enclosing the nucleus pulposes (see Fig. 1-2).

The anulus fibrosus consists of about 12 to 16 concentric lamellae, the outer lamellae being fibrous and the inner ones fibrocartilaginous. These have an outwardly convex arrangement around the circumference of the nucleus and are arranged in spiralling sheets. The parallel fibers of each successive sheet of collagen bundles, cross the fibers of the next sheet at an interstriation angle of about 57 degrees.[20] The arrangement is not unlike that of the layering of an onion. In the intervertebral disc the arrangement gives the anulus great strength. The outer fibrous lamellae of the anulus are firmly embedded in the bony vertebral rim. The inner fibrocartilaginous lamellae of the anulus are shown by polarized light studies[21] (see Figs 1-2 and 1-15) to be directly continuous with the horizontal lamellae of the "hyaline" cartilage plates above and below the nucleus. The inextensible but deformable envelope formed by the anulus and the cartilage plates encloses the elliptical sphere, which is the nucleus pulposus.

The cartilage plates not only form an essential part of the envelope containing the nucleus, they are also firmly bound to the end-surface of the vertebral body, of which they are developmentally a part. In the growing individual, growth plates at the junction of the bony vertebral body and the cartilage plate ensure growth in vertebral height. The cartilage plates are best regarded, not as belonging to the disc or as a part of the vertebra, but as the part where the two structures interlock.

The infant nucleus pulposus is a viscous-fluid structure with a clear, watery matrix.[21] Its appearance and consistency are quite changed in the adult when the nucleus contains many randomly oriented collagen bundles, has a reduced water content, and is difficult to dissect clear of its envelope. However, the healthy adult nucleus still behaves hydrostatically as a viscous fluid, which is incompressible and changes shape freely.[22] By changing shape the disc acts as a joint; by receiving axial loads and redistributing them outwards to the anulus, vertebral rims, and cartilage plates, it acts as a shock absorber. In this way, it dissipates vertical forces a horizontal directions.

The outer layers of the anulus are innervated, but no nerves penetrate beyond its outer third; no nerves have been demonstrated in the nucleus or the cartilage plates.[23–25] The outer anulus and cartilage plates are quite vascular in the fetus and infant, but vascularity is progressively reduced with maturation.[21] In the adult a few vessels penetrate the calcified cartilage layer binding the cartilage plate to the bony centrum and a few small blood vessels persist in the surface layers of the anulus.[26–28] The avascular nucleus contains a sparse cell population in a watery matrix rich in glycosaminoglycans (GAGs). The sparse cell population of the adult nucleus receives its nutrition by diffusion from the surrounding envelope (i.e., from the few vessels in the outer anulus) and from the vascular buds that extend into the cartilage plates for a short distance from the vertebral marrow-spaces.[28]

The nucleus is held under tension within the envelope formed by the anulus and cartilage plates. This tension, or turgor is dependent on the inextensibility of the envelope, and is produced by the chemical force resulting from the water-attracting capacity of the GAG macromolecules. These macromolecules "imbibe" water when the disc is not mechanically compressed (e.g., in recumbent posture when the disc tends to swell) and lose some of it during the course of each day when the disc is compressed by axial loading and "creeps" to become slightly thinner. Thus all individuals lose height due to axial weight bearing during the day, and regain height when recumbent at night.[21]

Zygapophyseal (Facet) Joints. Further stability is provided by the guiding and restraining mechanism of the two zygapophyseal joints, which permit movement to occur in the sagittal and coronal planes, restrain axial rotation, and bring flexion to a halt at the end of the physiologic range.[11,29,30] They protect the intervertebral disc from excessive strain and also widen the weight-bearing base. In normal, erect posture they bear a significant proportion (about 20 percent) of axial loading.[22] This weight-bearing function is larger in the flexed spine, particularly when lifting loads.

Joint Anatomy

The zygapophyseal joints are formed between the medially facing superior articular processes and the laterally facing inferior articular processes of the vertebra above. They are generally described as plane synovial joints, i.e., flat, but the superior articular facet is usually concave in the horizontal plane, enclosing the smaller convex inferior articular facet. Both articular surfaces are vertically oriented, so that they resemble segments of the surface of a cylinder. From the functional point of view, it is best to consider them as biplanar (see Fig. 1-3), with a small anterior coronal component, which controls flexion, and a larger posterior sagittal component, which controls and restrains rotation (Fig. 1-9). Not infrequently they have two distinct parts meeting at an angle greater than 90 degrees and in transverse sections, the joints resemble a boomerang. The sagittal component is largest in L1-2 and the coronal component is largest in L5-S1, with a gradual change in orientation from above down. The upper lumbar joints are also the joints that best show the biplanar or curved

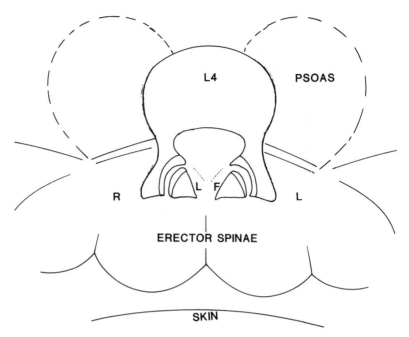

Fig. 1-9.   This tracing from a CT scan shows soft-tissue outlines of psoas, lateral and medial parts of erector spinae, and the outlines of the L3-4 zygapophyseal joints. The "joint space" (articular cartilage) and the compact bone of the subchondral bone plate with its coronal and sagittal components are distinguished. LF = ligamentum flavum.

nature of the facets, while the lower joints are more often truly planar (Fig. 1-10).

The joint is enclosed by a fibrous capsule posteriorly, and by the elastic ligamentum flavum, which forms the anteromedial capsule (see Fig. 1-3). The posterior capsule is frequently directly continuous with the posterior margin of the articular cartilage lining the concave superior articular facet. This gives the appearance of the capsule extending the concave socket with which the convex inferior facet articulates. The capsule is not tight posteriorly, depending on multifidus for "tensioning" (Fig. 1-11), and it is quite loose above and below at the superior and inferior joint recesses.[31] A neurovascular bundle lies close to, and may be seen entering, each joint recess where a large synovial-lined fat-pad lining the inside of the fibrous capsule extends for a short distance between the articular surfaces. These vascular fat-pads are mainly space fillers in the young, adapting easily to the changing shape of the joint cavity in movement, but in older people, they become fibrous at the tips where they have been repeatedly compressed between the articular surfaces.[32] A variety of synovial, fibrofatty, or fibrous fringes extend around each joint as space fillers extending from a base on the articular capsule to an apex projecting between the articular surfaces. The fat-pads in the articular recesses of the lower lumbar and lumbosacral joints are particularly large, and current investigations in our

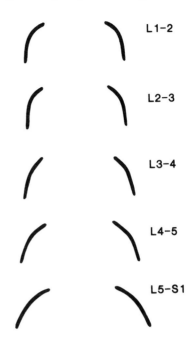

Fig. 1-10. The segmental variation in the orientation of lumbar zygapophyseal-joint planes is shown based on tracings from CT scans. It should be noted that there is a good deal of variation in structure between individuals. (Taylor JR, Twomey LT: Structure, function, and age changes in the lumbar zygapophyseal joints. Spine 11:739, 1986.)

laboratories show that, contrary to popular belief[33], these are innervated by small nerves that are probably sensory, as well as vasomotor.[34]

A vertical lip close to the posterior articular margin of each superior articular process, termed the mamillary tubercle, is formed by a lumbar attachment of multifidus. A lumbar fascicle of multifidus descends from the base of a spinous process two segments above, to the lateral margin of each joint (see Fig. 1-11). It uses this attachment to control joint posture, and maintain congruity in the posterior sagittal component of the zygapophyseal joint.[31] This action is analogous to the rotator-cuff function at the shoulder joint. Like the rotator-cuff muscles, multifidus is partly inserted into the joint capsule. Observations on postmortem lumbar spines suggest that its activity is essential to maintenance of joint congruity, since the capsule is slack and the joint gapes open posteriorly when the muscle is removed.[29,31]

The sagittal component of the joints appears well designed to block axial rotation around the usual axis of rotation near the posterior surface of the intervertebral disc, but some axial rotation is possible, as measurement studies show.[35] The function of the coronally oriented anterior components of the joints in limiting flexion is less well known. Posterior-release studies show that loading of these joints by the forward translational component of flexion is more important than tension in the posterior ligaments in bringing flexion to a halt.[1] The selective nature of age changes in the coronal components of the joints confirm that these are subject to greater compressive loading than the sagittal components.[31]

Lumbosacral Joints.   The anterior surface of the sacrum is normally in-

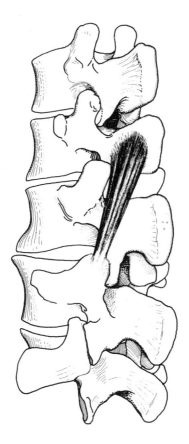

Fig. 1-11. Based on dissection studies, a single fascicle of the lumbar multifidus is shown descending from the spinous process of L2 to the mamillary tubercle on the superior articular process of L4, with some capsular insertion at the superior part of the L3-4 joint. This is one unit of a larger, more complex muscle, which is the lumbar representative of the transversospinalis muscle group. This fascicle is capable of both extension and rotation at the two mobile segments it crosses, but it is probably a fixator or stabilizer; a rotator-cuff muscle at the L3-4 zygapophyseal joint. This view contrasts with most textbook descriptions. (Taylor JR, Twomey LT: Structure, function, and age changes in the lumbar zygopophyseal joints. Spine 11:739, 1986.)

clined at an angle of about 60 degrees to the vertical plane, giving a sharp change in direction from the approximately vertically oriented lumbar spine. This angulation involves a division of the vertical weight-bearing force through the lumbar spine into two vectors, one obliquely downward and backward through the sacrum, and the other obliquely downward and forward parallel to the upper surface of S1. There is considerable shearing stress through the lumbosacral joints due to the anteriorly directed vector of the vertical weight-bearing force.[2] This shearing force is resisted by: (1) the lumbosacral intervertebral disc; (2) the two lumbosacral zygapophyseal joints; and (3) the iliolumbar ligaments.

The "line of force" transmission to the lumbosacral facets passes through the *pars interarticularis* of L5, a narrow isthmus of bone between its superior and inferior articular facets. Since this is the weakest link in the chain, it is the part most likely to break under stress. This is quite common and is called *spondylolysis*. The lumbar column, is now supported by ligamentous structures only, principally the lumbosacral disc. It may slip forwards (*olisthesis*) due to creep, stretch, and damage to the tissues of the disc. The displacement is termed *spondylolisthesis*.

Spondylolisthesis is more likely to follow spodylolysis in young people (under 25 years) with compliant discs, than in older people with stiff discs. Spondylolysis is not the only possible result of the particular stresses at the lumbosacral joints and in the lower lumbar spine. Degenerative changes in the lumbosacral articular triad and in the L4-5 articular triad are also common. Intervertebral disc rupture with nuclear extrusion is most common in the lowest two intervertebral discs[36], and zygapophyseal joint arthritis is also most common in the lumbosacral joints.[37]

DEVELOPMENT AND GROWTH OF THE LUMBAR SPINE AND RELATED PATHOLOGY

General Principles

The processes of development and growth influence structure, function, and pathology of the lumbar vertebral column in a number of important areas. Malformations result from abnormal genetic, chemical, or mechanical influences on growth.

By growth we mean measurable increase in size. This involves increase in cell numbers and cell size, increased production of matrix and fibers, or any combination of these. Prenatal growth is characterized by cell multiplication and postnatal growth principally, but not entirely, by increases is cell size and cell products. Development also involves differentiation of cells (i.e., cells become more specialized and less versatile in their function as they multiply). Connective tissue cells have a self-differentiating capacity depending on their genetic program, position in the developing embryo, and contact and interaction with other cells or tissues and on local and systemic hormonal influences. Some cells produce diffusible chemical substances, which influence the development of neighboring tissues. Other tissues influence the development of neighboring tissues by mechanical pressure, but the control mechanisms for many aspects of growth are still incompletely understood.[38]

Summary of Early Development

Before there is any vertebral column, in the third week of embryonic life the axis of the flat embryonic disc is determined by the appearance and growth of the notochord between the ectoderm and the endoderm. The appearance and growth of the notochord defines the axis of the flat embryonic disc, and it can now be described as having headward and tailward ends. At about the same time, mesoderm, the third primary layer of the embryo, develops on each side of the notochord, between the ectoderm and the endoderm.

The notochord is a long, thin rod of primitive cells, which have the potential to influence the development of other cells around them. They induce thickening of the ectoderm dorsally to begin neural tube formation, and attract the

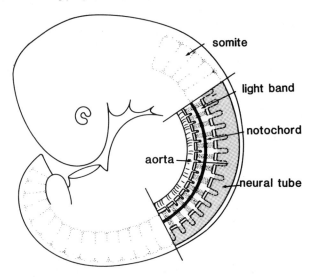

Fig. 1-12. A diagram of a 7 mm crown–rump length (CRL) human embryo shows somites on the external surface. The center section shows median plane axial structures at the blastemal stage of vertebral development. The intersegmental branches of the aorta pass around the light bands, which are the promordia of the vertebral bodies. Neural processes grow around the neural tube to form the vertebral arches. The cylindrical notochord (black) passes through the centers of the light bands (primitive vertebrae) and dark bands (primitive intervertebral discs). (Taylor JR, Twomey LT: The role of the notochord and blood vessels in vertebral column development and in the aetiology of Schmorl's nodes. Ch. 2. In Grieve GP (ed): Modern Manual Therapy of the Vertebral Column. Churchill Livingstone, Edinburgh, 1986.)

migration and condensation of mesodermal cells around them in order to form the blastemal vertebral column.

The ectodermal thickening appears dorsal to the notochord and folds longitudinally to form the neural tube. The columns of mesoderm alongside these primary axial structures are the paraxial mesoderm. The notochord, the neural tube, and the columns of paraxial mesoderm on each side of them, are essential for the formation of the vertebral column. Both the notochord and the neural tube have the potential to induce formation of a blastemal vertebral column around them from the surrounding mesoderm. As the embryo grows, it folds and bends; the transverse folding of the flat disc encloses the endoderm to form a primitive gut tube and the longitudinal bending forms a ventral concavity with the primitive axial structures curved in a bow around the gut tube. The paraxial mesoderm alongside the notochord and neural tube segments into a large number of somites or blocks of mesoderm. These blocks are destined to form a vertebral column with its associated muscles around the notochord and neural tube. Anterior to these structures, the primitive aorta runs down in the midline with blood already circulating to the area where the blastemal vertebral column will be formed (Fig. 1-12).

Three Developmental Stages

The vertebral column will pass through three developmental stages designated the blastemal stage, the cartilaginous stage, and the osseous stage.

Blastemal Stage

The blastemal or mesenchymal column is formed around the notochord by the mesoderm from the ventromedial portions of the somites.[39-42] Although formed from segmented mesoderm, this original mesodermal condensation around the notochord is continuous and unsegmented. It resegments into alternate light and dark bands all the way along its length. Neural processes grow around the neural tube from each light band. The aorta, which lies immediately in front of the blastemal column, sends intersemental branches around the middle of each light band. The light bands grow in height four times more rapidly than the adjacent dark bands.

Cartilaginous Stage

Each light band with its associated neural processes differentiates into a cartilaginous vertebra at the beginning of the fetal stage of development (2 months gestation). This differentiation takes place throughout all the tissue of the light band at about the same time.[41] There is no evidence that there are two centers of chondrification as described by Schmorl and Junghanns.[43] The rapid differentiation and growth of the fetal cartilage models of vertebral bodies is accompanied by notochordal segmentation (Fig. 1-13). Each notochordal segment will form a nucleus pulposus at the center of a dark band.[21] At the periphery of this primitive intervertebral disc, fibroblasts and collagen bundles appear in lamellar form. The cartilaginous stage of vertebral development is a short one. Soon, blood vessels grow into the cartilaginous vertebra, as centers of ossification appear.

Osseous Stage

Three primary centers of ossification are formed in each vertebra. Bilateral centers for the vertebral arch appear first, one for each half arch. The earliest vertebral-arch centers are in the cervicothoracic region, but the process rapidly extends up and down the column. The appearance of arch centers is generally sequential, with the most caudal appearing last, except that the appearance of midthoracic centers is delayed till all lumbar centers have appeared.[44] A single primary center for each vertebral body, forms the *centrum*. There is no evidence that double centers appear in normal development of the centra, but a bilobed appearance is common in vertical sections through the plane of the

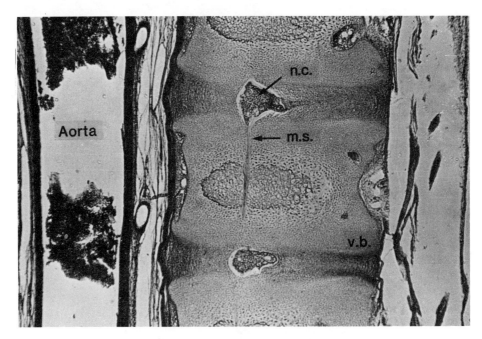

Fig. 1-13. Diagram of a median sagittal section of the thoracic spine of a 75 mm CRL (11th week) human fetus shows the cartilaginous stage of vertebral column development. At the center of each cartilage model of a vertebral body, calcified zones with hypertrophied chondrocytes herald the formation of centers of ossification (centra). The dark anterior rim around the calcified zone represents the first bone formation within the vertebral body. Vascular buds are seen within the posterior parts of the cartilaginous vertebrae. The notochord has segmented into notochordal aggregations (*nc*), which will each form a nucleus pulposus. All that remains of the notochordal track through the vertebra is the mucoid streak (*ms*).

notochord, due to a temporary inhibition of ossification in the immediate vicinity of the notochord.[21,45] The centra appear earliest near the thoracolumbar junction and then appear in sequence up and down the column.

The process of ossification extends through the cartilage model of each vertebra except for Growth plates, which persist to ensure continuing growth, and cartilage plates, which persist permanently on the upper and lower vertebral surfaces.

Dorsal–Midline Growth Plate.   A single growth plate in the midline dorsally between the two 'half-arches' (Fig. 1-14), persists till about 1 year postnatally.

Neurocentral Growth Plates.   These persist on each side, between the arch and the centrum, until 3 to 7 years, ensuring adequate growth of the vertebral canal to accommodate continuing growth of the spinal cord and cauda equina.

Cartilage-Plate Growth Plates.   Growth plates at the upper and lower (cephalic and caudal) surfacs of the centrum remain till completion of growth in height of the vertebra. These growth plates form parts of the cartilage plates capping the cephalic and caudal surfaces of each vertebral body (Fig. 1-15).

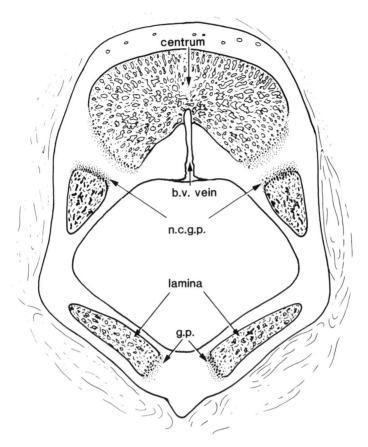

Fig. 1-14. This tracing of a horizontal section of a human fetal lumbar vertebra (28.5 cm CRL, 32nd week) shows the centrum and vertebral arches and the growth plates (*ncgp*) between the centrum and the arches and between the two halves of the arch (*gp*). There is only one center of ossification for each side of the vertebral arch, but the plane of the section has missed the middle part of each half arch.

The other part of each cartilage plate (see Fig. 1-2) persists unossified through-out life, except for a bony rim around its peripheral margin. The bony rims, or ring apophyses, can be clearly seen on lateral radiographs of the spines of older children and adolescents. They appear between 9 and 12 years, and fuse with the vertebral bodies at 18 to 20 years in males,[46] and 2 years earlier in females (Fig. 1-16). An apophysis is comparable to an epiphysis, except that it does not itself contribute to growth.[39]

Growth in Length of the Vertebral Column as a Whole

Growth is most rapid prenatally, decreasing exponentially throughout in-fancy and childhood. Sitting height and thoracolumbar spine length have been used as measures of postnatal growth in length of the spine.[29] The spine con-

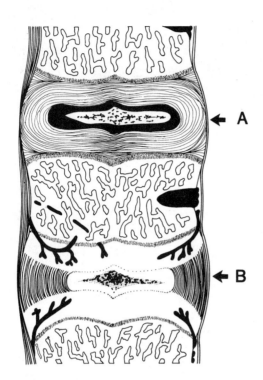

Fig. 1-15. (A) The intervertebral disc as it would appear in the median section of a full-term fetus when viewed by polarized light. There is direct continuity of the inner two-thirds of the anulus with the similar lamellar structure of the cartilage plates. (B) The outlines of the blood vessels supplying the lower disc as seen by normal transmitted light. The angular indentations of the cartilage plates from the nucleus pulposus are at the points where the notochordal track originally passed through the column. The growth plates of the cranial and caudal surfaces of the vertebral bodies may be seen. The black area at the posterior vertebral margin is the basivertebral vein. (Taylor JR, Twomey LT: The role of the notochord and blood vessels in vertebral column development and in the aetiology of Schmorl's nodes. Ch. 2. In Grieve GP (ed): Modern Manual Therapy of the Vertebral Column. Churchill Livingstone, Edinburgh, 1986.)

tributes 60 percent of sitting height. Sitting-height growth rate declines from 5 cm per annum in the second year of life, to 2.5 cm per annum at 4 years. It remains steady at this rate till 7 years, then declines further to 1.5 cm per annum just before adolescence. The adolescent growth spurt for the spine begins at 9 years in females, lasting till 14 years, and peaking at 12 years with a sitting-height growth velocity of 4 cm per annum. In males the growth spurt lasts from 12 to 17 years with a peak growth velocity of 4 cm per annum at 14 years.

Growth spurts in the thoracolumbar spine begin slightly earlier than for sitting height as a whole, and regional growth varies in that the lumbar spine grows more rapidly than the thoracic spine before puberty, but the thoracic spine grows more rapidly after puberty. The cervical and sacral regions mature latest.

Growth in length of the thoracolumbar spine is 60 percent more rapid in the female than in the male between the ages of 9 and 13 years (Fig. 1-17). After this the male spine grows more rapidly, but in adult females, the spine usually forms a greater proportion of the total stature than in males. Sitting height and thoracolumbar spine length both reach 99 percent of their maxima

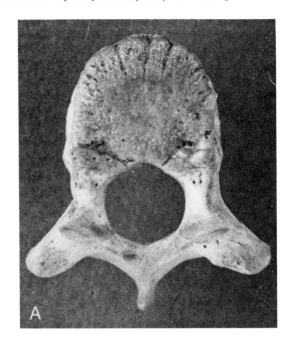

Fig. 1-16. (A,B) The superior and anterior surfaces, respectively, of a juvenile thoracic vertebra show the radial grooves due to the cartilage-plate blood vessels (see **Fig. 1-15B**). The lines of neurocentral fusion can also be seen in part A. (C) A young adult vertebra shows the ring apophysis fusing with the centrum. Small foramina for vascular canals run between the apophysis and the centrum. (Taylor JR, Twomey LT: The role of the notochord and blood vessels in vertebral column development and in the aetiology of Schmorl's nodes. Ch. 2. In Grieve GP (ed): Modern Manual Therapy of the Vertebral Column. Churchill Livingstone, Edinburgh, 1986.)

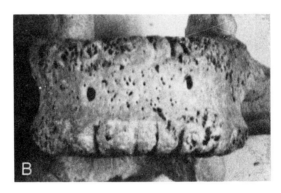

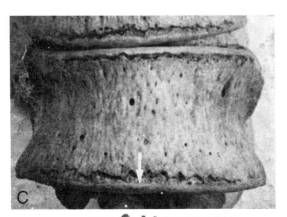

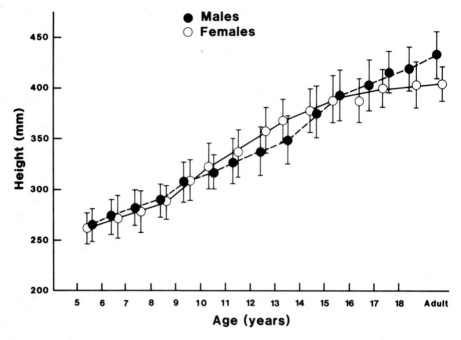

Fig. 1-17. Graphs show cross-sectional data for male and female growth in thoraco-lumbar spine length based on measurements in 1500 subjects.

by 15 years in girls and 17 years in boys, but individual variation is so wide that Risser's sign is used to judge individual completion of spinal growth. Risser's sign involves lateral appearance, medial excursion, and then fusion of the iliac apophyses. The whole process takes about 2 years from first appearance to fusion of the apophysis.[29]

Control Mechanisms in Normal and Abnormal Development

Notochordal, Neural, Vascular, and Mechanical Influences

A summary of normal and abnormal aspects of development follows:

1. The notochord and neural tube together induce formation of the blastemal vertebral column around them from the mesenchyma of the adjacent somites.[21]
2. Segmentation of the mesenchymal column is probably determined by the regular arrangement of intersegmental arteries within it.[47]
3. Anomalous development of the notochord or of segmental blood vessels is associated with developmental anomalies of the vertebral column.[29]
4. The notochord forms the original nucleus pulposus, but after rapid

growth in fetal life and infancy, notochordal tissue in the nucleus atrophies and disappears during childhood.[21]

5. Persistence of live notochord cells in vertebrae may lead to the formation of *chordomas* in adults.[21] These rare, malignant tumors are usually seen at the cephalic and caudal ends of the original notochord track, i.e., in a high retropharyngeal or sacrococcygeal situation.

6. Normal attrition (disappearance) of the notochordal track and of vascular canals from the cartilage plates of developing vertebrae leave weak areas, which are the sites of potential prolapse of disc material[40] into vertebral bodies (*Schmorl's nodes*).

7. Growth of the spinal cord and cauda equina influence growth of the vertebral arches and canal, just as brain growth is the most important influence on skull-vault growth. An enlarged spinal cord would result in an enlarged canal.[48] *Spina bifida* is a developmental anomaly, which varies from simple splitting of the skeletal elements of the vertebral arch (*spina bifida occulta*), which is common and innocuous, to complete splitting of skin, vertebral arch, and underlying neural tube (rachischisis) with associated neurologic deficits. In the more severe forms, abnormal development of the neural tube is probably the primary event, and the skeletal defects are secondary.[48]

8. Asymmetric growth of right and left halves of the vertebral arches is very common. It results in unequal pedicle lengths, producing slight rotation of the anterior elements away from the longer pedicle. This probably determines the laterality (direction of curvature) of both physiologic scoliosis and of progressive forms of scoliosis.[44]

9. Growth in lumbar zygapophyseal joint facets, changes them from a planar–coronal orientation in infants, to a biplanar or curved orientation, predominantly in the sagittal plane, in older children and adults. The coronal and sagittal components of the joint facets have different functions in controlling movements.[29,31]

10. Assumption of the erect posture in infants is associated with an increase in the lumbosacral angle, increased lordosis, related changes in the shapes of intervertebral discs, and the position of the nuclei pulposi. There are related changes in the shape of the vertebral bodies, which increase their anteroposterior growth rate, and of the vertebral end-plates. These vertebral end-plates are convex in fetal and infant vertebrae, and become concave in children, adolescents, and adults. The effect of the nucleus pulposus in weight bearing is important in this regard, as the end-plate concavity is opposite the maximum bulge of the nucleus.[49] Asymmetric weight bearing, as in leg-length discrepancy, is associated with asymmetric concavities in the vertebral end-plates.

11. Sexual dimorphism in vertebral-body shape and vertebral-column posture develops in later childhood and adolescence in association with different hormonal influences and differences in muscle development.[50] These differences contribute to the greater prevalence of progressive scoliosis in females than in males.

12. Deformity of the vertebral end-plates in adolescence associated with

multiple Schmorl's nodes, is related to the development of Scheuermann's disease.[29]

Some of these topics will be discussed in more detail below.

Segmentation, Segmental, and Other Vertebral Anomalies

Normal Segmentation. A condensation of mesenchyma is formed around the notochord by the medial migration of cells from the ventromedial portions of the somites, termed *sclerotomes*. The perichordal blastemal column formed from these segmented blocks of mesoderm is continuous and unsegmented. It resegments into alternate light and dark bands in such a way that the light bands, which will form cartilaginous vertebrae, are at the level of the inter-segmental branches of the aorta (see Fig. 1-12). Thus the muscles, derived from the remaining tissue of the adjacent somites, termed *myotomes*, alternate with the skeletal elements and are attached to upper- and lower-vertebral borders, rather than the middle of the vertebrae. This alternation of muscle and bone is essential to the proper function of the locomotor system.[41]

The intersegmental branches of the dorsal aorta have an important influence in vertebral-column resegmentation by virtue of their placement around the centers of the light bands where they provide nutrition for the more rapid growth of the primitive vertebrae.[29] They are the only constant and regularly recurring structures in the blastemal vertebral column, and vascular anomalies may result in anomalies of segmentation.[47]

Segmental Anomalies. A unilateral *hemivertebra* results if one side of the vertebral body fails to develop. Since normally there is only one primary center of ossification for the centrum, the anomaly must originate during a preosseous stage of development. Absence of an intersegmental vessel on one side may conceivably give rise to a unilateral hemivertebra, which will be associated with a sharply angled congenital scoliosis after assumption of erect posture. Absence of the anterior part of a vertebral body is also termed hemivertebra. The origin of this anomaly is difficult to explain. It may be related to congenital absence or failure of growth of a centrum, but it is likely that there would be an earlier anomaly, before appearance of the ossification centers. It gives rise to a congenital kyphosis (Fig. 1-18).

As the light bands grow rapidly, they appear to expel notochordal tissue into the more slowly growing intervertebral discs. Each notochordal segment forms a nucleus pulposus. Notochordal tissue grows rapidly by cell multiplication and production of mucoid matrix at the center of the fetal disc. Absence of a notochordal segment probably gives rise to congenital *block vertebrae* as adjacent centra fuse when no nucleus pulposus forms to separate them.

Later Notochordal Development, Chordoma, and "Butterfly Vertebra." The invasive nature of notochordal cells is important in growth of the noto-chordal nucleus pulposus, which grows rapidly in the fetus and infant, not only by multiplication of its cells but also by liquefaction of the surrounding fibers

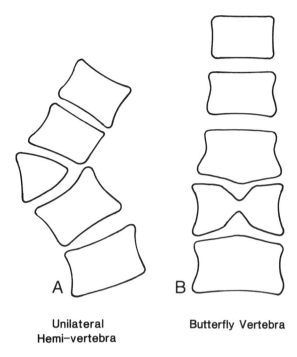

Fig. 1-18. (A) A tracing of vertebral-body outlines from an anteroposterior radiograph shows the appearance of a unilateral hemivertebra, with a consequent angled scoliosis. (B) A tracing from an anteroposterior radiograph shows a butterfly vertebra. Soft tissues are continuous through the vertebral body from one intervertebral disc to the next.

A   Unilateral
Hemi-vertebra

B   Butterfly Vertebra

and matrix.[21] The notochordal cells appear to produce substances that loosen and digest the inner margins of the surrounding envelope, incorporating these tissues into the expanding nucleus. The tissues of the envelope have to grow rapidly just to keep pace with the "erosion" of their inner margins by the rapidly expanding nucleus. It is fortunate that notochordal cells do not normally survive the end of the period of rapid growth—in fetal life, infancy, and early childhood—except perhaps deeply buried in the developing sacrum. Their demise during childhood is probably due to the progressive decrease in vascularity of the surrounding tissues. If some cells do survive, they may rarely be "released" by an incident such as trauma to the containing tissues, and begin to multiply again. The cells of malignant chordomas strongly resemble the embryonic notochordal cells.[21]

The acellular notochordal track, called the *mucoid streak*, persists for a while in the cartilage models of the vertebrae, but when ossification commences, it is usually obliterated. The notochordal track (mucoid streak) has a temporary inhibiting effect on ossification of the centrum, which may have a bilobed appearance in vertical sections through the plane of the notochord. Persistence of the notochordal track through the centrum is quite common until infancy[21], but rarely persists till adult life. If a complete notochordal track does persist, a *butterfly vertebra*, with a deep angled concavity in both vertebral end-plates, is the result. Partial persistence of the notochordal track in infancy produces a nipple-shaped deformity (Fig. 1-19) of vertebral end-plates, and may be responsible for the "Cupid's bow" appearance frequently seen in lower-lumbar vertebral bodies in adults.[45,51]

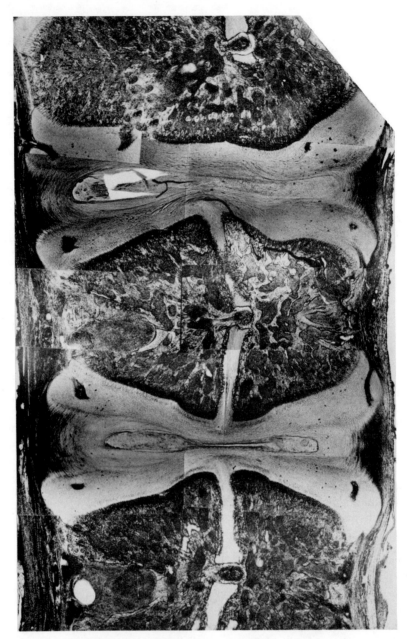

Fig. 1-19. A montage of a median sagittal section of part of a spine in a 1-month-old infant demonstrates continuity of the notochordal track through mid thoracic vertebral bodies. The notochordal track normally disappears from the vertebrae at about 20 weeks gestation. The track temporarily inhibits ossification, but in this case the nipple-shaped deformities of the vertebral end-plates appear to result from attempts by the bone to "grow around" it. The nucleus pulposus is bilocular because of the bony deformity. (Taylor JR: Persistence of the notochord canal in vertebrae. J Anat 111:211, 1972.)

Other Vascular and Notochordal Influences

Disappearance of Notochordal Cells from the Nucleus Pulposus. The cartilage plates of infants have an excellent blood supply from the adjacent vertebral periosteum. This brings nutrition to the rapidly growing intervertebral disc.[21] The capillary plexuses of the vascular arcades approach close to the growing notochordal nucleus pulposus (see Fig. 1-15B). When the vessels in these vascular arcades are gradually occluded during childhood and adolescence, the notochordal cells die off to be replaced by chondrocytes, cells better adapted to an avascular environment.

Schmorl's Nodes. The vascular canals are plugged by loose connective tissue, forming channels of reduced resistance from near the nucleus to the peripheral vertebral spongiosa.[40] These connective-tissue channels, arching around the advancing ossification front of the centrum, inhibit ossification locally, causing a toothed or grooved surface on the vertebral end surfaces of adolescents (see Fig. 1-16A,B).

The cartilage plates also have a consistently situated funnel-shaped defect on their nuclear aspect, where the notochordal track formerly penetrated the column, just behind the center of each vertebral end-plate (see Fig. 1-15). These notochordal and vascular weak points are the sites of two varieties of central and peripheral (mainly anterior) Schmorl's nodes (Fig. 1-20). They occur almost as frequently in adolescents and young adults as in older adults[43] indicating their probable developmental origin.

Schmorl's nodes occur in thoracic and lumbar vertebrae of 36 percent of adult spines. The central nodes are an incidental finding, and may not cause any symptoms, but the anterior nodes are not infrequently associated with a traumatic incident. Prolapse may stretch the pain-sensitive anterior longitudinal ligament, and the patient may complain of localized somatic back pain.[29]

Scheuermann's Disease. Multiple Schmorl's nodes, both large and small, are seen in Scheuermann's juvenile kyphosis, with a radiologic appearance of irregularity of the vertebral end-plates. Large anterior nodes are frequently seen, and are sometimes associated with anterior vertebral body collapse and wedging. The cause of the multiple Schmorl's nodes is uncertain, but one suggestion is that there may be an associated osteoporosis predisposing to vertebral end-plate weakness.[52] Alternatively, an "abnormally" vascular end-plate would have a correspondingly large number of "weak points" on attrition of the vessels, predisposing to a larger number of Schmorl's nodes than usual.

Scoliosis and Growth

In the growing fetus when centers of ossification appear in the thoracic vertebral arches, the right centers commonly appear before the corresponding left ones. Taylor[53] advanced the hypothesis that in the fetal circulation better oxygenated blood from the left ventricle through the aortic arch supplies the axial and paraxial structures on the right side in the thoracic region. It is pos-

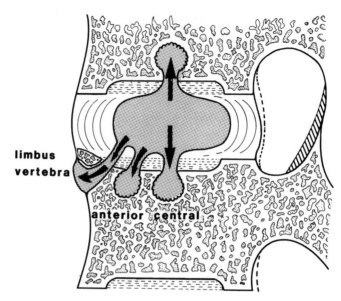

limbus
vertebra

anterior   central

Fig. 1-20.   Varieties of Schmorl's nodes (intraspongious prolapse of disc tissue). Central nodes are the most common and occur through weaknesses in the cartilage plates left by the notochordal track (see Fig. 1-15). Peripheral nodes are seen less frequently than central nodes. They occur along the lines of vascular canals. Blood vessels atrophy during maturation and the vascular canals are plugged by loose connective tissue (see Figs. 1-15 and 1-16). Prolapse of disc material between the centrum and the ring apophysis is termed a "limbus vertebra." Of the peripheral prolapses, anterior prolapse is more common than posterior prolapse, because vascular canals are more plentiful anteriorly. Note: Central nodes are usually slightly posterior of center. (Modified from Taylor JR, Twomey LT: The role of the notochord and blood vessels in vertebral column development and in the aetiology of Schmorl's nodes. Ch. 2. In Grieve GP (ed): Modern Manual Therapy of the Vertebral Column. Churchill Livingstone, Edinburgh, 1986.)

tulated that less-well-oxygenated blood from the right ventricle, passing through the ductus arteriosus, does not immediately mix with the stream from the aortic arch, but supplies the left side. This could account for the common observation that right arch primary centers appear before corresponding left arch centers in midthoracic vertebrae.[44,53] This asynchrony in appearance of paired ossification centers, correlates with measured asymmetry in pedicle lengths in infant vertebrae, and with the observation that infantile thoracic scoliosis tends to be convex to the left (Fig. 1-21).

The asynchronous maturation and growth of vertebral arches seen in fetuses and infants persists until the time of closure of the neurocentral growthplates (6 to 7 years in the midthoracic spine) but reverses its direction in older children by catch-up growth in the left side of the arch. In children and adolescents where the lines of neurocentral fusion are still evident, left pedicles tend to be longer than the corresponding right pedicles.[44] The consequent vertebral-body rotation gives a twist of the anterior elements to the right in mid-

0-5 years   **6-7 years**   **7-12 years**

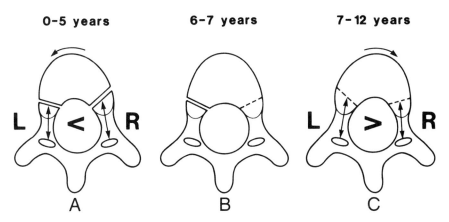

Fig. 1-21. Diagram representing the normal asynchrony in growth of thoracic verte-brae: (A) In later fetal and infant life, the right neural arch generally matures earlier than the corresponding left arch and therefore is slightly larger. (B,C) At neurocentral closure this symmetry is "reversed" by earlier closure on the right (see text). (Taylor JR, Twomey LT: Vertebral column development and its relation to adult pathology. Aust J Physiother 31:83, 1985.)

thoracic vertebrae. This change in the direction of rotation of the anterior elements at 7 years and hence in the direction of any spinal curvature, is related to asynchrony of closure of the neurocentral growth-plates. At the same time, flattening of the anterior surfaces of midthoracic vertebrae on the left begins to appear where they are in contact with the aorta. It is suggested that the aortic pressure, which flattens the anterior left surfaces of thoracic vertebral bodies, also supplies the force that twists these vertebral bodies to the right.[29,44,53] The different position of the lumbar aorta on the anterior surfaces of L2–4 and the different shape of the lumbar vertebral bodies, may be related to the observation that twisting to the left is more common here.[53,54] The asym-metries described accompany normal growth and probably determine the side of scoliosis, whether it be physiologic or progressive, and whatever other causes may operate in the multifactorial etiology of structural scolioses.

Growth of Lumbar Zygapophyseal Joints

Lumbar zygapophyseal joints are oriented in a coronal plane in fetuses and infants, similar to thoracic joints, but the lumbar articular facets grow in a posterior direction from their lateral margins so that they change in both their shape and orientation. The original coronally oriented part remains antero-medial, but a progressively increasing posterolateral component of the joint is added in the sagittal plane (Fig. 1-22). In the adult joints, from L1-2 to L3-4, the posterior two-thirds of the joint is approximately sagittal and the anterior third is approximately coronal (see Fig. 1-10). A variable amount of remodelling

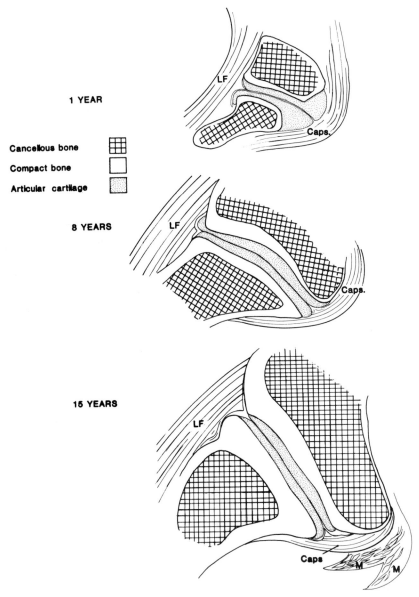

Fig. 1-22. Tracings from horizontal sections of three L4-5 zygapophyseal joints at 1 year, 8 years, and 15 years show the "rotation" of the joint plane from the coronal plane, towards the sagittal plane during growth. The concave anterior facet is on the superior articular process of the lower vertebra. The convex facet is on the inferior articular process of the upper vertebra. Note that the anteromedial capsule is formed by the ligamentum flavum (LF), and that multifidus (M) partly insets into the posterior fibrous capsule (Caps). Articular cartilage is seen (stippled), and deep to it the subchondral bone plate (white) becomes thicker with growth and is generally wedge-shaped and thus thicker anteriorly in the concave facet.

occurs at the juction of the two components so that the joints are either curved and hemicylindrical or biplanar. In transverse section or on CT scans the concavity of the superior articular facet is seen to "embrace" the smaller convex inferior facet (see Fig. 1-9). Both articular surfaces are inclined vertically so that their curves resemble segments of cylinders. The lower lumbar joints may also be biplanar, but are more nearly coronal in their overall orientation and tend to be flatter in an oblique plane, more often than in the upper joints.[55]

The coronal and sagittal components of the articular surfaces relate to two different functions. These are restraint of flexion and restraint of axial rotation respectively. The development of a wedge-shaped subchondral bone plate in the superior articular facet, much thicker in its anterior coronal part than in the sagittal part, reflects the greater physiologic compressive loading in flexion in the coronal part of the joint.[31] The subchondral bone plate (SCP) and articular cartilage reach their maximum thickness in young-adult life. The adult hyaline cartilage is about 1 mm thick on each facet. It has a very smooth surface and the matrix and cells stain lightly and evenly in the healthy young-adult joint. It is joined to the underlying SCP by a thin, regular calcified zone. In the growing joint the subchondral bone is very vascular, but with maturation this vascularity declines.

The articular cartilage is avascular and no nerves have been demonstrated, so that it is insensitive, except at its periphery, where it may be in continuity with the well-innervated joint capsule. It receives its nutrition from the synovial fluid that bathes it, circulation of the fluid being aided by movements of the joint. From the fourth decade onward, there are changes in the staining characteristics of the articular cartilage of the anteromedial coronal component of the joint, with hypertrophy of chondrocytes and increased intensity of staining of the matrix, reflecting the effects of stress in flexion in these parts of the joints.[31] This eventually progresses to splitting of the cartilage, or fibrillation, along lines parallel to the collagen framework (see Fig. 1-26).

Growth of Vertebral Bodies and Intervertebral Discs

Shape Changes on Assumption of Erect Posture

There are marked changes in the shape of lumbar vertebral bodies after infancy. These are closely related to a change in the position of the growing nucleus pulposus as lordosis is established. Fetal and infant lumbar vertebral bodies have convex upper and lower surfaces, so that the intervertebral discs are biconcave. With persistence of the primary fetal spinal curve, the appearance of each lumbar nucleus pulposus in median sagittal sections is wedge shaped with its main mass posteriorly situated. As the infant begins to sit up in the first year, and stand and learn to walk at the beginning of the second postnatal year, the secondary lumbar curvature appears, the disc changes its shape, and the nucleus pulposus moves forwards to a central position. Shallow

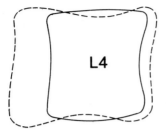

—— non-ambulant (14 year female)

--- ambulant (15 year female)

Fig. 1-23. Tracings from lateral radiographs show the effect of weight bearing on growth. In the absence of normal weight bearing in erect posture, no end-plate concavity appears and anteroposterior vertebral body growth is severely retarded. (Taylor JR: Growth of human intervertebral discs and vertebral bodies. J Anat 120:49, 1975.)

concavities begin to appear during childhood in the upper and lower vertebral body surfaces opposite the maximum bulge of the nucleus pulposus.[21,49]

The other important change in vertebral shape following assumption of the erect posture, is due to increased growth of the anteroposterior dimensions of the lumbar vertebral bodies and intervertebral discs. This change in the predominant direction of growth gives the lumbar spine more stability in the sagittal plane. The changes in vertebral-body shape on beginning weight bearing in the erect posture, reflect the plasticity of vertebral bone and its ready response to mechanical forces at this age. In nonambulatory children, these normal growth changes of early childhood do not appear in the anterior elements of the lumbar spine. Such children have very square vertebrae without the normal concavities in the endplates (Fig. 1-23). This strange shape is due to decreased horizontal growth rather than to any increase in vertical growth.[49] A similar square shape may also be seen when the posterior surfaces of vertebral bodies are scalloped by resorption in the presence of a tumor in the vertebral canal.

Sexual Dimorphism in Vertebral Body Shape

From the age of 8 or 9 years onward, normal lumbar vertebrae develop different shapes in males and females.[50] Female vertebrae grow in height more rapidly than male vertebrae; male vertebrae grow in girth more rapidly than female vertebrae. Male vertebrae grow more in both transverse and anteroposterior dimensions, particularly in transverse diameter, throughout the adolescent growth period, and appear wider and more squat than female vertebrae on radiographs (Fig. 1-24).[50] A measurement survey of a growing population showed that the thoracolumbar spine grows in height 1.7 times more rapidly in females than males between the ages of 9 and 13 years.[19] Thus the female spine is longer and more slender. Although the male spine grows in length more rapidly than the female spine after the age of 14 years, the greater transverse growth of male vertebrae maintains this shape difference. Accompanying these differences in vertebral growth patterns in males and females are differences in muscular support, since the effect of testosterone on muscle is to increase

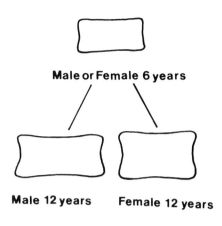

Fig. 1-24. The appearance of sex differences in vertebral-body shape is shown in tracings from anteroposterior radiographs of normal vertebrae. Male vertebral bodies grow more in width than female vertebrae, and female vertebral bodies tend to be relatively taller than male vertebrae. (Taylor JR, Twomey LT: The role of the notochord and blood vessels in vertebral column development and in the aetiology of Schmorl's nodes. Ch. 2. In Grieve GP (ed): Modern Manual Therapy of the Vertebral Column. Churchill Livingstone, Edinburgh, 1986.)

both its bulk and its strength-per-unit cross-sectional area. Thus the broader or thicker male vertebral column also has better muscular support than the average female column. When axially loaded, a slender column will buckle more easily than a wide column, particularly if it already has a slight bend in it (physiologic scoliosis). This may explain the greater tendency to progression of scoliosis in females than in males.[50]

The increased anteroposterior vertebral growth in both sexes in early childhood, and the greater increase in transverse vertebral growth in males than in females around puberty, both appear to relate to mechanical influences on bone growth. In the first case, the horizontal growth is the result of the stresses related to weight bearing in erect posture, and in the second case it is probably related to muscle activity on growing vertebrae. It is interesting to compare these growth changes in shape to the age changes in shape in elderly adults, where there is "thickening of the waist" of vertebral bodies, and loss of the sex difference in shape[1,3] associated with reduced physical stress, (and reduced sensitivity of osteoblastic activity to stress) and reduced estrogen levels in postmenopausal women (see Fig. 1-25 and the section Vertebral Bodies).

AGE CHANGES IN THE LUMBAR SPINE

Age Changes in the Anterior Elements

Vertebral Bodies

Measurement studies on a large series of lumbar vertebral columns of all ages[1,3,56] demonstrated that the length of the column decreases with aging, as expected, but the reason for this is not usually loss in disc height, but gradual collapse of vertebral end-plates, associated with reduced bone density. The

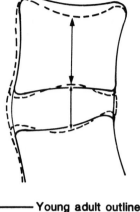

Young adult outline

– – – – Elderly adult outline

Fig. 1-25. A diagram based on tracings of vertebral bodies and on measurements of vertebral bodies and intervertebral discs[1] shows the changes in their shapes with age. "Ballooning" of the central part of the disc is related to collapse of the vertebral end-plates, and there is some increase in anteroposterior dimension with aging. (Twomey LT, Taylor JR: Age changes in lumbar intervertebral discs. Acta Orthop Scand 56:496, 1986.)

primary change is loss of horizontal trabeculae in vertebral bodies. This leads to buckling and breaking of the unsupported parts of vertical trabeculae or "beams" of bone, which hold up the vertebral end-plates (see the section Vertebral Bodies and Weight Bearing). A gradual increase in vertebral end-plate concavity is demonstrated with aging. This appears earlier in females than in males. In hemisected spines one notices a change in shape at the disc–vertebral junction, with "ballooning" of the center of each disc into the adjacent vertebral bodies. The traditional assumption that discs generally get thinner with aging is incorrect, as measurements of average disc thickness and mass show increases in the majority of old lumbar spines.[56]

There are also age changes in the horizontal dimensions of the anterior elements characterized as a "thickening of the waist" in vertebral bodies, as if loss of transverse trabeculae allowed horizontal spreading of the bone (Fig. 1-25). These changes in vertebral shape gradually eliminate the sex differences in vertebral-body shape that are seen from adolescence to middle age. Females' vertebrae are relatively taller and more slender during this child-bearing period. The effect of testosterone on muscle development may be a reason for the development of broader vertebrae in adolescent and young adult males, as the pull of muscle attachments affects bone shape. Other hormonal influences, such as estrogen loss at the menopause, relate to the earlier loss in bone density in aging females. It is unwise to regard bone loss with aging as inevitable. As noted in Chapter 2, regular exercise and adequate calcium intake may play a part in reducing or preventing the bone loss associated with aging.[57]

Intervertebral Discs

Contrary to popular belief, aging discs do not generally become thinner and bulge like underinflated car tires. However, a sizable minority of the population shows some evidence of disc thinning and degeneration with aging.

These changes particularly affect the L4-5 and L5-S1 levels where 30 percent of discs are classified as Rolander grade 3 in subjects over 60 years.[1,56] Aging of intervertebral discs is generally associated with a reduction in water content, particularly in the nucleus pulposus, though most of this loss occurs during maturation rather than in old age. The nucleus becomes less well differentiated from the anulus both in its water content and its histologic structure.[21] There are increases in the absolute amounts of collagen in the nucleus pulposus and changes in the types of collagen present. There are also changes in the proportions of keratan and chondroitin sulphate present, which probably relate to the decreased water-binding capacity of the disc. These changes are accompanied by increased disc stiffness and decreased ranges of movement, which will be fully discussed in Chapter 2.

Kissing Spines

With the collapse of vertebral end-plates allowing the discs to "sink into" shortened vertebral bodies, there is shortening of the column, and spinous processes, which were formerly well spaced, may come into contact with each other. Histologic studies on four cadaver specimens showing radiologic evidence of "kissing spines," revealed adventitious joints with a fibrocartilaginous covering on the bone and a bursa-like cavity, surrounded by fat and lined by synovial membrane, between the "kissing spines" (Taylor 1984, unpublished). In the view of Sartori et al[58] "kissing spines" are attributable to increased lordosis with aging.

Age Changes in Zygapophyseal Joints

Articular Surfaces and Subchondral Bone Plate (SCP)

The geometry of these biplanar joints at different lumbar levels has already been described (see Zygapophyseal (Facet) Joints). Age changes in young and middle-aged adults will be described first.[31]

Coronal Component (Anteromedial Third of Joint). The loading stress imposed on the anteromedial third of the joints by the forward translational component of flexion is reflected by changes to both the articular cartilage and the underlying SCP. In normal adolescents and young adults a thicker subchondral bone plate develops in the coronal component of the concave superior articular facet. Later, particularly in middle life, this subchondral bone in the coronal component of the concave facet also shows the intense hematoxylin staining suggestive of hypercalcification (sclerosis). From the beginning of the fourth decade, the articular cartilage lining this thicker part of the SCP in the anteromedial third of the joint, shows cell hypertrophy and increased staining of chondrocytes and matrix beginning in the mid-zone of the articular cartilage of the concave facet. These articular cartilage changes occur in the concave

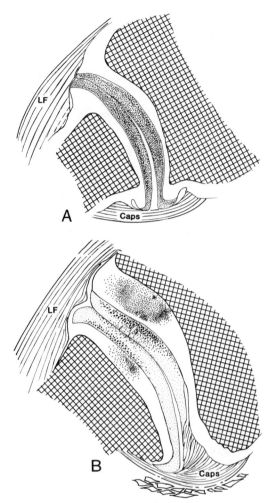

Fig. 1-26. Drawings of mid-joint horizontal sections of L3–4 zygapophyseal joints, which were stained by hematoxylin and light green. (A) A normal joint from a 20-year-old woman shows smooth articular cartilage with regularly distributed chondrocytes and even staining of the matrix. The subchondral bone plate (white) is thicker anteriorly than posteriorly in the concave facet. The elastic ligamentum flavum (LF) forms the anterior capsule, which maintains close apposition of the anterior articular surfaces, but, in the absence of multifidus, the posterior fibrous capsule (Caps) is lax and the posterior part of the joint is open. (B) A joint from a 37-year-old man shows chondrocyte hypertrophy in the articular cartilages of the coronal component. This is most evident in the concave facet of the superior articular process of L4 where two small splits in the articular cartilage are seen. There is thickening of the SCP, particularly in the coronal component, compared to the joint in (A). Increased staining of the thickened SCP suggests of hypercalcification or "sclerosis." The posterior fibrous capsule is covered by some fibers of multifidus. Note the continuity of the capsule with the posterior margin of the articular cartilage of the concave facet. Splitting of this cartilage away from the SCP is apparent *LF* = ligamentum flavum; *Caps* = posterior fibrous capsule. (*Figure continues.*)

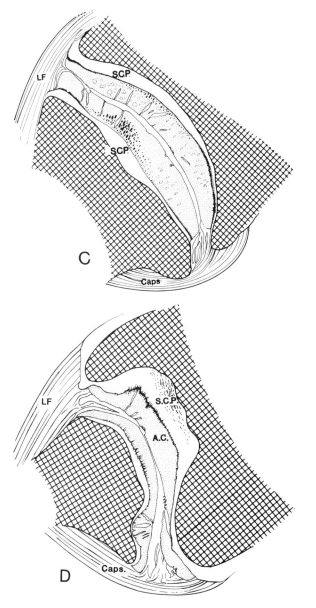

Fig. 1-26 (*Continued*).   (C) A joint from a 62-year-old man where there is some atrophy of chondrocytes and loss of staining in the concave facet, and some cell hypertrophy in the convex facet. Fibrillation of both articular cartilages, most marked in the coronal parts of the joint, may be seen. The SCP has lost thickness compared with the SCP in part B. There are osteophytes at the posterior joint margin. (D) A joint from a 61-year-old man showing advanced arthritic changes with widespread fibrillation of articular cartilage (*AC*). There are infractions and irregularity of the SCP. The coronal component of the SCP appears to have collapsed into the spongy bone of the concave facet. The SCP at this point shows local thickening and increased staining suggestive of "sclerosis."

facet first, in its coronal component, and at the deepest part of its concavity. They occur in the coronal component of the convex facet soon afterward, but generally do not affect the sagittal components of either facet. When the increased staining and chondrocyte hypertrophic changes are present concurrently in both facets, they are more advanced in the concave than in the convex facet. They appear in many adult joints in the fourth decade of life and progress to vertical splitting (fibrillation) of the cartilage (Fig. 1-26). The changes in bone and cartilage both appear to be reactions to the pressure or compression loading of the anteromedial parts of the joint, which would occur in flexion as a result of forward-translational movement of the inferior process of the vertebra above, against the superior facet of the vertebra below. In many respects these changes are analogous to those described in patellofemoral chondromalacia, where the stress also involves gliding movement accompanied by compression of the patella against the trochlea of the femur.

Sagittal Component (Posterior Two-thirds of Joint). The age changes in the posterior, sagittally oriented two-thirds of the zygapophyseal joints are quite different in character, and tend to occur later than the pressure changes described in the coronal component and at the center of the articular facets. The posterior, sagittally oriented parts of the SCPs are relatively thin, suggesting less pressure stress. However, in the fourth decade or later, the sagittal components of a number of joints show splitting of the articular cartilage at or parallel to the articular cartilage–SCP interface, near the posterior joint margin. This is related to a direct continuity of the posterior fibrous capsule with the posterior margin of the articular cartilage. This capsule–cartilage continuity is common, and is seen most often at the posterior margin of the concave superior articular facet. Multifidus is partly inserted through the capsule at this region, at the upper half of each joint (see Fig. 1-22C). Tension on the capsule transmitted to the cartilage and frequently repeated may shear it off. Either movement or muscle activity could exert this tension. The activity of axial rotation around an axis situated in the vertebral canal would exert an obliquely directed pressure on the sagittally oriented posterior part of the joint. However, the lack of a thick SCP here suggests that pressure-stress perpendicular to the articular surface is less here than anteromedially, and such pressure would not be likely to "shear off" the articular cartilage from the SCP. The curved nature of most lumbar zygapophyseal joint facets and the observation[59] that the center of axial rotation is usually close to the posterior disc margin, suggest that in axial rotation, some forward twisting and sliding movement of one joint may accompany backward twisting and sliding of the contralateral joint. This movement would produce tension on the articular cartilage from a capsule in continuity with it.

Meniscoid Inclusions, Back Pain, and "Locked Back"

In a previous section we described the different varieties of synovial lined fibrofatty pads, which project from the joint recesses between the articular surfaces, and from the anterior and posterior margins to a variable extent into the joint, up to 3 mm between the articulating surfaces. A survey of 80 adult joints found that there are larger fatty pads in the older joints, which show the wear and tear changes of osteoarthrosis, than in young-adult joints. They appear to act as cushions in lateral or medial joint recesses adjacent to osteophytes, and to extend further between articular surfaces where cartilage loss has occurred (Taylor and Connell, unpublished). These vascular structures are innervated, and also directly connected to the joint capsule, which has many pain-sensitive nerve fibers. They are particularly large in the inferior joint reseccus of the lowest two lumbar mobile segments.[32,34] They are capable of causing back pain if entrapped between articular surfaces, either due to direct stimulation of the innervated inclusions or due to traction on the innervated capsule. Their potential importance in this latter regard has been questioned by Engel and Bogduk[59] on the grounds that they are too friable to exercise tension on the capsule if caught between the articular surfaces.

In our most recent study,[31] we have found a number of instances of fibrocartilaginous inclusions projecting into the posterior aspect of zygapophyseal joints, which appear to be torn-off portions of articular cartilage that have remained attached to the fibrous capsule. Their origin in the articular cartilage is attested by their template-like fit on the underlying damaged cartilage, which is repairing (Fig. 1-27). They appear to be analogous to torn menisci in the knee joint. Like torn knee-joint menisci, they could be displaced in certain circumstances, and being firmer and more strongly attached to the capsule than other fibrofatty inclusions, their entrapment could cause a reduction in the normal range of spinal movement or even "locked back." It is highly likely that this would be painful because of traction on the joint capsule. In this regard, the action of multifidus in controlling the "posture" of the joint (see Zygapophyseal (Facet) Joints) would be important. If joint congruity is not maintained by tone in multifidus there would be an opportunity for the torn portions of cartilage to be displaced, particularly in sudden rotary movements. Manipulative techniques would be particularly successful in "freeing" such entrapped torn pieces of articular cartilage. On the other hand, strong manipulative techniques that attempt to "gap" these joints could conceivably exacerbate the damage due to "shearing off" of articular cartilage in a joint with capsule–cartilage continuity.

Age Changes in Middle-Aged and Elderly Zygapophyseal Joints

These include the pressure-related fibrillation in the anterior and central parts of the joints, particularly the concave facet, and also the splitting or "shearing off" of cartilage parallel to the cartilage bone interface as described above. They also include the more general age changes of osteoarthrosis, e.g., surface fibrillation and irregularity, osteophytic lipping, as seen in aging of other joints, but subchondral bone cysts are less common in the zygapophyseal joints than in the weight-bearing joints of the lower limb. "Wrap-around bumpers" of metaplastic cartilage appear at joint margins, under the posterior fibrous capsule. These may occur as a response to pressure of the capsule on underlying osteophytes projecting into the joint recess. Fibrillation of the articular cartilage

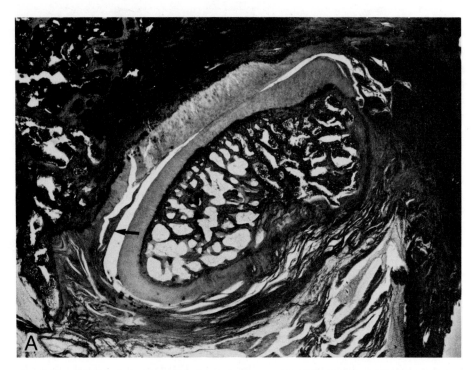

Fig. 1-27. (A) Horizontal section from the lower third of a left L3-4 joint in a 37-year-old man that shows a joint inclusion, which may be a torn-off portion of the damaged articular cartilage of the concave facet, attached at its base to the posterior fibrous capsule. There is continuity of the capsule with the posterior margin of the cartilage on the concave facet, and also metaplastic formation of articular cartilage around the posterior margin of the convex facet under the capsule in the form of a "wrap-around bumper" (×4). (*Figure continues.*)

is more often accompanied by thickening of the central parts of the articular cartilage[30] than by thinning (see Fig. 1-26C,D). The appearance often suggests disruption and swelling of the matrix. The underlying subchondral bone plate may show infractions and collapse of its anterocentral portion. Measurements of concavity indices in L1-2 joints, L3-4 joints, and L4-5 joints from 70 lumbar spines of all ages show increased concavity of the superior articular facets in old age. This index represents the degree of concavity of the bone–cartilage interface in the superior articular facet. The observed concurrent increase in central cartilage thickness may simply represent an attempt to maintain joint congruity. Some osteoporotic joints with very thin SCPs show a marked increase in concavity. Other arthritic joints show infractions or local collapse, at variable sites along the bone–cartilage junction. The increased concavity is a phenomenon similar to the collapse of the vertebral body end-plate at the disc–vertebral junction, which is also a result of loading of bone weakened by osteoporosis.

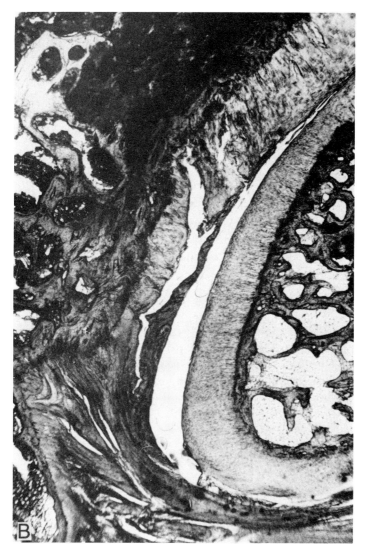

Fig. 1-27 (*Continued*).   (B) A higher-power view of the joint inclusion in (A) shows the template-like fit of the inclusion on the underlying damaged cartilage, which shows signs of repair ($\times 10$). (B from Taylor JR, Twomey LT: Structure, function, and age changes in the lumbar zygaphophyseal joints. Spine 11:739, 1986.)

Changes at Joint Margins: Tension Effects

Articular Cartilage.   While the initial and more dramatic age ch~ articular cartilage take place in the coronal and central parts of described, in the long term, the more destructive effects are at the jo particularly at the polar regions and at the posterior margins of the joi.

loss of cartilage is most common in these regions, probably due to the "shearing off" of cartilage by tension from capsular attachments.[31] This is often accompanied by the intrusion of enlarged fat pads into the defect.

Bone Changes.   In middle-aged joints, osteophytes appear at the joint margins in addition to the subchondral bony sclerosis previously described in the coronal components of the superior articular facets. They are another manifestation of response to tension, both by extension of ossification from the laminae into the ligamenta flava, and at the posterior articular margins with associated enlargement of the mamillary processes.

Radiologic Diagnosis.   The assumption that subchondral bone thickening and sclerosis are reliable indicators of wear and tear changes may be valid in the joints of middle-aged active patients, but in elderly osteoporotic joints there may be many false negative diagnoses. Our studies show that many elderly subjects with advanced fibrillation and cartilage loss have extremely thin subchondral bone plates due to concomitant osteoporosis.

Relation of Age Changes in Discs and Facet Joints

It is commonly stated[61] that disc degeneration (as a primary change) leads to secondary zygapophyseal-joint degeneration. This is not always so. Thus, for example, in spondylolysis, when the protective influence of the zygapophyseal joint is removed, damage to the intervertebral disc will ensue. The view has been advanced here that the anterior, coronally oriented parts of lumbar zygapophyseal joints exercise a protective influence on intervertebral discs when they bring flexion to a halt at the end of the physiologic range (see Articular Surfaces and Subchondral Bone Plate (SCP) and Age Changes in Middle-aged and Elderly Zygapophyseal Joints). These joints also limit the range of extension. The observation of a build-up of sclerotic compact-bone in the laminae of the inferior joint recesses in adults of all ages, is witness to the effect of impingement of the tips of the inferior articular processes on the subjacent laminae, in bringing extension to a halt. The important protective effects of the zygapophyseal joints on the intervertebral discs are largely substantiated by the evidence we have presented.[3,11,29,31] The increased ranges of movement amounting to instability that result from experimental sectioning of pedicles would place additional stress on the intervertebral discs. It is apparent from our studies of discs and zygapophyseal joints from the same individuals that in some cases the zygapophyseal joints show more advanced degeneration than is apparent in the intervertebral discs. However, the mobile segments interact in a mutually dependent way and it is likely that any defect in one joint of the articular triad would adversely influence the other joints of the triad.

SUMMARY

Age changes in both discs and zygapophyseal joints reflect the stresses imposed on these joints by weight bearing and movement. These include:

1. *Pressure* at the center of the vertebral-body end-plates producing a gradual increase in end-plate concavity;

2. *Pressure* on the coronal components of the zygapophyseal joints and at the centers of the concave zygapophyseal-joint facets, giving SCP thickening and sclerosis, and articular cartilage changes leading to cartilage fibrillation.

3. *Tension* at the vertebral-body margins and at the zygapophyseal-joint margins, where osteophytes appear and "shearing off" and splitting of cartilage in the synovial facet joints lead to cartilage loss or formation of cartilaginous inclusions due to capsule–cartilage continuity.

4. Osteoporosis adds to the above changes in the elderly, with vertebral endplate collapse and "balooning" of discs into veretebral bodies, and infractions and central collapse in the concave zygapophyseal SCP, with subsequent thickening of the central cartilage to "fill in the deficit."

REFERENCES

1. Twomey LT: Age changes in the human lumbar vertebral column. Ph.D. thesis, University of Western Australia, 1981
2. Davis PR: Human lower lumbar vertebrae. J Anat 95:337, 1961
3. Twomey LT, Taylor JR, Furniss B: Age changes in the bone density and structure of the lumbar vertebral column. J Anat 136:15, 1983
4. Knutsson F: Growth and differentiation of postnatal vertebrae. Acta Radiol 55:401, 1961
5. Eisenstein S: The morphometry and pathological anatomy of the lumbar spine in South African negroes and caucasoids with special reference to spinal stenosis. J Bone Joint Surg 59B:173, 1977
6. Parkin IG, Harrison GR: The topographical anatomy of the lumbar epidural space. J Anat 141:211, 1985
7. Sunderland S: Meningeal-neural relationships in the intervertebral space. J Neurosurg 40:756, 1974
8. Crock HV, Yoshizawa H: The blood supply of the lumbar vertebral column. Clin Orthop 115:6, 1976
9. Romanes GJR: The arterial blood supply of the human spinal cord. Paraplegia 2:199, 1965
10. Dommisse GF: The blood supply of the spinal cord. J Bone Joint Surg 56B:225, 1974
11. Twomey LT, Taylor JR: A quantitative study of the role of the posterior vertebral elements in sagittal movements of the lumbar vertebral column. Arch Phys Med Rehabil, 64:322, 1983
12. Ramsey RH: The anatomy of the ligamenta flava. Clin Orthop 44:129, 1966
13. Yong-Hing MD, Reilly J, Kirkaldy-Willis WH: The ligamentum flavum. Spine 1:226, 1976
14. Heylings DJA: Supraspinous and interspinous ligaments of the human lumbar spine. J Anat 125:127, 1978
15. Bowen V, Cassidy JD: Macroscopic and microscopic anatomy of the sacro-iliac joint from embryonic life until the eighth decade. Spine 6:620, 1981
16. Palfrey AJ: The shape of the sacroiliac joint surfaces. J Anat 132:457, 1981
17. Clayson SJ et al: Evaluation of mobility of hip and lumbar vertebrae of normal young women. Arch Phys Med Rehabil, 43:1, 1962
18. Bourdillon JF: Spinal Manipulation. 2nd Ed. William Heinemann Medical Books, London, 1973

19. Taylor JR, Slinger BS: Scoliosis screening and growth in Western Australian students. Med J Aust 1:475, 1980
20. Horton WG: Further observations on the elastic mechanism of the intervertebral disc. J Bone Joint Surg 40B:552, 1958
21. Taylor JR: Growth and development of the human intervertebral disc. Ph.D. thesis, University of Edinburgh, 1973
22. Nachemson A, Elfstrom G: Intravital dynamic measurements in lumbar discs. Scand J Rehabil Med suppl 1:1, 1960
23. Taylor JR, Twomey LT: Innervation of lumbar intervertebral discs. Med J Aust 2:(13)701, 1979
24. Taylor JR, Twomey LT: Innervation of lumbar intervertebral discs. NZ J Physiother 8:36, 1980
25. Bogduk N: The innervation of the lumbar spine. Spine 8:286, 1983
26. Hirsch C, Schazowicz F: Studies on structural changes in the lumbar anulus fibrosus. Acta Orthop Scand 22:184, 1953
27. Walmsley R: The development and growth of the intervertebral disc. Edin Med J 60:341, 1953
28. Maroudas A, Nachemson A, Stockwell RA, Urban J: Factors involved in the nutrition of the adult human lumbar intervertebral disc. J Anat 120:113, 1975
29. Taylor JR, Twomey LT: Vertebral column development and its relation to adult pathology. Aust J Physiother 31:83, 1985
30. Twomey LT, Taylor JR: Age changes in the lumbar articular triad. Aust J Physiother 31:106, 1985
31. Taylor JR, Twomey LT: Structure, function and age changes in lumbar zygapophyseal joints. Spine 11:739, 1986
32. Giles L, Taylor JR: Intra-articular synovial protrusions in the lower lumbar apophyseal joints. Bull Hosp Dis Orthop Inst 42:248, 1982
33. Wyke B: The neurology of joints: a review of general principles. Clin Rheum Dis 7:223, 1981
34. Giles L, Taylor JR, Cockson A: Human zygapophyseal joint synovial folds. Acta Anat 126:110, 1986
35. Taylor JR, Twomey LT: Sagittal and horizontal plane movement of the human lumbar vertebral column in cadavers and in the living. Rheumatol Rehab 19:223, 1980
36. Spangfort EV: The lumbar disc herniation. Acta Orthop Scand, suppl. 142:1, 1972
37. Weinstein PR, Ehni G, Wilson CB: Lumbar Spondylosis: Diagnosis, Management and Surgical Treatment. Year Book Medical Publishers, Chicago, 1977
38. Wolpert L: Cellular basis of skeletal growth during development. Br Med Bull 37:215, 1981
39. Taylor JR, Twomey LT: Factors influencing growth of the vertebral column. Ch. 1. In Grieve GP (ed): Modern Manual Therapy. Vol. 1. Churchill Livingstone, Edinburgh, 1986
40. Taylor Jr, Twomey LT: The role of the notochord and blood vessels in vertebral column development and in the aetiology of Schmorl's nodes. Ch. 2. In Grieve GP (ed): Modern Manual Therapy of the Vertebral Column. Churchill Livingstone, Edinburgh, 1986
41. Verbout AJ: The Development of the Vertebral Column. Springer-Verlag, Berlin, 1985
42. O'Rahilly R, Meyer DB: The timing and sequence of events in the development of the human vertebral column during the embryonic period proper. Anatomy Embryol 157:167, 1979

43. Schmorl G, Junghanns H: The Human Spine in health and Disease. 2nd American Ed. Grune & Stratton, New York, 1971
44. Taylor JR: Scoliosis and growth. Acta Orthop Scand 54:596, 1983
45. Taylor JR: Persistence of the notochordal canal in vertebrae. J Anat 111:211, 1972
46. Dale-Stewart TD, Kerley ER: Essentials of Forensic Anthropology. p. 136. Charles C Thomas, Springfield, Illinois, 1979
47. Tanaka T, Uhthoff HK: The pathogenesis of congenital malformations. Acta Orthop Scand 52:413, 1981
48. Watterson RL, Fowler I, Fowler BJ: The role of the neural tube and the notochord in development of the axial skeleton of the chick. Am J Anat 95:337, 1954
49. Taylor JR: Growth of human intervertebral discs and vertebral bodies. J Anat 120:49, 1975
50. Taylor JR, Twomey LT: Sexual dimorphism in human vertebral body shape. J Anat 138:281, 1984
51. Dietz GW: Christensen EE: Normal Cupid's bow contour of the lower lumbar vertebrae. Radiology 121:577, 1976
52. Bradford DS, Moe JH: Scheuermann's juvenile kyphosis: a histologic study. Clin Orthop 110:45, 1975
53. Taylor JR: Vascular causes of vertebral asymmetry and the laterality of scoliosis. Med J Aust 144:533, 1986
54. Dickson RA, Lawton JO, Butt WP: The pathogenesis of idiopathic scoliosis. p. 17. In Dickson RA, Bradford DS (eds): Management of Spinal Deformities. Butterworth, London, 1984
55. Van Shaik JPJ, Verbiest H, Van Shaik FDJ: The orientation of laminae and facet joints in the lower lumbar spine. Spine 10:59, 1985
56. Twomey LT, Taylor JR: Age changes in lumbar intervertebral discs. Acta Orthop Scand 56:496, 1986
57. Twomey LT, Taylor JR: Old age and physical capacity: use it or lose it. Aust J Physiother 30:115, 1984
58. Sartoris DJ, Resnick D, Tyson R, Haghighi P: Age-related alterations in the vertebral spinous processes and intervening soft tissues: radiologic–pathologic correlation. AJR 145:1025, 1985
59. Engel R, Bogduk N: The menisci of the lumbar zygapophyseal joints. J Anat 135:795, 1982
60. Pope MH, Wilder DG, Matteri RE, Frymoyer JW: Experimental measurements of vertebral motion under load. Orthop Clin North Am 8:155, 1977
61. Vernon-Roberts B: The pathology and interrelation of intervertebral disc lesions, osteoarthrosis of the apophyseal joints and low back pain. p. 83. In Jayson MI (ed): The Lumbar Spine and Back Pain. 2nd Ed. Pitman, London, 1980

2 | Lumbar Posture, Movement, and Mechanics

Lance T. Twomey
James R. Taylor

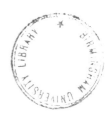

The adult vertebral column is a segmented, jointed, flexible rod, which supports the loads of weight bearing in the erect posture, protects the spinal cord and emerging spinal nerves, allows a considerable range of movements in all directions, and serves as the axial support for the limbs. The vertebral column's capacity to fully subserve these functions alters through the different phases of the life cycle. The extremely malleable C-shaped column of the neonate remains almost as flexible and mobile in childhood as it grows and develops its finely balanced curves. Further growth and maturation are associated with progressive increases in the strength and "dynamic" stability of the adolescent and young-adult columns, and with a continuing small decline in its mobility. The middle years demonstrate an increasing incidence of minor traumatic and degenerative pathology, with a further decline in range of movement. In old age with osteoporotic decrease in bone strength, there is progressive increase in joint stiffness with a considerable decline in movement ranges, and a flattening of the lumbar spine. The lumbar spine is markedly lordotic in children, with a small decline in lordosis in adolescents and young adults, and a pronounced flattening of the region in middle life and old age.

Posture is a term that indicates the relative position of the body segments during rest or activity, while *stature* indicates the height of a subject. In most individuals their resting supine length exceeds their standing height (or stature) by about 2 cm.

51

line of gravity

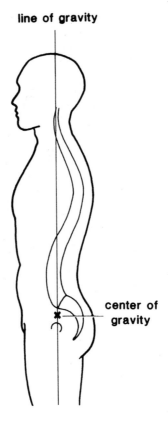

center of gravity

Fig. 2-1. The relationship between the vertebral column and the line of gravity.

POSTURE

Posture refers to a composite of the positions of all of the joints of the body at any given moment.[1] A minimum of muscle work is required for the maintenance of good posture in any human static or dynamic situation. In good standing posture, the head is held tall and level, while the spine is nicely balanced so that its sagittal curves allow free movement of the chest and abdomen, and prevent the shoulders from sagging forward. The lower limbs serve as balanced support. In a side view of most individuals, a plumb line would intersect the mastoid process, the acromion process, and the greater trochanter. It would pass just anterior to the center of the knee joint and through the ankle joint.

The usual static posture for the lumbar spine is that of lordosis. Normal spinal posture is expressed as a balanced series of curves when viewed from the side (Fig. 2-1). The adult spine is supported on a symmetrical level pelvis by two equal-length lower limbs. In normal sitting posture, the level pelvis is supported with body weight distributed equally through both ischial tuberosities. There is no discernable lateral curvature or rotation of the spine when viewed from the front or behind.

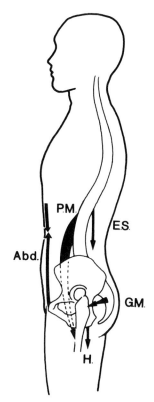

Fig. 2-2. The muscles responsible for the maintenance of pelvic tilt. *Abd* = abdominal muscles, *ES* = Erector spinae, *GM* = gluteus maximus, *H* = hamstrings, *PM* = psoas major.

The cervical lordosis begins to appear at birth and develops as a permanent curve at about three months of age, while the permanent lumbar lordosis appears with the extension of the legs and weight bearing in the erect posture, usually between 12 and 18 months of age. These curves continue to change until the completion of spinal growth, usually between the ages of 13 and 18 years.[2–4]

Sagittal Pelvic Tilt and Muscle Action

Pelvic tilt in the sagittal plane and lumbar lordosis are inextricably linked together, as the lumbar spine and the sacrum are united at the strong, relatively immobile sacroiliac joints. Thus, when the pelvis is tilted further forward, it brings about an increase in lordosis, and when tilted backward, the lumbar spine flattens. The muscles responsible for pelvic posture include erector spinae (sacrospinalis), abdominals (recturs abdominus and oblique muscles), psoas major and iliacus, gluteus maximus, and hamstrings (Fig. 2-2).

It is the interaction between these muscles that is the major factor determining pelvic tilt and lumbar lordosis at any point in time. Thus, while the back extensor muscles primarily increase lumbar lordosis, the abdominal muscles,

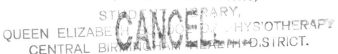

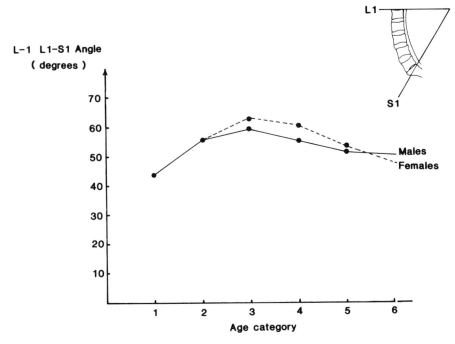

Fig. 2-3.   Changes that occur through life to the lumbosacral angle.

gluteals, and hamstrings act together to flatten lumbar lordosis by their action about the lever of the pelvis. The psoas muscles, which attach to the lateral margins of the lumbar vertebrae, can also increase lumbar lordosis when the lower limbs are extended by pulling the lumbar vertebrae forward around the "pulley" of the hip joint (Fig. 2-2). In this way they pull the pelvis and lumbar vertebrae ventrally. In the course of everyday activity we are constantly adjusting our posture to allow for comfort, ergonomic advantage, and in response to our environment. Muscle tightness affecting any of the muscle groups listed can change both habitual resting posture and the total range of dynamic postures available. Tightness of psoas major and hamstring muscles is associated with increased lordosis in some individuals. Shortened hamstrings should pull down on the pelvis and flatten the lumbar spine. For this reason, it is possible that tight hamstrings are the *result* of lordotic posture rather than its cause.

Analysis of the Lumbar Curve

The lumbosacral lordosis is a compound curve (Fig. 2-3) with the degree of curvature greatest at the L5-S1 level, and least at the L1-2 level. In general, at all ages the intervertebral discs contribute to a greater proportion of the lordosis in both sexes than do the vertebrae. However, at the lumbosacral junction, the L5 vertebral body makes a significant contribution. The L5-S1 disc is also more wedge-shaped than any of the higher discs.

Sexual Dimorphism

During the childbearing years (i.e., between adolescence and middle age) the L1-S1 angle of lumbar lordosis is greater in women than in men.[5] This sexual dimorphism is not apparent in childhood and disappears again in old age. Although the reasons for this difference remain obscure, its place in the life cycle suggests that it has a hormonal basis. One of the hormones that may be involved consists of three closely related polypeptides collectively called *relaxin*. Relaxin is secreted by the ovary and has been shown to relax the symphysis pubis, sacroiliac joints, and spinal ligaments.[6] These hormones, which are secreted in relatively large amounts by the corpus luteum of pregnancy, are also found in small amounts in the circulating blood of nonpregnant women of childbearing age.[7] It is suggested that the effects of relaxin in "loosening" pelvic and lumbar ligaments may coincidentally allow an increase in the lumbar curve during that period in the female life cycle (adolescence and early-adult life) when the hormones are present in relatively large amounts.

Another suggestion advanced to explain the gender differences in lordosis relates to Treanor's[8] demonstration that the wearing of high-heel shoes tips the body's center of gravity forward and brings about an associated increase in pelvic tilt and an increase in lumbar lordosis as lumbar lordosis is dependent on pelvic posture (Fig. 2-4). The habitual wearing of high heels (predominantly a female fashion) in the "developed" countries, may contribute to a difference in lordosis between men and women in Western societies. This is less likely to be a feature in societies where outdoor activity in bare feet or soft-heel shoes is possible for most of the year.

A recent study[9] showed that an increase in pelvic tilt due to high heels does not always bring about an increase in lumbar lordosis in nonpregnant young women. An equal number of women demonstrated a flattening of their lumbar curve as showed an increase. However, pregnant women showed a significant increase in lordosis when wearing 2-inch-high heels. The response of the lumbar spine to changes in pelvic posture would appear to relate to the location of the center of gravity. In pregnancy, the center of gravity is displaced ventrally and is balanced by an increase in lumbar lordosis.

An analysis of the components of the L1-S1 angle in a major cadaveric study[5] showed that the principal difference between the lumbar posture of females and males occurs at the lumbosacral junction, as the composite L1–5 angles are similar throughout life in both sexes (Fig. 2-5). Thus, it is the increased sacral and pelvic tilt of females that is primarily responsible for the difference in lordosis during adolescence and early-adult life. In this regard, it is interesting to note that anatomists such as Romanes[10] consider that in normal erect posture, the antero superior iliac spines and the symphysis pubis lie in the same plane. This was confirmed in a measurement study of 39 nonpregnant

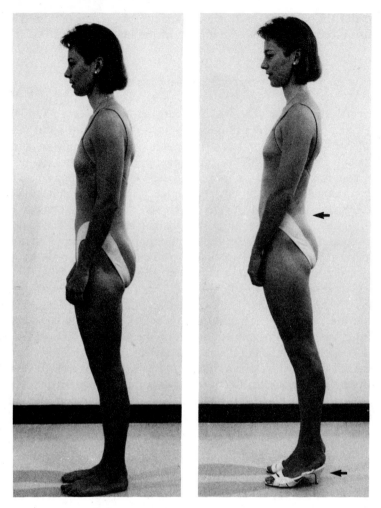

Fig. 2-4.   The increase in lumbar lordosis due to wearing high-heel shoes.

females by Taylor and Alexander.[11] Obstetric experience suggests that the symphysis pubis lies in a more anterior plane than do the iliac spines.[12] The greater L5-S1 angle in females may well be related to a greater degree of pelvic tilt during the childbearing years.

Variations in Lumbar Lordosis

Lumbar lordosis is maintained by intrinsic features such as the shape of the vertebrae, discs, and the sacrum, and by extrinsic factors such as position of center of gravity, body weight and its distribution, muscle strength, and sociocltural preferences. In regard to sociocultural preferences, it is commonly

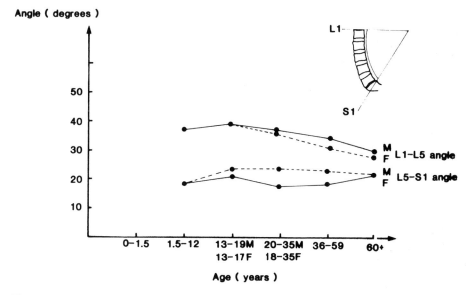

Fig. 2-5. An analysis of the change in L1–L5 and L5–S1 angles with increasing age.

observed that an individual's lumbar lordosis and thus habitual posture is based on factors such as fashion (e.g., wearing high heels), repetitive daily activity (e.g., a schoolchild carrying a heavy schoolbag), life-style (e.g., the "typical" military posture), affect and attitude (e.g., depression or elation), and aesthetics or training (e.g., swayback model's posture).

Prolonged Maintenance of the Static Erect Posture

Standing in the upright position for long periods of time tends to produce an increase in lumbar lordosis as muscles begin to fatigue and as the slow "creep" of the soft tissues often emphasizes the natural tendency towards extension of the region. This occurs because the center of gravity is usually ventral to the sacral promontory in most adults.[13] The effect of gravity acting through this center pulls the lumbar spine into a more lordotic posture in those individuals. This postural change accompanies the diurnal decline in height (see Diurnal Variation in Stature). Vertebral column posture is ideally dynamic rather than static, as the tissues adapt to prolonged static loading by further "creep" of the column.

The Effects of Age on Lumbar Lordosis

The lumbar spinal lordosis flattens considerably in old age in both sexes (Fig. 2-5),[2,5] although a few individuals do show small increases in lordosis. Increases are usually associated with increased abdominal girth and weight and declines in abdominal-muscle strength, so that their physique approximates that of a pregnant female. Thus, the explanation for an increase in lordosis is the same as that for pregnant women (see above). However, Twomey's[5] large study of a typical Australian society clearly shows a significant decrease in lumbar lordosis with increasing age after adolescence of 32 percent in females and 20 percent in males.

Lumbar Lordosis in Association with Back Pain

Clinicians often report a flattening of the lumbar lordosis during episodes of back pain. However, a recent study of 600 men between the ages of 23 and 60 years has shown that the distribution and range of lordosis (as viewed on radiographs) does not vary in acute or chronic low-back pain more than it does in men without back pain.[14]

Leg-Length Inequality and Pelvic Obliquity

While pelvic tilt in the sagittal plane is inextricably linked with lumbar lordosis, coronal-plane obliquity of the pelvis is associated with lumbar scoliosis. The most common cause of this functional situation is leg-length inequality.[15] Functional scoliosis must be distinguished from idiopathic structural scoliosis. Structural scoliosis progresses during the growth period, is seen most frequently in girls,[16] and is usually convex to the left in the lumbar spine. Leg-length inequality and postural scoliosis have been associated with low back pain, degenerative changes in the intervertebral discs and zygapophyseal joints, and with a higher incidence of osteoarthritic changes in hip and knee joints. Interestingly, it is most often the left leg that tends to be longest, particularly in men,[17] since most right-handed people put more weight on their left foot.[18]

Unequal leg length may be associated with pathologic conditions (e.g., Perthes' disease, previous fracture), but in the vast majority of situations, it accompanies normal growth. In most of this latter group, the degree of asymmetric growth of the lower limbs is very common. It is associated with "out of phase" growth, where one of a pair of bones is more advanced than the other at maturity.[17] A leg-length difference of 1 cm or greater is twice as common at the peak of the adolescent growth spurt (13 percent) than at maturity (7 percent).[19] Indeed, it is very rare to find exactly equal leg lengths in normal communities.

Giles and Taylor[20,21] showed that unequal leg length and the associated "postural" scoliosis are linked with minor structural changes in lumbar discs and vertebral end-plates, and with asymmetric changes to the articular cartilage and subchondral bone of the of the lumbar zygapophyseal joints. The joints on the convex side of the scoliotic curve show thicker subchondral bone plates and thinner articular cartilage than those from the concave side, suggesting greater loading on the convex side of the curve. This may be related to the greater postural muscle forces necessary on the convex side to prevent buckling of the scoliotic column under axial loading. A number of surveys have shown a statistical association between leg-length inequality and low back pain.[15,22,23] Leg-length inequality is twice as common in low back pain patients (13–22 percent) than in control populations (4–8 percent). Giles and Taylor[15] also suggested that the response to manipulative therapy in low back pain associated with leg-length inequality is much improved when a foot-raise shoe insert is provided as part of the treatment.

STATURE

Effects of Variations in Stature

The topics of stature and posture are closely related. Stature is affected by posture in a number of ways.

Postural Fatique

Laxity in posture causes "creep" of soft tissues (see Prolonged Maintenance of the Static Erect Posture).

Diurnal Variation in Stature

In 1777, Buffon noted that a young man was considerably shorter after spending the night at a ball but he regained his previous height after a rest in bed. Merkel (1881) measured his own daily loss in height (2 cm standing, 1.6 cm sitting) by measuring the height of his "visual plane" from the floor. He found that half his loss in stature occurred in the first hour after rising, and that a greater loss occurred after vigorous exercise.

De Puky[24] measured diurnal variation in stature and found the daily loss in height to average 15.7 mm. Diurnal variation as a percentage of total body height decreases steadily with increasing age. Blackman[25] showed a decrease in stature of 0.76 cm one hour after rising and 1.77 cm four hours after rising and this order of decrease was confirmed by Stone and Taylor,[26] who showed that loss in sitting height was equivalent to 80 percent of the loss in standing height.

In a recent study, Tyrrell, Reilly, and Troup[27] showed that average daily variation in stature was about 1 percent of normal stature, and that the greatest loss occurred in the first hour after rising in the morning. Approximately 70 percent of this lost stature was gained during the first half of the night. The carrying of heavy loads increased the rate of shrinkage loss (i.e., by "creep"). Interestingly, rest with the lumbar spine in full flexion produced more rapid gains in stature than in other positions. This also suggests that the diurnal loss involves "creep" into extension (see Prolonged Maintenance of the Static Erect Posture). Adams and Hutton[28] have recently demonstrated that the flexed position induces the transport of metabolites and fluids into the intervertebral discs. If most of the diurnal loss in stature is a loss of trunk length due to small diurnal reductions in disc height,[26] then the use of flexion as a tool to maintain disc height and to preserve normal erect posture without excessive lordosis becomes of clinical interest for physical therapists.

The mechanism involved in diurnal variation in stature is discussed further under later sections on "creep" of vertebral structures.

The Influence of Changes in Posture on Stature

When parents measure their child's stature as a record of their growth rate the usual instructions given are to "stand tall, like a soldier." This implies a general understanding that stature is dependent in part on a person's posture. When "standing tall," the child flattens the spine as much as possible, tucks the chin in, and attempts to push the top of the head as far upward as possible. Similarly, after surgical correction of moderate to severe scoliosis, when the spine is surgically "straightened," children can gain up to 8 cm in height.

The thoracic spine makes the largest contribution to spine length. The lumbar spine constitutes one-third, the cervical spine one-fifth, and the thoracic spine the remainder of the total length of the presacral spine in the adult.[29]

The Effect of Growth and Aging on Stature

The rates of growth and decline in stature are described in Chapter 1. The spinal component in the decline in stature that occurs in old age is much more a result of a decrease in vertebral height than it is a decrease in intervertebral disc height.[30,31] An increasing thoracic kyphosis (particularly in women) also contributes significantly to the loss of stature in old age.

MOVEMENTS OF THE LUMBAR VERTEBRAL COLUMN

At each level in the vertebral column there are three interacting joints allowing and controlling movement. This unique combination is known as the *articular triad* or as the *mobile segment* (Ch. 1). Each articular triad allows only a few degrees of movement. However, lumbar movement usually involves a complex interaction of mobile segments at multiple levels. The thickness of each intervertebral disc, the compliance of its fibrocartilage, and the dimensions and shape of its adjacent vertebral end-plates are of primary importance in governing the extent of movement possible. The shape and orientation of

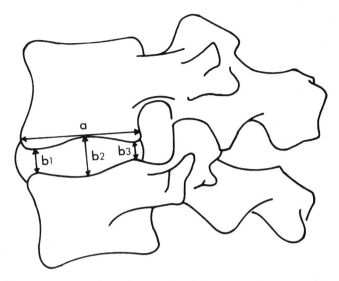

Fig. 2-6. The anterior vertebral elements (mobile segment): a = vertebral end-plate and b = disc thickness.

the vertebral-arch articular facets, with the ligaments and muscles of the arch and its processes, guide the types of movement possible and provide restraints against excessive movement.

Ranges of Disc Movement

The anterior elements (vertebrae and discs) of the articular triads are capable of certain ranges in movement depending on disc dimensions (thickness and horizontal dimensions) and disc stiffness.

Disc Dimensions

A large range of movement would occur when disc height was relatively great and vertebral end-plate horizontal dimensions relatively short (Fig. 2-6). Adolescent and young-adult females have shorter vertebral end plates (a) than males, while disc height ($b1$, $b2$, and $b3$) and disc stiffness are substantially the same. Thus, females possess the necessary combination of dimensions for a larger range of movements than is possible in males.[5,32] In old age when male and female vertebrae and disc shapes become very similar and hormonal dif-

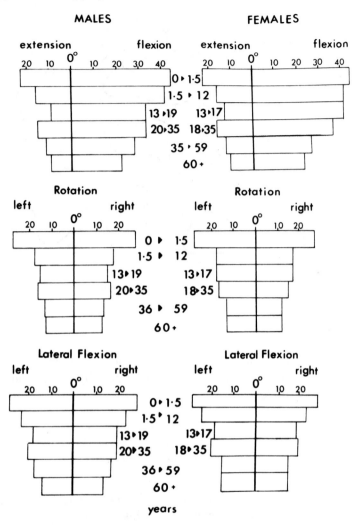

Fig. 2-7. Age changes in the range of lumbar movements in both sexes. (Taylor JR, Twomey LT: Sagittal and horizontal plane movement of the human vertebral column in cadavers and in the living. Rheumatol Rehabil 19:223, 1980.)

ferences are reduced the range of movement of men and women become almost identical (Fig. 2-7).

Disc Stiffness

The general reduction in movement ranges in both sexes is attributable to increased disc stiffness. This has been demonstrated by the posterior release experiment of Twomey and Taylor,[33] which demonstrates a 40 percent increase in disc stiffness in the elderly.

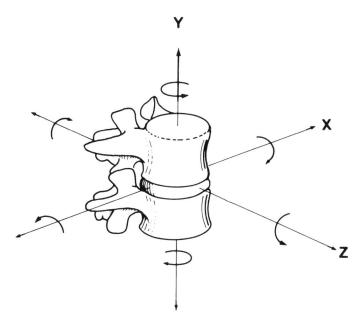

Fig. 2-8. Planes and axes of movement: sagittal plane movements occur along the *X* axis: rotational plane movements occur along the *Y* axis; and coronal plane movement occurs along the *Z* axis.

Planes of Movement

The movements possible at each lumbar-motion segment are traditionally described as being in the sagittal (flexion-extension), coronal (lateral flexion), and horizontal (axial rotation) planes. Each movement occurs along one of three coordinate axes *x*, *y*, and *z* (Fig. 2-8). Thus, all mobile segments of the lumbar spine possess 6 degrees of freedom and each movement consists of an angular or rotary displacement together with translation of a vertebra on its subjacent vertebra. It is rare for movement to occur exclusively in a single plane. Movements are generally "coupled" in habitual movement,[34] and occur across the standard descriptive planes of motion.

Ranges of Lumbar Movement

Despite the availability of simple, reliable methods for measuring spinal mobility these have not been applied to studies of normal lumbar spine movement until recently. The literature records considerable variation in the values given for the ranges of movements of the lumbar spine. This variation stems largely from the different measurement methods used and the differences in age, sex, race, and numbers of subjects studied. The clinical measurements most frequently used include indirect estimates of spinal mobility from measurement of (1) the distance from the fingertips to the floor when the patient bends forward and (2) the use of a tape measure to measure the increase in distance between two skin landmarks, often the S1 and L1 spinous processes. These methods are most inaccurate, and give no direct measure of the range (angular deflection) of spinal movement. The former is dependent on hamstring muscle length and the latter fails to show a reasonable level of consistency between repeated measures. Published studies of lumbar spinal movement have mostly concentrated on sagittal and coronal plane movements and include:

1. Direct measurement in living subjects, utilizing a wide variety of equipment[32,35–43]
2. Radiographic studies[44–51]
3. Cadaveric studies that have mostly involved a single mobile segment in a small number of specimens[3,49,52–64]
4. Photographic techniques[65,66]
5. Theoretical studies based on mathematical models.[67–72]

Estimates of the range of sagittal motion of the lumbar region vary widely from 121 degrees in a young male acrobat,[44] to 21.8 degrees in elderly women.[47] However, Begg and Falconer[73] considered 70 degrees to be the "normal" average total range of lumbar flexion-extension. Few studies have attempted to measure axial rotation in the lumbar spine, largely because of methodologic problems. It has proven difficult to measure lumbar rotation in the living either directly or radiographically with any degree of accuracy, and cadaveric studies have mostly been confined to motion segments rather than to the whole lumbar column. Some authorities maintain that rotary movement does not exist as a separate entity in the lumbar region,[74–76] or that if rotation does occur, it is in spite of the fact that the facets are designed to prevent it.[77] Other sources have assessed the total range of rotation as between 5 to 36 degrees of movement.[3,38,40,78–80]

Clinical Measurement

In an effort to provide instrumentation that would be relatively easily applied in the clinical situation and provide reasonably accurate objective data, two instruments have been devised to measure lumbar sagittal- and horizontal-plane movement, and have been tested in clinical trials.[32,64,81] The lumbar spondylometer is noninvasive, has good interperson and intertest reliability, and measures lumbar sagittal motion (Fig. 2-9). Since its base rests on the sacrum, the measurement is not confounded and invalidated by the inclusion of hip motion. Tests of its accuracy made by comparing living subjects with fresh, cadaveric specimens suggest that it underestimates the range of movement by an average of 1 degree.[32] Inter- and intraoperator repeatability trials show high correlations.[82] The lumbar spondylometer is comparable in accuracy and in some respects in principle to an inclinometer, but with a more complex

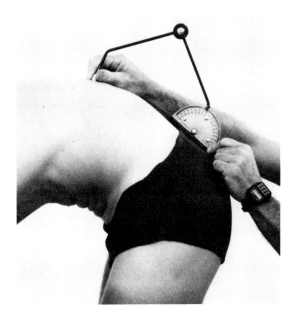

Fig. 2-9. The lumbar spondylometer.

geometry,[35] it is also easier to use in a clinical situation where separate readings from two inclinometers would be required. Its use requires a thorough knowledge of the surface anatomy of the lumbar region, with consistently accurate placement of the cushions, and the precise location of the L1 spinous process.

The cushions of the lumbar spondylometer rest on the dorsal surface of the sacrum, with the top cushion at the level of S1. The distal end of the instrument rests on the spinous process of L1 (Fig. 2-9). The physical therapist reads off the initial starting position in degrees, asks the subject to fully extend, and reads off the new position in degrees. The subject returns to the starting position (checked by the operator), and then moves into full-range flexion, with the operator recording the result. Thus, flexion, extension, and full-range sagittal motion are recorded. This entire process takes an experienced physical therapist less than 2 minutes to administer and record, and is a useful objective clinical measurement in the assessment of the progress of treatment for back conditions.[81]

The external measurement of rotation in the clinical situation has been made possible by the development of a lumbar rotameter.[32,64] The apparatus consists of a large protractor strapped at right angles to the subject's sacrum, and a belt with a pointer strapped around the trunk at L1. The tip of the pointer rests just above the protractor (Fig. 2-10). The subject is asked to rotate fully to the right and the left, angular deflections of the pointer being read off on the protractor. Intertrial and interoperator reliability tests show a maximum variation of 5 degrees in a range of 56 degrees, and these measurements correlate well with cadaveric motion.[32] The rotameter is relatively cumbersome, and it takes about 3 minutes for an experienced physical therapist to use it in

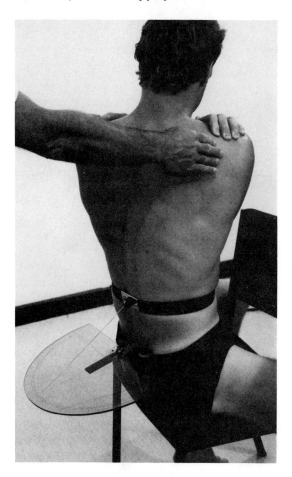

Fig. 2-10. The lumbar rotameter.

a clinical setting. For these reasons, it has proven less useful as a clinical tool. It has the additional disadvantage that its reading may be influenced to a minor degree by lower rib cage movements.

Ranges of lumbar movements, for both sexes in six age-group categories using the spondylometer and the rotameter, and the gravity inclinometer[37] for side flexion are listed in Table 2-1.

Age Changes in Ranges of Movements

Table 2-1 clearly demonstrates a decline in the ranges of all lumbar movements in the living with increasing age. This decline parallels the reductions observed in cadaveric studies by other authors.[5,47,48,83,84]

In old age the ranges of lumbar movement in men and women become almost identical. It would appear that when hormonal differences are reduced, sexual differentiations in vertebral shape, posture, and spinal-movement ranges

Table 2-1. The Mean and Standard Deviation for the Total Ranges of Sagittal, Horizontal and Coronal Plane Movements in Living Subjects (population 960 persons)

	Ranges of Movements					
	Sagittal Range (flexion-extension)		Horizontal Range (rotation to both sides)		Coronal Range (side flexion)	
Age	male	female	male	female	male	female
5–12 years	58° ± 9°	58° ± 9°	34° ± 6°	34° ± 6°	47° ± 6°	47° ± 6°
13–19 years	45° ± 10°	57° ± 8°	30° ± 4°	34° ± 4°	38° ± 5°	37° ± 4°
19–35 years	42° ± 6°	42° ± 7°	33° ± 6°	33° ± 6°	40° ± 5°	40° ± 5°
35–59 years	38° ± 7°	38° ± 7°	26° ± 6°	27° ± 6°	32° ± 4°	30° ± 3°
60+ years	30° ± 7°	28° ± 6°	22° ± 5°	20° ± 4°	28° ± 4°	30° ± 5°

disappear. The general reduction in ranges in both sexes occurs as a result of increased "stiffening" of the intervertebral disc in association with disc-shape changes involving increases in the anteroposterior length and concavity of the vertebral end-plate.[33] A reason often provided for the decline in average ranges of movements in aging populations (i.e., a general tendency to thinning of intervertebral discs in old age) has recently been shown to be false.[30,31] In old age most discs increase in volume and become thicker and more convex at the disc–vertebral interface. Only about 30 percent of discs become thinner. The principal reason for decreased range of movement is increased disc stiffness.[33]

The 40 percent increase in disc stiffness with age is associated with well-documented histologic and biochemical changes. These include an increase in the total number of collagen fibers and in the ratio of Type I to Type II collagen; a decrease in water content; and a change in the proteoglycan ratios where the proportion of keratan sulfate:chondroitin sulfate increases.[85,85] There is also an associated increase in "fatigue failure" of collagen in older cartilage. It is uncertain whether it is collagen fibers that undergo "fatigue" or splitting or whether it is the bonds between adjacent collagen fibers that separate (Stockwell, 1979). Collectively, these changes and the associated decrease in compliance render the disc fibrocartilage less capable of acting efficiently as a shock absorber or joint, and of transmitting loads along the vertebral column.[33,87]

Lumbar Intersegmental Motion

It is an essential part of a physical therapist's examination to determine ranges of movement of the whole lumbar spine. In addition to measurement of these physiologic ranges of movements, the manipulative physical therapist always conducts a manual assessment of lumbar intersegmental motion. This involves the displacement of a lumbar motion segment by the application of an external, manual force applied directly through the spinous processes, or indirectly via the ligaments and joints of the adjacent vertebrae. Small rotations and translations about and along the axes of movement can be achieved in this way (Fig. 2-8). No techniques are currently available for objective clinical measurement of mobile-segment range of motion, but in experienced hands local anomalies (increases or decreases in movement) can be confidently diagnosed. While these techniques involve subjective evaluation of vertebral motion, it is interesting to note its current excellent correlation with other diagnostic studies.[88]

Many clinical reports have associated either hypo- or hypermobility with a variety of lumbar disorders and low back pain.[34] At this point in time, there is very little real evidence linking ranges of motion and back pain, although anecdotal and clinical stories abound. However, Farrell and Twomey[81] in a study of acute low-back pain and manipulative therapy did show an improvement in lumbar sagittal motion (measured manually) associated with improvement in back pain symptoms. Giles and Taylor[15] also showed increased lumbar range of movement following recovery from episodes of low back pain, but this increase was only in patients under the age of 50 years. Similarly, Jull[88] has shown an increase in intersegmental motion associated with remission of symptoms in patients with low back pain. It is likely that current research may throw further light on this question over the next few years.

BIOMECHANICS

The orientation of the lumbar articular processes facilitates sagittal movement and allows for a considerable range of motion in this plane. From the "normal" erect standing posture, flexion usually comprises about 80 percent and extension 20 percent of the total range of sagittal movement. Flexion ceases due to apposition of lumbar zygapophyseal joint surfaces and tightening of posterior ligaments and muscles, while extension is blocked by bone contact when the inferior joint facets come into contact with the laminae of the vertebra below or the spinous processes meet.[33]

Control of Flexion

Muscular Control of Flexion

The lumbar back muscles exert considerable control over active ranges of lumbar movement (Ch. 4). Erector spinae and multifidis are principally responsible for all movements by exerting an eccentric control (i.e., by paying out) on movements that are gravity assisted. Thus trunk flexion in standing or sitting is controlled by an eccentric contraction of these muscle groups. In exerting this control, the muscles tend to restrict the total range of movements possible, particularly in the sagittal plane.[32] This helps explain why cadaveric studies show a slightly greater range of lumbar sagittal movement than is usually recorded in the living.[5]

It has been shown that after suitable warm-up exercises, ranges of lumbar flexion increase by a few degrees,[32] and that a change in posture from the upright to the side-lying position brings about an additional increase, which equates with the ranges observed in the cadaveric studies. It would appear that warm-up exercises achieve their effect by relaxation or stretching of the sacrospinalis muscle group and it is not unreasonable to assume that the slightly larger increase obtained in side lying is due to the elimination of antigravity activity in the long back muscles. Kippers and Parker[13] have shown an "electrically silent" phase in the back muscles at the limit of lumbar flexion. While they conclude that the spine is supported passively by tension in postvertebral connective tissue structures at this point, it may also be due in part to passive elastic tension of the posterior muscles themselves. Indeed, the apposed zygapophyseal facets play the greater restraining role.[33]

Each lumbar multifidus muscle attaches strongly to a mamillary process on a superior articular process and also into the capsule of a zygapophyseal joint. It acts as a rotator cuff muscle and maintains the approximation and congruity of the zygapophyseal facets on the posterolateral aspect of the joint (the ligamentum flavum maintains the articular surfaces in close apposition on the anteromedial side of the joint). The close relation of this muscle to the joint capsule and its similar innervation would readily explain how with other postvertebral muscles it would severely limit flexion and rotation in any painful condition of the joints.

Other Factors Controlling Lumbar Flexion

In addition to the postvertebral muscles, the posterior elements of the lumbar spine consist of a complex ligamentous system and the articulating bony arches. Over the years there have been a number of conflicting views on the relative roles played by these posterior elements in limiting and controlling the range of lumbar flexion. In general, it has been considered that the interspinous and supraspinous ligaments and the strong elastic ligamentum flavum served principally to act as a "brake" to flexion.[89] In this regard, the elasticity of the ligamentum flavum was seen as important because tension increased as the movement continued, while the dense, strong, and inelastic inter- and supraspinous ligaments acted as a physical barrier to the movement.

Adams, Hutton, and Stott[90] in a sequential posterior release experiment quantitated the relative parts played by the supraspinous-infraspinous ligaments, the ligamentum flavum, the zygapophyseal joint fibrous capsule, and the intervertebral disc in resisting flexion of individual motion segments. They showed that the joint fibrous capsule and intervertebral disc play the more important roles, with the ligamentum flavum and spinous ligaments making lesser contributions. They found it most surprising that the relatively unimpressive fibrous capsule should exert such large restraining forces, and noted that technical problems in sectioning all capsular fibers made it difficult to distinguish the role of capsular forces from articular facet forces exerted through the articular processes.

In the authors' study[33] of the role of the posterior elements, each of the posterior ligaments was sectioned in turn (supraspinous and interspinous, li-

Table 2-2. Average Increases (degrees) in Sagittal Range following Section

Section	Flexion Increase	Extension Increase	Sagittal Range Increase
Supraspinous and interspinous ligaments	2.0	1.5	3.5
Ligamenta flava	2.5	1.0	3.5
Joint capsules	3.0	2.0	5.0
Pedicles	14.0	3.0	17.0

gamentum flavum and capsule), as was the bony arch to assess the influence of each on the range of lumbar flexion. The range of flexion was measured before and after sectioning of each of the elements and the results are listed in Table 2-2. Analysis demonstrated small regular increases in sagittal range on each successive ligamentous release and a large abrupt increase in range following section of the vertebral arches. Young and middle-aged subjects showed almost a 100 percent increase in lumbar sagittal range after removal of all posterior elements, while elderly subjects showed a 60 percent increase (Fig. 2-11).

This study confirms that all the ligamentous elements offer some resistance to lumbar flexion, with the joint capsules having the greatest influence, as suggested by Adams, Hutton, and Stott.[90] However, by far the greatest restraining influence on flexion is the pressure between the apposed articular facets of the zygapophyseal joints. Radiographic analysis of flexion in a young cadaveric lumbar spine showed that the movement includes both forward rotation of a vertebra on the vertebra beneath along an axis in the posterior part of the intervertebral disc, and an associated forward translation or slide of the superior vertebrae on the inferior vertebra (Fig. 2-12). The zygapophyseal joints

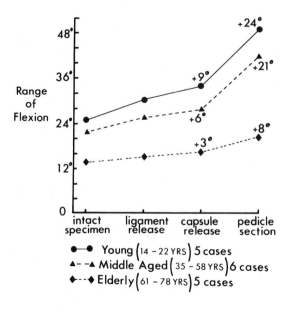

Fig. 2-11. The effects of the release of the posterior vertebral elements on the range of lumbar flexion. (Twomey LT, Taylor JR: Sagittal movements of the human lumbar vertebral column: A quantitative study of the role of the posterior vertebral elements. Arch Phys Med Rehabil 64: 322, 1983.)

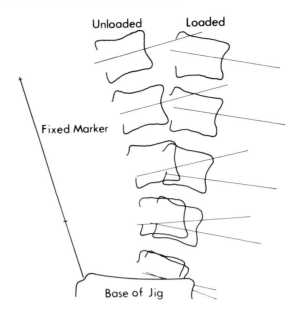

Fig. 2-12. Tracings of super-imposed radiographic plates showing the range of flexion produced and indicating the types of movement involved. (Twomey LT, Taylor JR: Sagittal movements of the human lumbar vertebral column. A quantitative study of the role of the posterior vertebral elements. Arch Phys Med Rehabil 64:322, 1983.)

guide the plane of rotation and resist the forward slide. The coronally oriented anterior component of each articular facet bears the resultant stress. When the pedicles are cut, a greater degree of forward slide permits further rotation.

Joint loading in axial weight bearing has been described by Nachemson[91] and by Shah, Hampsom, and Jayson.[92] It seems clear from our studies that flexion involves progressive joint loading to the point where the horizontal moment prevents further rotation from occurring. The lumbar vertebral arches through the zygapophyseal joints thus provide an essential restraint limiting or preventing the transmission of shearing forces to the intervertebral discs. This could lead to instability (as in spondylolisthesis) with danger to the cauda equina and to the nerve roots in the intervertebral canals.

Age differences in response to the posterior sectioning procedure cited above throw light on the effect of increased stiffness with aging in the intervertebral discs. Following ligamentous release and also more dramatically following pedicle section, the available increase in movement range is much reduced in elderly subjects compared to young subjects. This demonstrates that the increased stiffness or the reduction in disc compliance with aging is the principal reason for the observed decrease in lumbar range of movement. The important conclusions drawn from the studies described above are summarized below:

1. Lumbar sagittal movement involves both forward rotation and slide of one vertebra on the vertebra beneath around a coronal axis located in the posterior anulus of the intervertebral disc.

2. Sagittal movement of the vertebral column is restricted more by pro-

gressive increase in loading of apposed facetal joint surfaces in flexion than by tension or compression in posterior ligaments.

3.   The decline in sagittal range of movement in old age is principally due to increasing stiffness in the intervertebral disc.

"Creep" in the Lumbar Spine

We have argued above that the stiffness in intervertebral discs and the progressive loading of the zygapophyseal joints are the factors bringing the normal range of flexion to a halt. However, prolonged loading in flexion (10 minutes or more) *does* produce further flexion of the spine. This movement is due to "Creep," which is the progressive deformation of a structure under constant load when the forces are not large enough to cause permanent damage to the vertebral structures.

Axial "Creep"

In the normal erect posture, approximately 16-20 percent of axial compressive load on the lumbar spine is borne by the zygapophyseal joints, while the rest is carried by the intervertebral discs,[91,93] which are well suited to this purpose. When axial loads to intervertebral discs are maintained, the discs progressively lose height until the chemical forces developed within them equal those mechanical forces applied externally.[94] Provided that the forces used are below the levels that would cause permanent damage, the greater the external force then the greater the loss of height that occurs.[95]

During the day, a person's body weight acts as an axial compression force through the vertebral column, and the subsequent "creep" brings about a reduction in stature. When body weight is relieved (e.g., at night in bed) and axial loads reduced, the intervertebral discs and other soft tissues are able to rehydrate and stature increases.[96] It has recently been demonstrated that a period of rest in full flexion brings about a more rapid increase in stature than does rest in the fully extended position.[27] This presumably occurs because flexion acts as a distracting force on the lumbar region, causing the discs to "suck in" water at a greater rate.

"Creep" in Flexion

When full range lumbar flexion is maintained under load for a period of time, the articular triad is distorted so that the anterior disc region is "squeezed" while the posterior region is stretched; the zygapophyseal joint surfaces are compressed tightly together as the coronal part of the articular surfaces bear most of the load; and the soft tissues adjust by "creep."[94,97]

"Creep" in flexion is observed as progressive ventral movement into further flexion, so that the end point of flexion is increased (i.e., range increases). The amount of "creep" in the elderly is greater than in the young and both the "creep" and the recovery from "creep" take place over a longer period of time. During the process fluid is extruded from the soft tissues and they become relatively deprived of their nutrition.[98] Repetitive loading causes cartilage degeneration and bone hypertrophy in the various elements of the articular triad.[99]

If the amount of "creep" involved after prolonged load bearing in flexion is considerable, then recovery back to the original starting posture (hysteresis) is extremely slow. It takes considerable time for the soft tissues to imbibe fluid after it has been expressed during prolonged flexion loading. Many occupational groups (e.g., stonemasons, bricklayers, roofing carpenters, and the like) regularly submit their lumbar spines to this category of insult. They work with their lumbar column fully flexed and under load for considerable periods of time. There is often little movement away from the fully flexed position once it has been reached and little opportunity for recovery between episodes of work in this position. It is therefore not at all surprising to find so many bricklayers, for instance, with chronic back pain and with occasional episodes of acute pain. These occupational groups need considerable ergonomic advice and require alterations to their working conditions if this situation is to be rectified.

Control of Extension

The Role of Muscles

The control of lumbar extension has not been investigated and analyzed to the same extent as flexion. In the erect standing or sitting postures, the movement is initiated by contraction of the long back-extensor muscles, and then controlled by the eccentric contraction of the abdominal muscle group once the movement has begun. The range of extension from the neutral erect standing position is much less than the range of flexion, but the muscular control mechanisms are very similar.

Other Contributing Factors

It seems probable that the range of extension is not controlled by ligamentous tension, but that it ceases when the two inferior articular processes at any level are forced against the laminae of the vertebrae below or perhaps when the spinous processes "kiss." This is witnessed by the build-up in compact bone, which is evident in the lamina beneath the inferior process. Extension occurs along an axis in the posterior part of the intervertebral disc at that level. This position probably does not place the soft tissues under the same constant strain as flexion does except at the limits of lordosis after prolonged standing when zygapophyseal joints probably take a larger amount of the load of body weight. When hyperextension occurs, it is likely that the axis of movement shifts even further posteriorly and is located where the tips of the inferior facets articulate with the laminae. This would cause stretching of the anterior soft tissues, notably the anterior longitudinal ligament and the anterior anulus fibrosus, which are extremely strong and capable of withstanding such forces. It is apparent from our investigations that considerable osteoarthritic change takes place in the articular cartilage and subchondral bone. This change occurs at the polar region of the inferior recesses of the zygapophyseal joints corresponding to the areas of extension impact and compression.[99]

"Creep" in Extension

Prolonged maintenance of an extended posture or of loading in extension are rare, and few if any occupational groups have such a working situation. Brunnstrom[100] describes the position of the line of gravity as passing anterior to the thoracic vertebrae and through the lumbar vertebrae. Theoretically, prolonged standing, (i.e., axial loading with body weight) would tend to increase thoracic kyphosis (by "creep"), but not alter lumbar lordosis. However, present evidence indicates that in prolonged standing there is a tendency for the axial load of body weight to increase lumbar lordosis. In this way, the zygapophyseal joints will take an increasing proportion of the load of body weight. Although long, continued lordotic posture and loading are rare, a number of sports activities involve full extension movements of an explosive nature. These may be repetitive movements and may involve high peaks of loading in full extension. Thus, fast bowlers in cricket, gymnasts, and high jumpers are three groups who place tremendous impact forces through this posterior arch complex. At heel strike during these sports, the chisel-like inferior articular processes are forced down suddenly into the laminae of the vertebrae below. The forces involved are very considerable, as the load borne by the facets increases dramatically with the amount of extension of the region.[101] Repetition over long periods of time results in soft-tissue inflammation and bone sclerosis that may become obvious on radiographic examination, but which may later result in fracture and perhaps displacement. The bone area that absorbs this force is the isthmus between the zygapophyseal facets, i.e., the pars interarticularis. As is well known, this is the site at which spondylolysis occurs. It is even more likely that the repetitive combination of alternative explosive full extension followed suddenly by full flexion places enormous strain on the pars interarticularis region. This extension/flexion repetition moment at the pars may cause fatigue fracture in a similar way to that of fatigue in metal caused by successive opposite movements.

Considerable research on the mechanics of this region has taken place in recent years and the reader is referred to the series of papers on the posterior vertebral elements in the journal *Spine*, Volumes 3 and 4, 1983.

VULNERABILITY OF THE DISC TO LOADING: INTRADISCAL PRESSURE

The nucleus of the intervertebral disc is contained under pressure within its protective fibrous and cartilaginous envelope. Intradiscal pressure is a useful index of disc function and it has been shown to vary according to posture, movement, and age. Nachemson's[91] comprehensive study on lumbar intradiscal pressure in 128 discs from 38 cadavers of both sexes from 6 to 82 years concluded the following:

1. The loaded disc behaves hydrostatically in that the nucleus acts as a fluid, distributing external pressures equally in all outward directions to the anulus.
2. Axial loading produces lower pressure readings in children below the age of 16 years than in adults.
3. The level of the lumbar spine does not influence the pressures recorded in "loaded" or resting discs (the L5-S1 disc was not included in the study).
4. The posterior vertebral structures (pedicles and articular processes) absorbs 16 to 20 percent of the vertical loading forces.
5. "Moderately degenerated" discs (as suggested by disc "thinning") show similar pressure behavior to "intact" discs, and the mechanical behavior of a lumbar disc does not change appreciably provided "degeneration" is not advanced.

Since Nachemson's[91] original study, it has been shown in living subjects that: intradiscal pressures are higher in the sitting than the standing posture[102,103]; they are less in the physiologic lordotic posture than in the straight or kyphotic positive[103] posture; pressures are increased with passive lumbar flexion of 20 degrees[104]; they are further increased during active trunk flexion exercises[105]; and the largest increases accompany heavy lifting particularly when the valsalva maneuver is performed.[106] Nachemson, Schultz, and Berkson[30] and Merriam et al[107] showed that abnormal degenerated discs did not behave in a consistent way, as they showed patterns of pressure changes in different postures often dissimilar from that shown by normal discs. Similarly, other studies have shown that the ability of the disc to withstand compressive forces depends on both the integrity of the disc envelope and the turgor of the contained nucleus pulposus.[55,108,109] This contrasts with the claim of Belytschko et al[110] that in a theoretical model anular tears would reduce intradiscal pressures more than degenerative nuclear lesions.

Clinical Considerations

The effects of different postures, exercises, and loading conditions on intradiscal pressure are of concern to the physical therapist as an indicator of what activities are likely to be safe or dangerous in the presence of disc degeneration. Exercise prescription needs to take into account specific disc as well as zygapophyseal joint pathology.

It is clear that movements such as lumbar flexion and lateral bending and tasks such as lifting heavy weights increase intradiscal pressure. Thus, this information needs to be carefully conveyed to those patients with proven or suspected disc problems. Similarly, because it is known that intradiscal pressure is lowest in supine and prone lying, is lower in sitting than standing, and low in activities involving lumbar extension and rotation, this information should be utilized in the physical treatment of the same patients. Similarly ergonomic advice as to lifting, seat design (including car seat design), working posture, and daily activities needs to emphasize the maintenance of a lordosis and the care to be taken whenever disc lesions are suspected (Ch. 11).

THE PROTECTIVE INFLUENCE OF INTRATRUNKAL PRESSURE

Intrathoracic and intraabdominal pressure have been shown to be most important in relieving the spine of part of the axial compression and shear loads by converting the trunk into a more solid cylinder and transmitting part of the load over the wider area. It is likely that intraabdominal pressure exerts a major force in this regard and involves simultaneous contraction of abdominal muscles, the diaphragm, and the muscles of the pelvic diaphragm. These are mostly transverse and obliquely oriented muscles, all capable of exerting considerable torque.

The thoracic spine bears less weight than the lumbar spine and therefore does not require as large a supportive force as that developed in the abdomen. The role of intraabdominal pressure in reducing forces acting on the spine and protecting vulnerable vertebral bodies and intervertebral discs was initially investigated by Bartelink[111] and has since excited the imagination of other researchers.[106,112-116]

Contraction of the muscles of the trunk cavity to raise intraabdominal pressure probably functions as a protective reflex mechanism, both to protect abdominal viscera from damage by a blow and to protect the vertebral column from excessive loading. Thus, when loads are placed on the vertebral column, the muscles are involuntarily called into action to fix the rib cage and to restrain and compress the contents of the abdominal cavity so that it becomes like a "balloon".[115] The positions of the trunk and the load influence the extent of any rise in intraabdominal pressure. The greater the spine is flexed and the further the load is away from the body the greater is the increase in intraabdominal pressure required to balance the load and distribute the compression forces.

The mechanism may be compared to an inflated balloon, which acts on an anterior moment arm two or three times the length of the posterior moment arm of the back extensor muscles. Pressures generated in the abdominal cavity will produce a net positive moment, and tend to restore the lordotic curvature of the lumbar spine. This will counteract the flexion moments produced by the upper body and the anterior load carried. Eie[114] described the relieving force of intraabdominal pressure as reducing by about 40 percent the required compressive effect of the contraction force of the erector spinae muscles.

Intraabdominal pressure thus plays a major role in stabilizing the spine and pelvis at the onset of the lift by resisting trunk flexion and reducing intervertebral compression forces. This allows the pelvis to be rotated backward and the lumbar curve flattened by the powerful gluteal and hamstring muscles, which have a longer moment arm and a greater crosssectional area (and thus power) than do the spinal extensors. Thus, they are the most suitable and capable muscles to be recruited in initiating the task of heavy lifting[117] and to reduce the moment of the load, thereby allowing the erector spinae muscles to take over and extend the spine on a stable pelvis. Raised intraabdominal pressure was able to reduce the reaction forces at the lumbosacral junction by approximately 30 percent during heavy lifting[112,118] and 10 percent when light loads were involved.[119]

Andersson, Ortengren, and Nachemson[106] showed in a small study of four adults that there was no significant correlation between high intradiscal and intraabdominal pressures in experiments where small loads were lifted. However, a linear relationship exists between intraabdominal and intradiscal pressure when the weight of the upper body and the load is moved further forward from the spine. Thus, they demonstrated that a simultaneous increase in intradiscal and intraabdominal pressures (doubled) and myoelectric back muscle activity when a 50 kg weight was moved horizontally outward from shoulder level and the effective load was greatly increased.

The lowest intraabdominal pressures have been recorded in the smallest people while largest pressures are evident in taller, heavier subjects. Strong athletes are able to produce enormous rises in intraabdominal pressure.[120] Gait shows phasic changes in this pressure, with increases as the speed of the activity increases. Jumping in place or from a height raises the pressure, as do pushing and pulling activities. It is uncertain whether or not the valsalva maneuver or the use of a lumbosacral corset does any more than produce marginal increases in intraabdominal pressure.

Clinical Considerations

Intraabdominal pressure is a potent influence for reducing the loads applied to the spine. The prime requirement necessary to develop high intraabdominal pressure is strong muscles surrounding the abdominopelvic cavity. Thus, not only the abdominal muscles, but also the thoracic and pelvic diaphragms need to be strong. It is likely that the oblique and transverse abdominal muscles have an important role in bringing about intraabdominal pressure increases without increasing the axial loading on the spine.[116,117] Gracovetsky, Farfan, and Lamy[72] imply that subjects with weak abdominal muscles would be less able to control their vertebral lever system, and that this would force their extensor musculture to work harder placing the region at greater risk. Further studies need to be performed to clarify this situation. However, it is likely that a close relationship exists between the strength of the abdominal musculature and the ability to increase intraabdominal pressure, and thus protect the spine during heavy activities.

ZYGAPOPHYSEAL JOINT INTRACAPSULAR PRESSURE

In 1983, physical therapists Giovanelli, Thompson, and Elvey[121] conducted a pilot trial investigating lumbar zygapophyseal intracapsular joint pressures in living subjects. They placed two needles within the joint under radiographic control, one needle to inject saline and the other to record pressure changes. They showed that there is no intracapsular pressure at rest. Once fluid was injected into the joint, most active and passive movements caused a drop in the pressure produced by the injection, the pressure rising again on return to the starting position. The greatest drops in pressure occurred when passive techniques were directed specifically to the joint concerned. This highlighted a possible mechanism of pain relief by the use of localized manipulative and mobilizing techniques because raised intracapsular pressure with outpouring of fluid may result from some forms of joint pathology. This pilot trial needs to be extended considerably before much regard can be placed on its conclusions, but it does provide interesting information useful to the manipulative physical therapist on the ways in which manipulative techniques directly influence the joints moved.

SKELETAL HEALTH AND EXERCISE

As described in Chapter 1, the internal architecture of lumbar vertebrae consists of vertical bony trabeculae (beams or struts of bone) supported by horizontal trabeculae, which are aligned parallel to the lines of stress. Thus, the vertical trabeculae absorbs the axial loads of weight bearing, and transmit the load downwards and outwards to the vertebral shell via the transverse trabeculae, which resist buckling of the vertical weight-bearing beams. It is likely that the horizontal trabeculae are also important in absorbing and transmitting the lateral forces applied through the body as a consequence of muscular activity. Old age is associated with a significant selective decline in the numbers of horizontal trabeculae. The compressive load of body weight, which is usually maintained in old age, brings about fractures of the now less-well-supported vertical trabeculae, and collapse of the vertebral end-plate. Lumbar vertebrae become shorter and wider in old age, and more concave at the disc–vertebral junction.[122]

This pattern of selective bone loss and associated changes in vertebral body shape is part of the general picture of osteopenia and osteoporosis seen in the elderly. In western society at age 65, radiographic comparison with a "standard" suggests that 66 percent of women and 22 percent of men have osteoporosis. In women the incidence increases by about 8 percent for each additional decade, whereas a large increase does not occur until after the age of 76 in men.[128] The principal sites of fracture and pain due to osteoporosis are the vertebral column, the distal radius, and the neck of the femur. It causes over 200,000 hip fractures annually in the United States, while pain and shortened stature accompanied by "dowager's hump" or hunchback in elderly women are major symptoms of advanced osteoporosis, which often lead to vertebral collapse and functional disability.[123]

The prevention of osteoporosis at present focuses on the need for relatively high levels of dietry calcium (1000–1200 mg per day), particularly in women and for estrogen replacement therapy in some women.[124,125] Recently, considerable attention has also been paid to the important role of exercise in prevention. Important studies by Aloia et al[126] and Smith et al[127] have shown bone gain to follow exercise even in the very elderly. Physical therapists concerned in the prevention and treatment of back pain and disability need to stress these factors with their middle-aged and elderly patients. There is no doubt that bone loss occurs in the absence of physical activity, and that bone hypertrophy

follows increased exercise activity. It is likely that the incidence of osteoporotic bone fractures in the elderly could be reduced if regular exercise was generally maintained into old age. This reduced risk of fracture may relate as much to the maintenance of muscle strength and neuromuscular coordination as to the associated maintenance of bone mass.

REFERENCES

1. Kendall FP, McCreary EK: Muscles, Testing & Function. 3rd Ed. Williams & Wilkins, Baltimore, 1983
2. Schmorl G, Junghanns H: The Human Spine in Health and Disease. 2nd Ed. Grune & Stratton, New York, 1971
3. Farfan HF: Mechanical Disorders of the Low Back. Lea & Febiger, Philadelphia, 1973
4. Taylor JR: Growth of human I/V discs and vertebral bodies. J Anat 120:1, 49, 1975
5. Twomey LT: Age changes in the human lumbar spine. PhD thesis, University of Western Australia, 1981
6. Landau BR: Essential Human Anatomy and Physiology. 2nd Ed. Scott, Foresman, Glenview, Illinois, 1980
7. Hytten FE, Leitch I: The Physiology of Human Pregnancy. 3rd Ed. Blackwell Scientific, Oxford, 1971
8. Treanor WJ: Motions of the Hand & Foot. In Licht SH (ed): Therapeutic Exercise. Waverly Press, Baltimore, 1965
9. Youngman A, Elliott M: The effect of high heel shoes on lumbar lordosis. BAppSc project, Western Australian Institute of Technology, 1985
10. Romanes CJ: Cunningham's Textbook of Anatomy. 11th Ed. Oxford University Press, Oxford, 1972

11. Taylor JR, Alexander R: BSc project, University of Western Australia (unpublished), 1983
12. Clayton SG: Obstetrics. 11th Ed. E Arnold, London, 1966
13. Kippers V, Parker AW: Hand positions at possible critical points in the stoop–lift movement. Ergonomics 26:9, 895, 1983
14. Hansson T, Sandstrom J, Roos B et al: The bone mineral content of the lumbar spine in patients with chronic low back pain. Spine 10:158, 1985
15. Giles LGF, Taylor JR: Low back pain associated with leg length inequality. Spine 6:5, 510, 1981
16. Willner S: A study of height, weight and menarche in girls with idiopathic structural scoliosis. Acta Orthop Scand 46:71, 1975
17. Taylor JR, Halliday M: Limb length asymmetry and growth. J Anat 126:634, 1978
18. Ingelmark BE, Lindstrom J: Assymetries of the lower extremities and pelvis and their relationship to lumbar scoliosis. Acute Morphol Neerl Scand 5/6:227, 1963
19. Taylor JR, Slinger BS: Scoliosis screening and growth in Western Australian students. Med J Aust May 17, 475, 1980
20. Giles LGF, Taylor JR: Intra-articular synovial protrusions. Bull Hosp J Dis Orthop Inst 42:2, 248, 1982
21. Giles LGF, Taylor JR: The effect of postural scoliosis on lumbar apophyseal joints. Scand J Rheumatol 13:209, 1984
22. Nichols PJR: Short leg syndrome. Br Med J Clin Res 1863, 1960
23. Sicuranza BJ, Richards J, Tisdall LH: The short leg syndrome in obstetrics and gynaecology. Am J Obstet Gynecol 107:217, 1970
24. De Puky MD: Diurnal variation in stature. Acta Orthop Scand 6:338, 1935
25. Blackman J: Experimental error inherent in measuring the growing human being. p. 389. In Boyd E (ed): Am J Phys Anthropol 13, 1924
26. Stone M, Taylor JR: Factors influencing stature. BSc anatomy dissertation, University of Western Australia, 1977
27. Tyrrell AR, Reilly T, Troup JDG: Circadian variation in stature and the effects of spinal loading. Spine 10:2, 161, 1985
28. Adams MA, Hutton WC: The effect of posture on the lumbar spine. Bone Joint Surg 67B:4, 625, 1985
29. Sullivan WE, Miles M: The lumbar segment of the vertebral column. Anat Rec 133:619, 1959
30. Nachemson AL, Schultz AB, Berkson MH: Mechanical properties of human lumbar spine motion segments. Spine 4:1, 1, 1979
31. Twomey LT, Taylor JR: Age changes in the lumbar intervertebral discs. Acta Orthop Scand 56:496, 1985
32. Taylor JR, Twomey LT: Sagittal and horizontal plane movement of the human lumbar vertebral column in cadavers and in the living. Rheumatol Rehabil 19:223, 1980
33. Twomey LT, Taylor JR: Sagittal movements of the human lumbar vertebral column: A quantitative study of the role of the posterior vertebral elements. Arch Phys Med Rehabil 64:322, 1983
34. White AA, Panjabi MM: The clinical biomechanics of the spine. JB Lippincott Philadelphia, 1978
35. Dunham WF: Ankylosing spondylitis: measurement of hip and spine movements. Brit J Phys Med 12:126, 1949
36. Lindahl O: Determination of the sagittal mobility of the lumbar spine: A clinical method. Acta Orthop Scand 37:241, 1966

37. Leighton JR: The Leighton flexometer and flexibility test. J Assoc Phys Ment Rehabil 20:3, 86, 1966
38. Gregersen G, Lucas DB: An in vivo study of the axial rotation of the human thoraco-lumbar spine. J Bone Joint Surg 49A:2, 247, 1967
39. Loebl WY: Measurement of spinal posture and range of spinal movement. Ann Phys Med 9:103, 1967
40. Loebl WY: Regional rotation of the spine. Rheumatol Rehabil 12:223, 1973
41. Macrae IF, Wright V: Measurement of back movement. Ann Rheum Dis 28:584, 1969
42. Moll JMH, Liyanage SP, Wright V: An objective clinical method to measure spinal extension. Rheum Phys Med 11:293, 1972
43. Moll J, Wright V: Measurement of Spinal Movement. p. 93. In Jayson M (ed): The Lumbar Spine and Back Pain, Pitman Medical, Kent 1976
44. Wiles P: Movements of the lumbar vertebra during flexion and extension. Proc R Soc Med 28:647, 1935
45. Gianturco C: A roentgen analysis of the motion of the lower lumbar vertebrae. Am J Roentogenol 52:3, 261, 1944
46. Hasner E, Schalintzek M, Snorrason E: Roentgenological examination of the function of the lumbar spine. Acta Radiol 37:141, 1952
47. Tanz SS: Motion of the lumbar spine. A roentgenologic study. Am J Roentgenol 69:3, 399, 1953
48. Allbrook D: Movements of the lumbar spinal column. J Bone Joint Surg 39B:2, 339, 1957
49. Rolander SD: Motion of the lumbar spine with special reference to the stabilising effect of posterior fusion. Acta Orthop Scand suppl 90, 1966
50. Troup JDG, Hood CA, Chapman AE: Measurements of the sagittal mobility of the lumbar spine and hips. Ann Phys Med 9:308, 1967
51. Froning EC, Frohman B: Motion of the lumbosacral spine after laminectomy and spine fusion. J Bone Joint Surg 50A:5, 897, 1968
52. Virgin WJ: Experimental investigations into the physical properties of the intervertebral disc. J Bone Joint Surg 33B:4, 607, 1951
53. Hirsch K: The reaction of the intervertebral discs to compression forces. J Bone Joint Surg 37A:1188, 1955
54. Hirsch K, Nachemson A: A new observation on the mechanical behaviour of lumbar discs. Acta Orthop Scand 23:254, 1954
55. Brown T, Hansen RJ, Yorra AJ: Some mechanical tests on the lumbosacral spine with particular reference to the intervertebral discs. J Bone Joint Surg 39A:5, 1135, 1957
56. Evans FG, Lissner HR: Biomechanical studies on the lumbar spine and pelvis. J Bone Joint Surg 41A:278, 1959
57. Roaf, R: Vertebral growth and its mechanical control. J Bone Joint Surg 42B:40, 1960
58. Galante JO: Tensile properties of the human lumbar annulus fibrosis. Acta Orthop Scand suppl 100:1, 1967
59. White AA: Analysis of the mechanics of the thoracic spine in man. Acta Orthop Scand suppl 127, 1969
60. Farfan HF, Cossette JW, Robertson GH et al: The effects of torsion on the lumbar intervertebral joints: The role of torsion in the production of disc degeneration. J Bone Joint Surg 52A:468, 1970
61. King AI, Vulcan AP: Elastic deformation characteristics of the spine. J Biomech 4:413, 1971

62. Kazarian L: Dynamic response characteristics of the human lumbar vertebral column. Acta Orthop Scand suppl 146:1, 1972

63. Panjabi MM: Experimental determination of spinal motion segment behaviour. Orthop Clin North Am 8:1, 169, 1977

64. Twomey LT: The effects of age on the ranges of motions of the lumbar region. Aust J Physiother 25:6, 257, 1979

65. Keegan JJ: Alterations of the lumbar curve related to posture and seating. J Bone Joint Surg 35A:589, 1953

66. Davis PR, Troup JDG, Burnard JH: Movements of the thoracic and lumbar spine when lifting: A chrono-cyclophotographic study. J Anat 99:1, 13, 1965

67. Schultz AB, Belytschko TP, Andriacchi TP et al: Analog. studies of forces in the human spine: Mechanical properties and motion segment behaviour. J Biomech 6:373, 1973

68. Panjabi MM: Three-dimensional mathematical model of the human spine structure. J Biomech 6:671, 1973

69. Belytschko TB, Andriacchi TP, Schultz AB et al: Analog. studies of forces in the human spine: Computational techniques. J Biomech 6:361, 1973

70. Panjabi MM, Brand RA, White AA: Mechanical properties of the human thoracic spine. J Bone Joint Surg 58A:5, 642, 1976

71. Panjabi MM, Krag MH, White AA: Effects of preload on load displacement curves of the lumbar spine. Orthop Clin North Am 8:1, 181, 1977

72. Gracovestky S, Farfan HF, Lamy C: A mathematical model of the lumbar spine using an optimized system to control muscles and ligaments. Orthop Clin North Am 8:1, 135, 1977

73. Begg AG, Falconer MA: Plain radiographs in intraspinal protrusion of lumbar intervertebral discs: A correlation with operative findings. Br J Surg 36:225, 1949

74. Lovett RW: A contribution to the study of the mechanics of the spine. Am J Anat 2:457, 1902

75. Tondury G: Functional anatomy of the small joints of the spine. Ann de Med Phys 15:2, 1971

76. Kapandji IA: The Physiology of the Joints. 2nd Ed. Vol. 3. Trunk and Vertebral Column. Churchill Livingstone, London, 1974

77. Lewin T, Moffett B, Viidik A: The morphology of lumbar synovial intervertebral joints. Acta Morphol Neerl Scand 4:229, 1961

78. Rissanen PM: The surgical anatomy and pathology of the supraspinous and interspinous ligaments of the lumbar spine with special reference to ligament ruptures. Acta Orthop Scand suppl 46, 1960

79. Hollingshead WH: Textbook of Anatomy. 2nd Ed. Harper & Row, New York, 1967

80. Lumsden RM, Morris JM: An in vivo study of axial rotation and immobilisation at the lumbosacral joint. J Bone Joint Surg 50A:1591, 1968

81. Farrell JP, Twomey LT: Acute low back pain: Comparison of two conservative treatment approaches. Med J Aust 1:160, 1982

82. Farrell J: A comparison of two conservative treatment approaches to acute low back pain. MAppSc thesis, Western Australian Institute of Technology, 1982

83. Hilton RC, Ball J, Benn RT: In-vitro mobility of the lumbar spine. Ann Rheum Dis 38:378, 1979

84. Nachemson A: Lumbar spine instability: A critical update and symposium summary. Spine 10:3, 290, 1985

85. Adams P, Eyre DR, Muir H: Biomechanical aspects of development and ageing of human lumbar intervertebral discs. Rheum Rehabil 16:22, 1977

86. Bushell GR, Ghosh P, Taylor TFK et al: Proteoglycan chemistry of the intervertebral disc. Clin Orthop 129:115, 1977
87. Nachemson AL: The lumbar spine: An orthopaedic challenge. Spine 1:1, 59, 1976
88. Jull G: The changes with age in lumbar segmental motion as assessed by manual examination. Master's thesis, University of Queensland, 1985
89. Ramsey RH: The anatomy of the ligamenta flava. Clin Orthop 44:129, 1966
90. Adams MA, Hutton WC, Stott MA: The resistance to flexion of the lumbar intervertebral joint. Spine 5:3, 245, 1980
91. Nachemson A: Lumbar intradiscal pressure. Acta Orthop Scand suppl 43, 1960
92. Shah JS, Hampson WGJ, Jayson MIV: The distribution of surface strain in the cadaveric lumbar spine. J Bone Joint Surg 60B:2, 246, 1978
93. Miller JAA, Haderspeck KA, Schultz AB: Posterior element loads in lumbar motion segments. Spine 8:3, 331, 1983
94. Kazarian LE: Creep characteristics of the human spinal column. Orthop Clin North Am 6:1, 3, 1975
95. Koreska J, Robertson D, Mills RH et al: Biomechanics of the lumbar spine and its clinical significance. Orthop Clin North Am 8:1, 121, 1977b
96. Koeller W, Meier W, Hartmann F: Biomechanical properties of human intervertebral discs subjected to axial dynamic compression. Spine 9:7, 725, 1984
97. Twomey LT, Taylor JR: Flexion creep deformation and hysteresis in the lumbar vertebral column. Spine 7:2, 116, 1982
98. Adams MA, Hutton WC: The effect of posture on the fluid content of lumbar intervertebral discs. Spine 8:6, 665, 1983
99. Twomey LT, Taylor JR: Age changes in the lumbar articular triad. Aust J Physiother 31:3, 106, 1985
100. Brunnstrom S: Clinical Kinesiology. 2nd Ed. FA Davis, Philadelphia, 1966
101. Yang KH, King AI: Mechanism of facet load transmission as a hypothesis for low back pain. Spine 9:6, 557, 1984
102. Nachemson A, Morris JM: In vivo measurements of intradiscal pressure. J Bone Joint Surg 46A:5, 1077, 1964
103. Andersson BJG, Ortengren R, Nachemson A et al: Lumbar disc pressure and myoelectric back muscle activity during sitting. Scand J Rehabil Med 6:104, 1974
104. Nachemson A: The effect of forward bearing on lumbar intradiscal pressure. Acta Orthop Scand 35:314, 1965
105. Nachemson A, Elfstrom G: Intravital dynamic pressure measurements in lumbar discs. Scand J Rehabil Med suppl 1:1, 1970
106. Andersson BJG, Ortengren R, Nachemson A: Quantitative studies of back loads in lifting. Spine 1:3, 178, 1976
107. Merriam WF, Quinnell RC, Stockdale HR et al: The effect of postural changes on the inferred pressures within the nucleus pulposus during lumbar discography. Spine 9:4, 406, 1984
108. Virgin WJ: Anatomical and pathological aspects of the intervertebral disc. Indian J Surg 20:113, 1958
109. Panjabi MM, Krag MH, Chung TQ: Effects of disc injury on mechanical behaviour of the human spine. Spine 9:7, 707, 1984
110. Belytschko T, Kulak RF, Schultz AB et al: Finite element stress analysis of an intervertebral disc. J Biomech 4:277, 1974
111. Bartelink DL: The role of abdominal pressure in relieving the pressure on the lumbar intervertebral discs. J Bone Joint Surg 39B:4, 718, 1957
112. Morris JM, Lucas DB, Bresler B: Role of the trunk in stability of the spine. J Bone Joint Surg 43A:3, 328, 1961

113. Davis PR, Troup JDG: Pressures in the trunk cavities when pulling, pushing and lifting. Ergonomics 7:465, 1964

114. Eie N: Load capacity of the low back. J Oslo City Hosp 16:73, 1966

115. Kumar S, Davis PR: Lumbar vertebral innervation and intra-abdominal pressure. J Anat 114:47, 1973

116. Grillner S, Nilsson J, Thorstensson A: Intra-abdominal pressure changes during natural movements in man. Acta Physiol Scand 103:275, 1978

117. Farfan HF: Muscular mechanism of the lumbar spine and the position of power and efficiency. Orthop Clin North Am 6(1):135, 1975

118. Davis PR, Stubbs DA, Ridd JE: Radio pills: Their use in monitoring back stress. J Med Eng Technol 1:4, 209, 1977

119. Ortengren R, Andersson GBJ: Electromyographic studies of trunk muscles, with special reference to the functional anatomy of the lumbar spine. Spine 2:1, 44, 1977

120. Eie N, Wehn P: Measurements of the intra-abdominal pressure in relation to weight bearing of the lumbo-sacral spine. J Oslo City Hosp 16:73, 1962

121. Giovanelli B, Thompson E, Elvey R: Measurement of variations in lumbar zygapophyseal joint intracapsular pressure: A pilot study. Aust J Physiother 31:3, 115, 1985

122. Twomey LT, Taylor JR, Furniss B: Age changes in the bone density and structure of the lumbar vertebral column. J Anat 136:1, 15, 1983

123. Pardini A: Exercise, vitality and aging, Age Ageing 344:19, 1984

124. Dixon AStJ: Non hormonal treatment of osteoporosis. Br Med J 286:999, 1983

125. Spencer H, Kramer L, Lesniak M et al: Calcium requirements in humans. Clin Orthop 184:270, 1984

126. Aloia JF, Cohn SH, Ostuni JA et al: Prevention of involutional bone loss by exercise. J Clin Endocrinol Met 43:992, 1978

127. Smith EL, Reddan W, Smith PE: Physical activity and calcium modalities for bone mineral increase in aged women. Med Sci Sports Exerc 13:60, 1981

128. Dent CE, Watson L: Osteoporosis. Postgrad Med J suppl Oct., 583, 1966

3 | Innervation, Pain Patterns, and Mechanisms of Pain Production

Nikolai Bogduk

Fundamental to the interpretation of lumbar pain syndromes is a knowledge of the mechanisms by which local and referred pain can be produced. If the mechanisms involved in a particular patient are properly understood, then treatment can be prescribed logically and appropriately. However, when interpretations are based on misconception or restricted knowledge, then there is a risk of treatment being inappropriate and unsuccessful.

What has compromised the evolution of thought on lumbar pain syndromes has been a tendency to simply infer or deem that a particular mechanism or cause is responsible for a particular syndrome, without actually proving it to be so. Indeed, if reiterated often and strongly enough, such inferences, even if incorrect, seem to gain the respectability of a "rule" or "dogma," and sometimes become so "sacred" as to be exempt from challenge. Yet in some instances, new facts or correct logic expose the limitations or errors in concepts evolved in this way.

As far as possible, concepts should be based on scientific fact, and it is the purpose of this chapter to collate those facts with experimental observations that are relevant to the comprehension of the mechanisms of lumbar pain syndromes. In this way, one can provide a rational basis for interpretation, while at the same time challenging or dispelling certain common misconceptions that are no longer tenable.

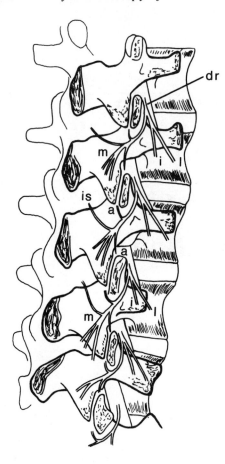

Fig. 3-1. A Sketch of a right posterolateral view of the lumbar dorsal rami showing the disposition of their branches. *dr:* L1 dorsal ramus; *m:* medial branches; *i:* intermediate branches; *l:* lateral branches; *is:* branch to interspinous muscle and ligament; *a:* articular branches of the medial branch, to the lumbar zygapophyseal joints.

INNERVATION

For any structure to be a source of pain it must be connected to the nervous system and, conversely, any structure that has a nerve supply is a potential source of pain. For this reason, the innervation of the lumbar spine has been the subject of several recent studies[1-3] and reviews.[4,5] Since details are available in these publications, only a summary need be provided here.

The posterior elements of the lumbar vertebral column are those parts that lie dorsal to the intervertebral foramina, and they are all innervated by branches of the dorsal rami of the lumbar spinal nerves. The dorsal rami themselves are very short nerves directed backward and caudally through the intertransverse spaces (Fig. 3-1). As each dorsal ramus approaches the subjacent transverse process, it divides into two or three branches.[3] Lateral branches are distributed to the lateral column of the lumbar erector spinae—the iliocostalis muscle.[6] The lateral branches of the L1-3 dorsal rami emerge from this muscle and cross the iliac crest to become cutaneous over the buttock.[3,7] Intermediate branches of the lumbar dorsal rami arise independently from each dorsal ramus or from

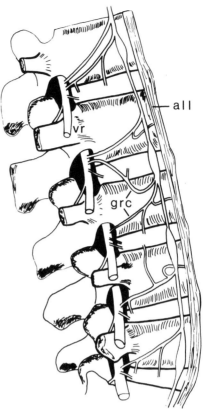

Fig. 3-2. Sketch of a lateral view of the lumbar vertebral column showing the nerves that supply the intervertebral discs. Branches of the gray rami communicans (*grc*) supply the lateral aspects of the discs, as well as the anterior longitudinal ligament (*all*). The posterolateral corner of each disc receives branches from a gray ramus or directly from a ventral ramus (*vr*).

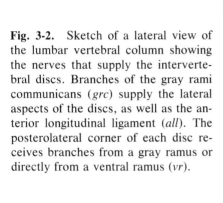

its lateral branch[3] and are distributed to the medial column of the lumbar erector spinae—the longissimus thoracis muscle.[6]

The medial branches of the lumbar dorsal rami have been considered the most relevant clinically for in addition to innervating the multifidus muscle and the interspinous muscles and ligaments they supply the lumbar zygapophyseal joints.[3,4,8–10]

The anterior elements of the lumbar vertebral column are the vertebral bodies and the intervertebral discs and their related ligaments (Ch. 1). These are innervated by branches of the lumbar ventral rami. Included among the anterior elements should be the anterior aspect of the lumbar dural sac, for not only does it lie anterior to the spinal nerves and their roots, but it is innervated by branches of the same nerves that innervate the other anterior elements. No nerve endings have been found in the posterior dura,[11] so for present purposes, no controversy need be raised as to whether the posterior dura should be classified as an anterior or posterior element.

The anterior longitudinal ligament and the lateral aspects of the intervertebral discs receive their innervation from branches of the gray rami communicantes[2] (Fig. 3-2). While it may appear that these structures are innervated by the sympathetic nervous system, this is not necessarily so, for it

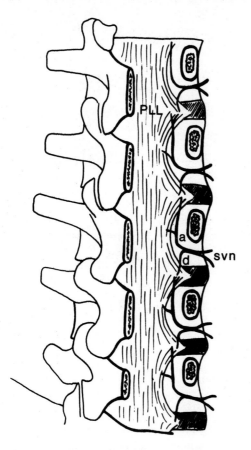

Fig. 3-3. Sketch of a posterior view of a lumbar vertebral column in which the right neural arches and dural sac have been removed to reveal the distribution of the lumbar sinuvertebral nerves (*svn*). Each nerve forms ascending (*a*) and descending (*d*) branches that supply the discs above and below, as well as the intervening posterior longitudinal ligament (*PLL*).

has been argued that the sensory fibers from the discs and anterior longitudinal ligament may simply use the course of the gray rami to reach the ventral rami, and thereby the somatic nervous system. To actually validate this interpretation would be difficult, but it should not be surprising. Sensory fibers from the vertebral artery run in the vertebral sympathetic plexus, but then enter the upper cervical ventral rami and dorsal root ganglia to return to the somatic nervous system,[12] and sensory fibers from viscera run in sympathetic nerves before reaching dorsal root ganglia.

The posterolateral angle of each intervertebral disc receives branches from the terminal portion of the adjacent gray ramus communicans and/or directly from the adjacent ventral ramus[2] (Fig. 3-2). The posterior aspects of the intervertebral discs and the posterior longitudinal ligament are innervated by the lumbar sinuvertebral nerves.[2,8,11,13]

The lumbar sinuvertebral nerves are recurrent nerves that enter the intervertebral foramina at each segmental level (Fig. 3-3). Each is formed by a branch of the gray ramus communicans and a branch of the ventral ramus. The main trunk passes into the vertebral canal just below the adjacent pedicle.[2,8,11,13] Descending branches of each nerve ramify in the intervertebral disc at the level of origin of the nerve while ascending branches supply the disc above and the intervening posterior longitudinal ligament.[2,8,13] Dorsally directed branches supply the anterior surface of the adjacent dural sac,[8,11,14] while vascular branches supply the vessels of the epidural space and vertebral bodies.[8,11,13]

Although it has long been held that the intervertebral discs lack an innervation,[15] this is manifestly not so. The description above of the sources of innervation of the lumbar discs is complemented by the results of histologic studies that have demonstrated nerve fibers and nerve endings not only in the superficial laminae of the anulus fibrosus,[16,18] but also as deeply as the outer third or outer half of the anulus.[1,2,19] A more comprehensive review of this issue is available elsewhere.[20]

This summary of neurologic anatomy establishes that the possible sources of lumbar pain are the lumbar zygapophyseal joints, the various back muscles, the interspinous ligaments (all innervated by dorsal rami), the vertebral bodies, intervertebral discs, longitudinal ligaments, and the dura mater (all innervated by ventral rami). Anatomy alone, however, does not prove that a structure can be a source of pain. It shows only that the necessary nerve supply is present. Additional physiologic evidence is needed to show that stimulation of a structure can actually cause pain.

Physiology

At one time or another, each of the structures listed above has been incriminated as source of low back pain. However, it has taken some 45 years to collect the experimental evidence that vindicates these incriminations. Thus, in 1938 and 1939, Kellgren[21,22] demonstrated that low back pain could be induced by noxious stimulation of the lumbar back muscles and interspinous ligaments while, reciprocally, Steindler and Luck[23] had shown that certain forms of low back pain syndromes could be relieved, at least temporarily, by anesthetizing these same structures. Although the term "facet syndrome" was introduced in 1933,[24] it was not shown until the last 10 years that experimental stimulation of lumbar zygapophyseal joints could cause low back pain in normal volunteers,[25,26] and that back pain stemming from these joints could be relieved by radiologically controlled blocks of the joints themselves[27-34] or their nerve supply.[35-38]

Two lines of evidence revealed that the intervertebral discs could be a source of back pain. Operating on patients under local anesthetic, Wiberg[39] showed that pressing on the posterior anulus fibrosus could evoke low back pain. Later, after the introduction of discography as a diagnostic procedure, it was recognized that back pain could be reproduced by injections of contrast medium into lumbar intervertebral discs.[40] Subsequent experience with provocation discography has confirmed that the injection of contrast medium or even normal saline into intervertebral discs can evoke back pain, even if the disc is structurally intact and appears normal on myelography.[41,45]

The dura mater has been shown to be capable of causing back pain in two types of clinical experiment. Firstly, it was shown that back pain could be evoked by traction on the dural sleeves of lumbar nerve roots by pulling on sutures threaded through the dura at operation for laminectomy.[46] More recently, it has been shown that chemical irritation of the dura in the form of injections of hypertonic saline can evoke back pain.[47]

There is, therefore, a wealth of clinical experimental data confirming that the ligaments, muscles, joints, discs, and dura mater of the lumbar spine are all capable of being a source of back pain. Of the innervated structures of the lumbar spine, only the epidural blood vessels and the vertebral bodies have not been subjected to experimental study to determine whether they too can be a source of pain. Circumstantial evidence, however, is conducive to the notion that distension of epidural veins can cause pain;[48] but while it is presumed that the pain of spinal osteoporosis arises from vertebral bodies, there have been no formal experimental studies of low back pain stemming from bone.

Pathology

Given that various structures in the lumbar spine have been shown to be capable of producing low back pain, it is important to realize that in each case, the mechanism involved is the stimulation of nerve endings in the affected structure. Lumbar nerve-root compression is in no way involved. To relate this to pathology, the possible causes of low back pain would be any pathologic process that stimulates the nociceptive nerve endings in one or other of the pain-sensitive structures of the lumbar spine and, in this respect, there are only two known mechanisms by which nerve endings may be stimulated: chemical or mechanical irritation.

Chemical irritation occurs in inflammatory diseases or follows tissue damage. Although it is very difficult to validate experimentally, the mechanism seems to involve the direct stimulation of nerve endings by chemicals. These may include hydrogen and potassium ions or proteolytic enzymes that are liberated from inflammatory cells or damaged tissue cells. Mechanical irritation, on the other hand, involves the stretching of connective tissue without the involvement of any chemical mediators. Exactly how mechanical irritation causes pain remains unclear, but a plausible explanation is that when an array of collagen fibers in a ligament, joint capsule, or periosteum is placed under tension, it deforms and closes the available space between individual collagen fibers. Nerve endings or perhaps nerve fibers within the array would then be stimulated by being squeezed between the encroaching collagen fibers.

It is beyond the scope of this chapter to expand on the pathology of the lumbar spine, but other publications have explored the pathomechanics of pain arising from discs,[2,20,49,50] dural pain,[49,50] and pain mediated by the lumbar dorsal rami.[2,51,52] However, it is worth elaborating on the issue of primary disc pain.

Primary Disc Pain

In contradistinction to pain caused by the compression of spinal nerves by herniated intervertebral discs, primary disc pain is pain that stems directly from the disc itself. It is caused by the stimulation of the nerve endings within the anulus fibrosus. Pathologic processes theoretically responsible for this stimulation include excessive mechanical strain of the anulus, chemical irritation as a result of inflammation following trauma to the anulus, and involvement of the anulus in the chemical degrading processes that occur in disc degeneration.

Logical deduction reveals that not every pathologic process affecting a disc will necessarily be painful, as only the peripheral anulus is innervated. Disc pain will occur only if a pain-producing process affects the innervated periphery of the disc. Processes like disc degradation or degeneration that are restricted to the nucleus and central portions of the anulus do not have access to the nerve supply of the disc, and therefore cannot directly cause pain. Thus, even severely degenerated discs may not be painful. However, should centrally located processes extend to the innervated periphery, as in a radial fissure,[53] or if the peripheral anulus itself is primarily damaged, as in a torsional strain,[53] then nerve endings may be affected, and if enough are stimulated, then pain may ensue. On the other hand, a healthy and innervated portion of an anulus could become painful if it is called upon to bear a greater mechanical load as a result of disease in other portions of the disc, and is thereby secondarily subjected to excessive strain. Variations and permutations like these explain why discs apparently affected by similar disease processes may be inconsistently painful or painless.

Referred Pain

Referred pain is pain perceived in a region topographically displaced from the area that is the source of the pain. In lumbar pain syndromes, referred pain is generated by lesions in the lumbar spine but is perceived in the buttocks and lower limbs or sometimes in the groin or abdominal wall.

There are two common types of referred pain from the lumbar spine. The mechanisms and their diagnostic and therapeutic implications are so different in each that the two must be recognized and distinguished. The first is somatic-referred pain. The other is radicular pain.

Somatic-Referred Pain

The term *somatic-referred* pain is used to emphasize the skeletal or "somatic" origin for this form of pain, and to distinguish it from radicular pain and referred pain caused by visceral or vascular disease.

Virtually any source of local lumbar or lumbosacral pain is also capable of producing somatic-referred pain. The mechanism appears to be that afferent impulses from the lumbar spine activate neurons in the central nervous system, which also happen to receive afferents from the lower limbs, buttocks, or groin. Stimulation of such central nervous system neurons by impulses from the lumbar spine results in the perception of pain arising from all the tissues subtended by these neurons. Thus the patient complains of pain in the lower limbs, as well as the back even though there is no signal actually emanating from the limbs.

The evidence for such a mechanism stems from several experimental and clinical studies. Kellgren[21,22] showed that low back pain experimentally induced by stimulating interspinous ligaments and back muscles could be accompanied by referred pain in the lower limbs. These observations were later corroborated by other investigators.[54,55] More recently it has been shown that in addition to back pain, experimental noxious stimulation of lumbar zygapophyseal joints can cause referred pain in various regions of the lower limbs, buttocks, and groin.[25,26] Traction on the dura mater has been shown to produce buttock and thigh pain,[46] and it has been reported, though not formally studied, that in some patients, disc stimulation can reproduce not only their back pain but their referred pain as well.[17,42–44] Complementing these experimental studies are the reports that anesthetizing intervertebral discs,[44] anesthetizing[23,25–28,30,32,33] or denervating[32,38,51] zygapophyseal joints in certain patients relieves not only their local pain but also their lower limb pain.

The critical feature of these various studies is that the stimuli used to evoke referred pain or the anesthetics used to relieve it were delivered directly to somatic elements of the lumbar spine. Nerve roots were not stimulated or anesthetized. The mechanism for the referred pain, therefore, must lie beyond the nerve roots, and the only possible site is in the central nervous system.

An overemphasized aspect of somatic referred pain is its apparent segmental distribution. Early investigators sought to establish charts of the segmental pattern of pain referral in the anticipation that the axial origin of referred pain could be diagnosed on the basis of its peripheral distribution, just as dermatomes are used to diagnose the segmental level of a root compression or spinal cord injury.[22,54,55] However, it is now evident that the fields of referred pain from individual segments overlap greatly within a given individual and the patterns exhibited by different individuals vary significantly.[51] These irregularities preclude the use of charts of so-called sclerotomes for any legitimate diagnostic purpose. Such charts serve only to illustrate that lumbar pain may be referred into the lower limbs, but not to pinpoint constant locations.

In this context, it is sometimes maintained that somatic-referred pain does not extend beyond the knee and that pain distal to the knee must be radicular in origin. However, while it is true that somatic-referred pain most commonly is distributed in the region of the buttock,[25,30,55] it nevertheless can extend as far as the foot.[22,25,54] Indeed, there is even some evidence that the distance of referral into the lower limb is proportional to the intensity of the stimulus to the spine.[25]

An important though overlooked legacy of the experimental studies on somatic-referred pain relates to its quality. All the studies showed that the referred pain was deep and aching in quality, and was hard to localize. This contrasts with the sharper, lancinating nature of radicular pain and putatively may be used to distinguish somatic-referred pain from radicular pain.[49]

Radicular Pain

The concept of "sciatica" stems from the coincidental similarity between the distribution of some forms of referred pain and the course of the sciatic nerve. Consequently, sciatica was originally ascribed to intrinsic disease of the sciatic nerve, then later to muscular compression, and eventually to compression of the lumbosacral nerve roots by disorders of the vertebral column; hence the term *radicular* pain.

These notions on the causation of sciatica, however, were based only on inference or circumstantial evidence. Thus, because arthritic changes could be demonstrated radiologically in patients with sciatic pain, the cause was deemed to be compression of the L5 spinal nerve by lumbosacral "arthritis."[56,57] Later, this notion was superceded by the revelation that herniated intervertebral discs could compress lumbosacral nerve roots.[58] The compressive causes of sciatica, however, were introduced without it being demonstrated that root compression could, in fact, cause pain.

Early investigators were probably drawn to their conclusions by the observations that most of their patients had weakness or numbness in association with their sciatic pain. Because weakness and numbness are features of nerve compression, it was understandably attractive to ascribe the pain to the same cause and mechanism. Moreover, these conclusions were made and the nerve root compression theory established before the earliest experiments on somatic-referred pain.[21,22]

It is surprising that nerve-root compression was sustained as the mechanism for referred pain, for it is known that compression of nerves elsewhere in the body does not cause pain.[59] Indeed, this paradox led to criticisms of the nerve-root compression theory.[60] However, subsequent clinical and laboratory experiments have helped resolve this paradox, albeit at the expense of raising new questions.

MacNab[61] reported that experimental compression of normal nerve roots using catheters inserted into intervertebral foramina, evoked paresthesiae and numbness, but did not cause pain. On the other hand, Smyth and Wright[46] demonstrated that pulling on nerve roots previously affected by disc herniation did evoke sciatic pain. Thus, clinically damaged, but not normal nerve roots are capable of generating pain.

These clinical observations have been corroborated by animal experiments, which showed that activity in nociceptive afferent fibers could be elicited by mechanical stimulation of previously damaged nerve roots, but not by stimulation of normal roots.[62] The questions raised by these experiments are (1) how do normal and damaged roots differ and (2) how soon after a compressive lesion is a normal root sufficiently damaged to become painful? These questions remain unanswered.

Another observation from these same animal experiments[62] is that nociceptive activity could be elicited by stimulation of dorsal root ganglia irrespective of whether they were normal or damaged. Thus, dorsal root ganglia are apparently more susceptible to mechanical stimulation than axons, and this difference may explain why root compression is capable of producing pain when compression of nerve trunks is not. Compression of the cell bodies in the dorsal root ganglia seems to be the key difference.

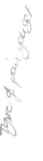

Other issues aside, there is no doubt that under the appropriate circumstances, compression of nerve roots can cause pain, but an unfortunate legacy of the concept of sciatica is the tendency in some circles to interpret all forms of pain in the lower limb as due to nerve-root compression. This is not justified.

The experiments of Smyth and Wright[46] showed that traction on nerve roots produced only a particular form of pain. It was lancinating or shooting in quality, and was felt along a relatively narrow band "no more than one-and-a-half inches wide."[46] This neuralgic type of pain is the only type that has been shown to be produced by root compression. Therefore, only this form of pain can legitimately be called *sciatica* and ascribed to root compression. In contrast, somatic referred pain is static, aching in quality, hard to localize, and should be recognized as a different entity.

There are two further irregularities concerning the concepts of sciatica and nerve-root compression. First, there is no known mechanism whereby a compressive lesion can selectively affect only nociceptive axons (i.e., without also affecting large-diameter afferent fibers that convey touch and other sensations). Therefore, there is no mechanism whereby root compression can cause pain without causing other neurologic abnormalities as well. Thus, for root compression to be deemed the cause, radicular pain must be accompanied by other features of nerve compression: numbness, weakness, or paresthesiae. In the absence of such accompanying features, it is very difficult to maintain that root compression is the cause of any pain. Pain in the lower limb in the absence of objective neurologic signs is most likely to be somatic-referred pain.

The second irregularity relates to back pain. All the experimental studies on radicular pain emphasize that root compression causes pain in the lower limb. Thus, although radicular pain may feel as if it starts in the back and radiates into the lower limb, there is no evidence that root compression can or should cause isolated low back pain. It is implausible that a compressive lesion could stimulate only those afferents in a root that come from the lumbar spine but spare those from the lower limb. Isolated low back pain suggests a somatic lesion, which should be sought, and the pain should not be dismissed as due to nerve-root compression when no evidence of compression can be found. One reservation, however, must be raised and that is that apparently local back pain may in fact be referred pain from pelvic or abdominal visceral or vascular disease. For this reason, abdominal and pelvic examinations are essential parts of the assessment of any patient presenting with low back pain.

Combined States

Whereas it is evident that back pain and referred pain may be caused by a variety of disorders and mechanisms, it is critical to realize that a patient's complaints may not be due to a single disorder or a single mechanism. Several disorders may coexist and different mechanisms may be coactive.

The simplest examples are the coexistence of zygapophyseal disorders and disc disorders at the same or different segmental levels; each disorder contributing separately to the patient's overall complaint. A more complex example relates to nerve-root compression syndromes.

The cardinal features of nerve root compression are the objective neurologic signs of weakness or numbness. In the presence of such signs accompanied by the lancinating pain that is characteristic of radicular pain, the syndrome may legitimately be ascribed to nerve-root compression. However, nerve-root compression may only be part of a patient's complaint. Local somatic and somatic-referred pain may occur in addition to the symptoms of nerve-root compression. In such cases, the most likely source or sources of the somatic pain are the structures immediately adjacent to the compressed root.

The closest relation of a nerve root is its dural sleeve, and it is obvious that any lesion that might compress a root must first affect its dural sleeve. Given that the dura is pain-sensitive,[46,47] it becomes a potent possible source of low back pain and even referred pain,[46] that can occur alone or be superimposed on any radicular pain. However, the mechanism involved is distinctly different from that of any radicular pain, for dural pain is caused by the stimulation of nerve endings in the dural sleeve, not by nerve compression.

Since the dura is mechanosensitive,[46] traction of the dura over a space-occupying lesion, like a herniated disc, could be the possible cause of dural pain. The dura is also chemosensitive,[47] so an additional or alternative process could be chemical irritation of the dura. With regard to the latter, it has been demonstrated that disc material contains potent inflammatory chemicals,[63] and when disc material ruptures into the epidural space it seems to elicit an autoimmune inflammatory reaction that can affect not only the roots but the dura as well.[64–67]

The other two possible sources of pain concurrent with root compression are the adjacent disc and zygapophyseal joint. Regardless of any herniation that compresses a root, a disc itself may be an intrinsic source of pain, the pain being mechanical in origin caused by strain of the anulus fibrosus of the diseased disc. In such cases, treating the nerve-root compression may relieve the objective neurologic signs and any radicular pain, but the discogenic pain may continue unless it is treated as well.

A zygapophyseal joint may compress or traumatize the underlying roots by developing osteophytes,[68] but a degenerative zygapophyseal joint may also be independently painful, causing both local and somatic referred pain. Thus, while resecting the osteophytes may decompress the roots, it may not relieve the intrinsic low-back pain and referred pain stemming from the diseased joint.

This concept has particular ramifications in the interpretation of spinal stenosis where not all the symptoms are necessarily due to the overt nerve-root compression.

PATTERNS

It might be expected that different causes of lumbar pain should be distinguishable from one another on the basis of differences in the distribution and behavior of symptoms. Frustratingly, however, this is not so. Because different structures in the lumbar spine share a similar segmental nerve supply, and because different disorders share similar mechanisms, no single disorder has a characteristic distribution of local or referred pain.

Even the classic syndrome of herniated lumbar disc is fraught with diagnostic pitfalls. The sensitivity of clinical examination in the diagnosis of this condition is about 77 percent,[69] meaning that using clinical features alone only 77 percent of actual disc herniations are accurately detected. Some 23 percent of cases are misdiagnosed. Other studies[70] suggest that the sensitivity of clinical examination may only be about 58 percent accurate meaning that up to 42 percent of cases are misdiagnosed. On the other hand, the specificity of clinical examination is high, 90 percent,[69] but even so, this figure indicates that some 10 percent of cases interpreted as disc herniation prove to be due to some other cause, like zygapophyseal osteophytes, spinal stenosis, and epidural varices.[69] Electromyography and myelography have sensitivities and specificities similar to those of clinical examination,[69,71] but even on the basis of these investigations a false-positive diagnosis of disc herniation is made in some 10 percent of patients.

With respect to zygapophyseal joint disorders, experimental studies have shown that local and referred pain patterns from joints at different levels vary considerably in different individuals and even in a given individual they overlap greatly.[25,26] Furthermore, the incidence of other clinical features in zygapophyseal syndromes, including various aggravating factors, is insufficiently different from their incidence in other syndromes. Fairbank et al[30] performed diagnostic joint blocks on patients presenting with back pain and referred pain, and analyzed the differences between those who responded and those who did not. Although certain features did occur more commonly in responders, they also occurred so frequently in nonresponders that no clinical feature could be identified that could be held to be indicative or pathognomonic of zygapophyseal-joint pain.

Other forms of pain, like disc pain and muscular-pain syndromes, have not been studied in this same rigorous way. Consequently, there is no scientific evidence that permits any claim that certain pain patterns are characteristic of these syndromes. Only the diagnosis of lumber-disc herniation has withstood scrutiny, while the diagnosis of zygapophyseal syndromes on the basis of conventional clinical signs has been shown to be impossible. Therefore, the diagnosis of lumbar-pain syndromes, other than those caused by disc herniation, relies on investigations outside the realm of symptomatic and conventional physical examination.

In this regard, plain radiography has little value as a diagnostic tool in low back pain,[44] while electromyography, myelography, and computed tomography are of relevance only in nerve-root compression syndromes. For conditions in which pain alone is the complaint, and there are no objective neurologic signs indicative of nerve-root compression, other investigations are required.

The mainstay for the diagnosis of lumbar pain in the absence of neurologic signs are diagnostic blocks and provocation radiology. These techniques are based on the principles that if a structure is the cause of pain, then stressing that structure should reproduce the pain and anesthetizing the structure should relieve it. Thus, zygapophyseal joints suspected of being the source of pain can be infiltrated with local anesthetic,[34] and relief of pain implicates the injected joint as the source. Similarly, intervertebral discs can be injected with saline or contrast medium to reproduce pain or with local anesthetic to relieve pain.[44] Radicular pain and dural pain can be diagnosed by infiltrating the root thought to be responsible with local anesthetic.[45] In all of these procedures, failure to provoke or relieve the pain excludes the investigated structure as the source of pain, whereupon other structures or other segmental levels in the lumbar spine may be investigated until the responsible site is identified. Although subject to certain technical limitations,[44,72] these techniques are the only available means of objectively confirming particular causes of pain suspected on the basis of clinical examination.

In conflict with this conclusion is the clinical evidence of manipulative therapists who maintain that they are able to diagnose the source of pain in the vertebral column by manual examination. Elaborate methods of assessment for this purpose have been described in a manipulative therapy texts.[73–75] However, little research has been undertaken to validate the purported accuracy of these methods. Thus, while perhaps attractive in principle, manual examination as a diagnostic effort is still open to scepticism from those unconvinced of a manipulative therapist's ability to detect changes in discrete components of the spine, and that these changes are at all diagnostic of any cause of pain.

The results of some research in this regard, however, have recently become available, at least with respect to the cervical spine. In a single-blind study, a manipulative therapist was required to determine the presence and location of symptomatic zygapophyseal-joint disease in patients otherwise evaluated by diagnostic zygapophyseal-joint blocks.[76] Complete concordance was found between the manipulative therapist's diagnosis and that made on the basis of diagnostic blocks, with no false-positive or false-negative observations. Thus, it was found that manual diagnosis can be as accurate as radiologically controlled blocks, for the diagnosis of pain stemming from the cervical zygapophyseal joints.

SUMMARY

What are required in the continuing study of the causes of back pain are similar studies addressing the manual diagnosis not only of zygapophyseal syndromes but of disc disease and other disorders throughout the vertebral column.

It appears not only that the long-held claims of manipulative therapists can be substantiated but also that segmental-manual examination can become a technique that obviates the need for invasive radiologic diagnostic procedures in the diagnosis of low back pain.

REFERENCES

1. Yoshizawa H, O'Brien JP, Smith WT, Trumper M: The neuropathology of intervertebral discs removed for low-back pain. J Pathol 132:95, 1980
2. Bogduk N, Tynan W, Wilson AS: The nerve supply to the human lumbar intervertebral discs. J Anat, 132:39, 1981
3. Bogduk N, Wilson AS, Tynan W: The human lumbar dorsal rami. J Anat 134:383, 1982
4. Paris SV: Anatomy was related to function and pain. Orthop Clin North Am 14:475, 1982
5. Bogduk N: The innervation of the lumbar spine. Spine 8:285, 1983
6. Bogduk N: A reappraisal of the anatomy of the lumbar erector spinae. J Anat 131:525, 1980
7. Johnston HM: The cutaneous branches of the posterior primary divisions of the spinal nerves and their distribution in the sin. J Anat 43:80, 1908
8. Pedersen HE, Blunck CFJ, Gardner E: The anatomy of lumbosacral posterior rami and meningeal branches of spinal nerves (sinu-vertebral nerves). J Bone Joint Surg 38A:377, 1956
9. Lazorthes G, Gaubert J: L'innervation des articulations interapophysaires vertebrales. CR Ass Anat 43e Reunion:488, 1956
10. Lazorthes G, Juskiewenski S: Etude comparative des branches posterieures des nerfs dorsaux et lombaires et de leurs rapports avec les articulations interapophysaires vertebrales. Bull Assoc Anat 49e Reunion:1025, 1964
11. Edgar MA, Nundy S: Innervation of the spinal dura mater. J Neurol Neurosurg Psychiatry 29:530, 1966
12. Kimmel DL: The cervical sympathetic rami and the vertebral plexus in the human fetus. J Comp Neurol 112:141, 1959
13. Lazorthes G, Pouhles J, Espagne J: Etude sur les nerfs sinu-vertebraux lombaires. Le nerf de Roofe existe-t-il? CR Ass Anat 34e Reunion:317, 1947
14. Kimmel DL: Innervation of the spinal dura mater and dura mater of the posterior cranial fossa. Neurology 10:800, 1961
15. Wyke B: Neurological aspects of low back pain. p. 189. In Jayson MIV (ed). The Lumbar Spine and Back Pain Sector, New York, 1976
16. Jung A, Brunschwig A: Recherches histolgiques des articulations des corps vertebraux. Presse Med 40:316, 1932
17. Hirsch C, Ingelmark B, Miller M: The anatomical basis for low back pain. Acta Orthop, Scand, 33:1, 1963
18. Jackson HC, Winkelmann RK, Bickel WH: Nerve endings in the human lumbar spinal column and related structures. J Bone Joint Surg 48A:1272, 1966
19. Malinsky J: The ontogenetic development of nerve terminations in the intervertebral discs of man. Acta Anat 38:96, 1959
20. Bogduk N: The innervation of the lumbar intervertebral discs. Ch. 14, p. 146, In Grieve GP (ed): Modern Manual Therapy of the Vertebral Column. Churchill Livingstone, Edinburgh, 1986

21. Kellgren JH: Observations on referred pain arising from muscle. Clin Sci 3:175, 1938
22. Kellgren JH: On the distribution of pain arising from deep somatic structures with charts of segmental pain areas. Clin Sci 4:35, 1939
23. Steindler A, Luck JV: Differential diagnosis of pain low in the back: Allocation of the source of pain by procain hydrochloride method. JAMA 110:106, 1938
24. Ghormley RK: Low back pain with special reference to the articular facets with presentation of an operative procedure. JAMA 10:1773, 1933
25. Mooney V, Robertson J: The facet syndrome. Clin Orthop 115:149, 1976
26. McCall IW, Park WM, O'Brien JP: Induced pain referral from posterior lumbar elements in normal subjects. Spine 4:441, 1979
27. Mehta M, Sluijter ME: The treatment of chronic back pain. Anaesthesia 34:768, 1979
28. Carrera GF: Lumbar facet joint injection in low back pain and sciatica. Radiology 137:665, 1980
29. Dory MA: Arthrography of the lumbar facet joints. Radiology 140:23, 1981
30. Fairbank JCT, Park WM, McCall IW, O'Brien JP: Apophyseal injection of local anaesthetic as a diagnostic aid in primary low-back pain syndromes. Spine 6:598, 1981
31. Destouet JM, Gilula LA, Murphy WA, Monsees B: Lumbar facet joint injection: indication, technique, clinical correlation, and preliminary results. Radiology 145:321, 1982
32. Rashbaum RF: Radiofrequency facet denervation. Orthop Clin North Am 14:569, 1983
33. Lippit AB: The facet joint and its role in spine pain. Spine 9:746, 1984
34. Carrera GF, Williams, AL: Current concepts in evaluation of the lumbar facet joints. CRC Crit Rev Diagn Imaging 21:85, 1984
35. Pawl RP: Results in the treatment of low back syndrome from sensory neurolysis of the lumbar facets (facet rhizotomy) by teral coagulation. Proc Inst Med Chgo 30:150, 1974
36. Lora J, Long DM: So-called facet denervation in the management of intractable back pain. Spine 1:121, 1976
37. Ogsbury JS, Simons H, Lehman RAW: Facet "denervation" in the treatment of low back syndrome. Pain 2:257, 1977
38. Sluijter ME, Mehta M: Treatment of chronic back and neck pain by percutaneous thermal lesions. p. 141. In Lipton S, Miles J (eds): Persistent Pain: Modern Methods of Treatment, Vol. 3. Academic Press, London, 1981
39. Wiberg G: Back pain in relation to the nerve supply of the intervertebral disc. Acta Orthop Scand 19:211, 1947
40. Lindblom K: Technique and results in myelography and disc puncture. Acta Radiol 34:321, 1950
41. Collis JS, Gardner WJ: Lumbar discography-An analysis of 1,000 cases. J Neurosurg 19:452, 1962
42. Wiley JJ, MacNab I, Wortzman G: Lumbar discography and its clinical applications. Can J Surg 11:280, 1968
43. Simmons EH, Segil CM: An evaluation of discography in the localization of symptomatic levels in discogenic disease of the spine. Clin Orthop 108:57, 1975
44. Park WM: The place of radiology in the investigation of low back pain. Clin Rheum Dis 6:93, 1980
45. White AH: Injection techniques for the diagnosis and treatment of low back pain. Orthop Clin North Am 14:553, 1983

46. Smyth MJ, Wright V: Sciatica and the intervertebral disc: An experimental study. J Bone Joint Surg 40A:1401, 1958
47. El Mahdi MA, Latif FYA, Janko M: The spinal nerve root innervation and a new concept of the clinicopathological interrelations in back pain and sciatica. Neurochirurgia 24:137, 1981
48. Boas RA: Post-surgical low back pain. p. 188. In Peck C, Wallace M (eds): Problems in Pain. Pergamon, Sydney, 1980
49. Bogduk N: The rationale for patterns of neck and back pain. Patient Management 13:17, 1984
50. Bogduk N: Low back pain. Aust Fam Physician 14:1168, 1985
51. Bogduk N: Lumbar dorsal ramus syndrome. Med J Aust 2:537, 1980
52. Bogduk N: Lumbar dorsal ramus syndromes. Ch. 38, p. 396. In Grieve GP (ed): Modern Manual Therapy of the Vertebral Column. Churchill Livingstone, Edinburgh, 1986
53. Farfan HF: A reorientation in the surgical approach to degenerative lumbar intervertebral joint disease. Orthop Clin North Am 8:9, 1977
54. Feinstein B, Langton JNK, Jameson RM, Schiller F: Experiments on pain referred from deep structures. J Bone Joint Surg 36A:981, 1954
55. Hockaday JM, Whitty CWM: Patterns of referred pain in the normal subject. Brain 90:481, 1967
56. Danforth MS, Wilson PD: The anatomy of the lumbosacral region in relation to sciatic pain. J Bone Joint Surgery 7:109, 1925
57. Williams PC: Reduced lumbosacral joint space: Its relation to sciatic irritation. JAMA 99:1677, 1962
58. Mixter WJ, Barr JS: Rupture of the intervertebral disc with involvement of the spinal canal. N Engl J Med 211:210, 1934
59. Fisher CM: Pain states: A neurological commentary. Clin. Neurosurg 31:32, 1984
60. Kelly M: Is pain due to pressure on nerves? Neurology 6:32, 1956
61. MacNab I: The mechanism of spondylogenic pain. p. 89. In Hirsch C, Zotterman Y (eds): Cervical Pain. Pergamon, Oxford, 1972
62. Howe JF, Loeser JD, Calvin WH: Mechano-sensitivity of dorsal root ganglia and chronically injured axons: A physiological basis for the radicular pain of nerve root compression. Pain 3:25, 1977
63. Marshall LL, Trethewie ER, Curtain CC: Chemical radiculitis: A clinical, physiological and immunological study. Clin Orthop 129:61, 1977
64. Gertzbein SD, Tile M, Gross A, Falk R: Autoimmunity and degenerative disease of the lumbar spine. Orthop Clin North Am 6:67, 1975
65. Gertzbein SD: Degenerative disk disease of the lumbar spine. Clin Orthop 129:68, 1977
66. Gertzbein SD, Tai JH, Devlin SR: The stimulation of lymphocytes by nucleus pulposus in patients with degenerative disc disease of the lumbar spine. Clin Orthop 123:149, 1977
67. Murphy RW: Nerve roots and spinal nerves in degenerative disk disease. Clin Orthop 129:46, 1977
68. Epstein JA, Epstein BS, Lavine LS, Carras R, Rosenthal AD, Sulner P: Lumbar nerve root compression at the intervertebral foramina caused by arthritis of the posterior facets. J Neurosurg 39:362, 1973
69. Knutsson B: Comparative value of electromyography, myelography and clinico-neurological examination in diagnosis of lumbar root compression syndrome. Acta Orthop Scand suppl 49:1, 1961

70. Kosteljanetz M, Espersen JO, Halaburt H, Miletic T: Predictive value of clinical and surgical findings in patients with lumbago-sciatica: A prospective study. (part I) Acta Neurochir 73:67, 1984
71. Espersen JO, Kosteljanetz M, Halaburt H, Miletic T: Predictive value of radiculography in patients with lumbago-sciatica: A prospective study. (part II) Acta Neurochir 73:213, 1984
72. Raymond J, Dumas JM: Intra-articular facet blocks: Diagnostic test or therapeutic procedure? Radiology 151:333, 1984
73. Maitland GD: Vertebral Manipulation. 4th Ed. Butterworth, London, 1977
74. Grieve GP: Common Vertebral Joint Problems. Churchill Livingstone, Edinburgh, 1982
75. Bourdillon JF: Spinal Manipulation. 3rd Ed. Heinemann, London, 1982
76. Jull GA, Bogduk N: Manual examination: An objective test of cervical joint dysfunction. In Proceedings of the Fourth Biennial Conference of the Manipulative Therapists' Association of Australia, Manipulative Therapists' Association of Australia:159, Brisbane, 1985

4

The Anatomy and Function of the Lumbar Back Muscles and Their Fascia

Janet E. Macintosh
Nikolai Bogduk

In undergraduate curricula the muscles of the back and their associated fascia are commonly dismissed as an area of anatomy that does not need to be known in the detail expected for the musculature of the limbs. Textbook descriptions of the anatomy of the back muscles and fascia are either very brief,[1-3] or details of attachments are presented in an overwhelming fashion without an explanation of the significance of this detail and without a similarly detailed discussion of function.[4] Nonetheless, a knowledge of the anatomy of the back muscles and fascia is integral to the practice of physical therapy, for the comprehension of spinal function, the assessment and interpretation of spinal disorders, and the proper prescription of therapeutic exercise. Moreover, there is a growing interest in the role of muscle dysfunction in the pathogenesis of spinal pain, and a proper knowledge of the back muscles must be fundamental to any theories in this regard.

This chapter focuses specifically on those muscles of the back that exert an action on the lumbar spine, and the generic term "lumbar back muscles" is used to refer to them. These muscles include those that are attached to the lumbar vertebrae and certain muscles that lack an attachment to lumbar vertebrae but nevertheless exert an indirect action on them. The descriptions differ

103

from conventional descriptions offered in textbooks, and are based on the results of recent and contemporary studies of these muscles.[5–14]

These studies have examined in detail the disposition and attachments of all the individual fascicles of the lumbar back muscles as determined by dissection in a total of 12 embalmed human adult cadavers. The principal difference in the descriptions provided as compared to textbook descriptions is that the muscles are described "upside down." The lumbar back muscles are viewed as a series of fascicles passing from rostral origins to caudal insertions, instead of the traditional approach in which the back muscles are considered to have a common caudal origin with diverse rostral insertions.

The justification for this inversion is that in the first instance, the rostrocaudal interpretation is consistent with the pattern of innervation of these muscles.[6,12] This view also clarifies the identity of certain muscles and the identity of the erector spinae aponeurosis, and reveals certain features germane to their biomechanical function.

The chapter is divided into three major sections. The first deals with the *morphology* of the lumbar back muscles and their fascia. In the second section the *actions* of the muscles are derived on the basis of their orientation and attachments, and in the third the *functions* of the muscles and their fascia are described.

ANATOMY

The lumbar spine is supported, stabilized, and moved by three groups of muscles. The first are the intersegmental muscles that connect consecutive lumbar vertebrae. These are represented by the intertransversarii and the interspinales. The second group may be considered the major intrinsic muscles of the lumbar spine. They are polysegmental muscles that attach to the lumbar vertebrae and anchor them to the iliac crest and sacrum. These are the multifidus and the lumbar components of longissimus and iliocostalis. The third group are the long, extrinsic, polysegmental muscles that for the most part do not attach to the lumbar vertebrae, but pass from thoracic levels to the iliac crest and sacrum, thereby spanning the lumbar region and covering the intrinsic lumbar back muscles. The thoracic components of longissimus and iliocostalis form this group.

Intertransversarii and Interspinales

In the lumbar region there are three types of intertransversarii. Intertransversarii mediales arise from an accessory process and insert into the subjacent accessory and mamillary processes. The intertransversarii laterales dorsales also arise from an accessory process, but insert into the subjacent transverse process. The intertransversarii laterales ventrales connect adjacent transverse processes.

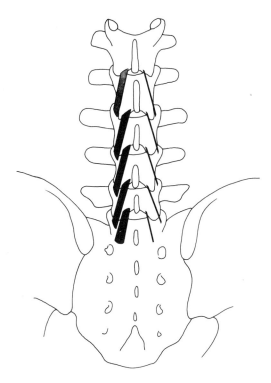

Fig. 4-1. The laminar fibers of multifidus. The appearance of the fascicles is depicted on the left; the scheme of attachments is depicted on the right.

Although all the lumbar intertransverse muscles act on the vertebral column, only the intertransversarii mediales can be considered to be true back muscles, for only they are innervated by the lumbar dorsal rami.[15] The intertransversarii laterales dorsales and ventrales are innervated by the lumbar ventral rami, and represent respectively, the lumbar homologues of the thoracic levatores costarum and intercostal muscles.[16]

The lumbar interspinales are short, paired muscles that lie on either side of the interspinous ligament and connect the spinous processes of adjacent lumbar vertebrae. There are four pairs in the lumbar region.

Multifidus

Multifidus is the largest and most medial of the lumbar back muscles, and recent studies reveal that it consists of a repeating series of fascicles, which stem from the laminae and spinous processes of the lumbar vertebrae and exhibit a constant pattern of attachments caudally.[12]

The shortest fascicles of the multifidus are the *laminar fibers* which arise from the caudal end of the dorsal surface of each vertebral lamina and insert into the mamillary process of the vertebra two levels caudad (Fig. 4-1). The L5 laminar fibers have no mamillary process into which they can insert and insert instead into an area on the sacrum just above the first dorsal sacral

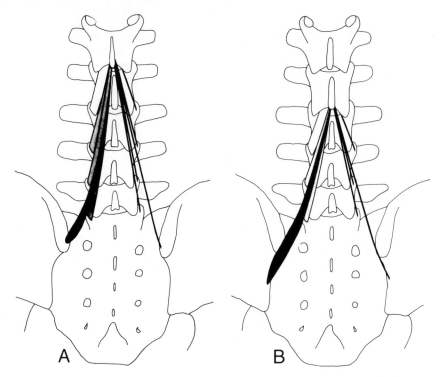

Fig. 4-2.   The fascicular organization of multifidus. (A) On the left, the fascicles from the L1 spinous process are shown in isolation. On the right the general scheme of their attachments is depicted. (B) The fascicles of the L2 spinous process. (*Figure continues.*)

foramen. Because of their attachments, the laminar fibers may be considered homologous to the thoracic rotatores.

The bulk of the lumbar multifidus consists of fascicles that radiate from the lumbar spinous processes. These fascicles are arranged in five overlapping groups such that each lumbar vertebra gives rise to one of these groups. At each segmental level a fascicle arises from the base and caudolateral edge of the spinous process, and several fascicles arise by way of a common tendon from the caudal tip of the spinous process. This tendon is referred to below as the *common tendon.*

Although confluent with one another at their origin, the fascicles in each group diverge caudally to assume separate attachments to mamillary processes, the iliac crest, and the sacrum (Fig. 4-2). The fascicle from the base of the L1 spinous process inserts into the L4 mamillary process, while those from the common tendon insert into the mamillary processes of L5, S1, and the posterosuperior iliac spine (Fig. 4-2A). The fascicle from the base of the spinous process of L2 inserts into the mamillary process of L5, while those from the common tendon insert into the S1 mamillary process, the posterosuperior iliac spine, and an area on the iliac crest just caudoventral to the posterosuperior iliac spine (Fig. 4-2B).

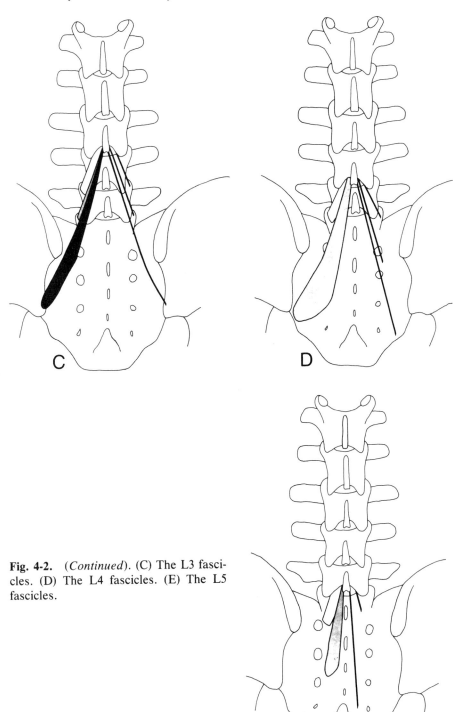

Fig. 4-2. (*Continued*). (C) The L3 fascicles. (D) The L4 fascicles. (E) The L5 fascicles.

The fascicle from the base of the L3 spinous process inserts into the mamillary process of the sacrum, while those fascicles from the common tendon insert into a narrow area extending caudally from the caudal extent of the posterosuperior iliac spine to the lateral edge of the third sacral segment (Fig. 4-2C). The L4 fascicles insert onto the sacrum in an area medial to the L3 area of insertion, but lateral to the dorsal sacral foramina (Fig. 4-2D), while those from the L5 vertebra insert onto an area medial to the dorsal sacral foramina (Fig. 4-2E).

It is noteworthy that while many of the fascicles of multifidus attach to mamillary processes, some of the deeper fibers of these fascicles attach to the capsules of the zygapophyseal joints next to the mamillary processes.[17] This attachment allows the multifidus to protect the joint capsule from being caught inside the joint during the movements executed by the multifidus.

The key feature of the morphology of the lumbar multifidus is that its fascicles are arranged segmentally. Each lumbar vertebra is endowed with a group of fascicles that radiate from its spinous process, anchoring it below to mamillary processes, the iliac crest, and the sacrum. This disposition suggests that the fibers of multifidus are arranged in a way that their principal action is focussed on individual lumbar spinous processes. This contention is supported by the pattern of innervation of the muscle. All the fascicles arising from the spinous processes of a given vertebra are innervated by the medial branch of the dorsal ramus that issues from below that vertebra.[6,12,15] Thus it is evident that, with respect to multifidus, the muscles that directly act on a particular segment are innervated by the nerve of that segment.

Lumbar Erector Spinae

The lumbar erector spinae lies lateral to the multifidus and forms the prominent dorsolateral contour of the back muscles in the lumbar region. It consists of two muscles, iliocostalis and longissimus, each of which has two components: lumbar fascicles arising from lumbar vertebrae; and thoracic fascicles arising from thoracic vertebrae or ribs.

In the lumbar region the longissimus and iliocostalis are separated from each other by the *lumbar intermuscular aponeurosis,* a posteroanterior continuation of the erector spinae aponeurosis.[5] It appears as a flat sheet of collagen fibers that extend rostrally from the medial aspect of the posterosuperior iliac spine for 6 to 8 c. It is formed mainly of the caudal tendons of the rostral four fascicles of the lumbar component of longissimus (Fig. 4-3).

Lumbar Longissimus

The lumbar longissimus is composed of five fascicles, each arising from the accessory process and the adjacent medial end of the dorsal surface of the transverse process of a lumbar vertebra.

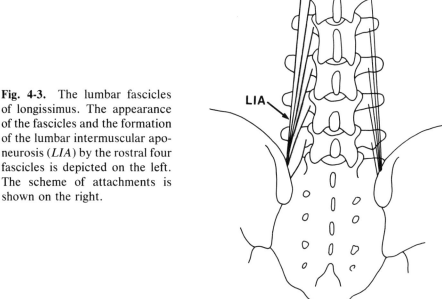

Fig. 4-3. The lumbar fascicles of longissimus. The appearance of the fascicles and the formation of the lumbar intermuscular aponeurosis (*LIA*) by the rostral four fascicles is depicted on the left. The scheme of attachments is shown on the right.

The fascicle from the L5 vertebra is the deepest and shortest. Its fibers insert directly into the medial aspect of the posterosuperior iliac spine. The fascicle from L4 also lies deep but lateral to that from L5. Succeeding fascicles lie in progressively more dorsal positions so that the L3 fascicle covers those from L4 and L5 but is itself covered by the L2 fascicle, while the L1 fascicle lies most superficially.

The L1–4 fascicles all form tendons at their caudal ends, which converge to form an aponeurotic sheet, the lumbar intermuscular aponeurosis. This eventually attaches to a narrow area on the ilium immediately lateral to the insertion of the L5 fascicle. The lumbar intermuscular aponeurosis thus represents a common tendon of insertion for the bulk of the lumbar fibers of longissimus.

Lumbar Iliocostalis

The lumbar component of iliocostalis consists of four overlying fascicles arising from the L1 through to L4 vertebrae. Rostrally, each fascicle attaches to the tip of the transverse process and to an area extending 2 to 3 cm laterally onto the middle layer of the thoracolumbar fascia (Fig. 4-4).

The fascicle from L4 is the deepest, and caudally it is attached directly onto the iliac crest just lateral to the posterosuperior iliac spine. This fascicle is covered by the fascicle from L3 that has a similar attachment to the iliac crest, located in a more dorsolateral position. In sequence, L2 covers L3 and

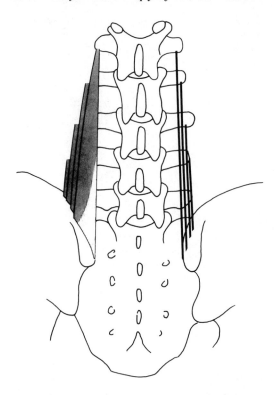

Fig. 4-4. The lumbar fascicles of iliocostalis. The disposition of the fascicles is shown on the left. The scheme of their attachments is depicted on the right.

L1 covers L2 with insertions on the iliac crest becoming successively more dorsolateral. The most lateral fascicles attach to the iliac crest just medial to the attachment of the lateral raphe of the thoracolumbar fascia.[7] The most medial fibers of iliocostalis contribute to the lumbar intermuscular aponeurosis, but only to a minor extent.

Although an L5 fascicle of lumbar iliocostalis is not described in the literature it does exist in the form of the iliolumbar "ligament." In neonates and children the "ligament" is completely muscular in structure. However, by the third decade of life the muscle fibers are entirely replaced by collagen giving rise to the familiar iliolumbar ligament.[18]

Thoracic Longissimus

The thoracic longissimus typically consists of 11 or 12 pairs of small fascicles arising from the ribs and transverse processes of T1 or T2 down to T12 (Fig. 4-5). At each level two tendons can usually be recognized; a medial one from the tip of the transverse process; and a lateral one from the rib, although in the upper three or four levels, this may merge medially with the fascicle from the transverse process. Each rostral tendon extends 3 to 4 cm before forming a small muscle belly measuring 7 to 8 cm in length. The muscle bellies from the higher levels overlap those from lower levels. Each muscle belly

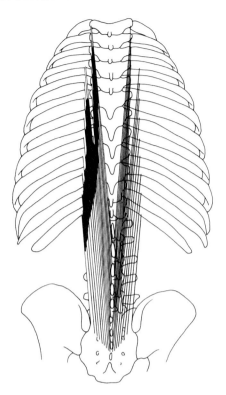

Fig. 4-5. The thoracic fascicles of longissimus thoracis. On the left, the disposition of the fascicles is shown. The parallel aggregation of the caudal tendons of each individual fascicle contributes to the formation of the erector spinae aponeurosis. The scheme of individual attachments is depicted on the right.

eventually forms a caudal tendon that extends into the lumbar region. The tendons run in parallel, with those from higher levels being most medial. The fascicles from the T2 level attach to the L3 spinous process, while the fascicles from the remaining levels insert into spinous processes at progressively lower levels. For example, those from T5 attach to L5 and those from T7 to S2-3. Those from T8 to T12 diverge from the midline to find attachment to the sacrum along a line extending from the S3 spinous process to the caudal extent of the posterosuperior iliac spine. The lateral edge of the caudal tendon of T12 lies alongside the dorsal edge of the lumbar intermuscular aponeurosis, which is formed by the caudal tendon of the L1 longissimus bundle.

The side-to-side aggregation of the caudal tendons of the thoracic components of longissimus form most of what is termed the erector spinae aponeurosis, which covers the lumbar fibers of longissimus and iliocostalis, but affords no attachment to them.

Thoracic Iliocostalis

The thoracic iliocostalis consists of fascicles from the lower seven or eight ribs that attach caudally to the ilium and sacrum (Fig. 4-6). It represents the thoracic component of the muscle traditionally known as iliocostalis lumborum,

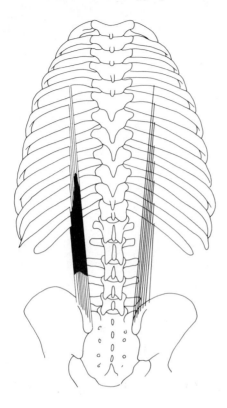

Fig. 4-6. The thoracic fascicles of iliocostalis lumborum. The caudal tendons of the muscle belly contribute to the formation of the erector spinae aponeurosis.

and should not be confused with the iliocostalis thoracis, which is restricted to the thoracic region between the upper-six and lower-six ribs.

Each fascicle arises from the angle of the rib via a ribbon-like tendon of 9 to 10 cm before forming a muscle belly of 8 to 10 cm. Thereafter, each fascicle continues as a tendon, contributing to the erector spinae aponeurosis, and ultimately attaching caudally to the posterosuperior iliac spine. The most medial tendons from the more rostral fascicles often attach more medially to the dorsal surface of the sacrum, caudal to the insertion of multifidus.

Erector Spinae Aponeurosis

The cardinal revelations of recent studies of the lumbar erector spinae[5,11] is that this muscle consists of both lumbar and thoracic fibers. Modern textbook descriptions largely do not recognize the lumbar fibers, especially those of iliocostalis.[5] Moreover, textbooks do not note that the lumbar fibers (of both longissimus and iliocostalis) have attachments quite separate to those of the thoracic fibers. The lumbar fibers of the longissimus and iliocostalis pass between the lumbar vertebrae and the ilium. Thus, through these muscles, the lumbar vertebrae are anchored directly to the ilium. They do not gain any attachment to the erector spinae aponeurosis, which is the implication of all modern textbook descriptions that deal with the erector spinae.

Classically, the erector spinae aponeurosis is described as a broad sheet of tendinous fibers that is attached to the ilium, the sacrum, and the lumbar and sacral spinous processes, and which forms a common origin for the lower part of erector spinae. However, as described above, the erector spinae aponeurosis is formed virtually exclusively by the tendons of the thoracic longissimus and thoracic iliocostalis.[5,11] The only additional contribution comes from the most superficial fibers of multifidus from upper lumbar levels, which contribute a small number of fibers to the aponeurosis.[12] Nonetheless, the erector spinae aponeurosis is essentially formed only by the caudal attachments of muscles acting from thoracic levels.

The lumbar fibers of erector spinae do not attach to the erector spinae aponeurosis, and indeed, the aponeurosis is free to move over the surface of the underlying lumbar fibers. This suggests that the lumbar fibers, which form the bulk of the lumbar back musculature, can act independently from the rest of the erector spinae.

Thoracolumbar Fascia

The thoracolumbar fascia consists of three layers: an anterior layer that arises from the anterior surface of the lumbar transverse processes and covers quadratus lumborum; a middle layer, from the tips of the lumbar transverse processes; and a posterior layer, which arises from the midline to cover the back muscles. Little is known about the biomechanical significance of the anterior and middle layers of thoracolumbar fascia but there has been considerable interest recently in the biomechanics of the posterior layer.[7,10,19,20]

The Posterior Layer of Thoracolumbar Fascia

The posterior layer of thoracolumbar fascia covers the back muscles from the lumbosacral region through to the thoracic region as far rostrally as the splenius muscle. In the lumbar region it is attached to the tips of the spinous processes in the midline, and lateral to the erector spinae. Between the twelfth rib and the iliac crest it unites with the middle layer of thoracolumbar fascia forming a raphe, referred to as the *lateral raphe*.[7] At sacral levels, the posterior layer extends from the midline to the posterosuperior iliac spine and the posterior segment of the iliac crest.

On close inspection, the posterior layer exhibits a cross-hatched appearance, manifest because it consists of two laminae: a superficial lamina with fibers oriented caudomedially; and a deep lamina with fibers oriented caudolaterally.[7]

The superficial lamina is formed by the aponeurosis of latissimus dorsi, but the disposition and attachments of its constituent fibers differ according to

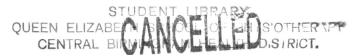

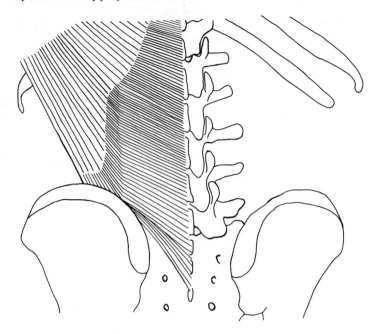

Fig. 4-7. The superficial lamina of the posterior layer of thoracolumbar fascia. (Bogduk N, Macintosh JE: The applied anatomy of the thoracolumbar fascia. Spine 9:164, 1984.)

the portion of latissimus dorsi from which they are derived. For descriptive purposes, four types of aponeurotic fibers can be recognized (Fig. 4-7). The first are those derived from the most lateral 2 to 3 cm of the muscle. They are short and insert directly into the iliac crest without contributing to the thoracolumbar fascia. The second type are derived from the next most lateral 2 cm of the muscle. These fibers approach the iliac crest near the lateral margin of the erector spinae, but then deflect medially, bypassing the crest to attach to the L5 and sacral spinous processes. These fibers form the sacral portion of the superficial lamina. The third type become aponeurotic just lateral to the lumbar erector spinae. At the lateral border of the erector spinae they fuse with the other layers of thoracolumbar fascia in the lateral raphe,[7] but then they deflect medially, continuing over the back muscles to reach the midline at the levels of the L3, L4, and L5 spinous processes. These fibers form the lumbar portion of the superficial lamina.

The rostral portions of the latissimus dorsi cross the back muscles and do not become aponeurotic until some 5 cm lateral to the midline at the L3 and higher levels. These aponeurotic fibers form the thoracolumbar and thoracic portions of the thoracolumbar fascia.

Beneath the superficial lamina, the deep lamina consists of bands of collagen fibers emanating from the midline, principally from the lumbar spinous processes (Fig. 4-8). The bands from the L4, L5, and S1 spinous processes

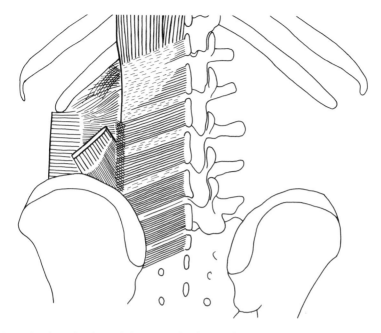

Fig. 4-8.   The deep lamina of the posterior layer of thoracolumbar fascia. (Bogduk N, Macintosh JE: The applied anatomy of the thoracolumbar fascia. Spine 9:164, 1984.)

pass caudolaterally to the posterosuperior iliac spine. Those from the L3 spinous process and L3-4 interspinous ligament wrap around the lateral margin of the erector spinae to fuse with the middle layer of thoracolumbar fascia in the lateral raphe. Above L3 the deep lamina progressively becomes thinner, consisting of sparse bands of collagen that dissipate laterally over the erector spinae. A deep lamina is not formed at thoracic levels.

Collectively, the superficial and deep laminae of the posterior layer of thoracolumbar fascia form a retinaculum over the back muscles. Attached to the midline medially and the posterosuperior iliac spine and lateral raphe laterally, the fascia covers or ensheaths the back muscles preventing their dorsal displacement. Additionally, the deep lamina alone forms a series of distinct ligaments. When viewed bilaterally, the bands of fibers from the L4 and L5 spinous processes appear like alar ligaments anchoring these spinous processes to the ilia. The band from the L3 spinous process anchors this process indirectly to the ilium via the lateral raphe. Finally, the lateral raphe forms a site where the two laminae of the posterior layer fuse not only with the middle layer of thoracolumbar fascia but also with the transversus abdominis whose middle fibers arise from the lateral raphe. The posterior layer of thoracolumbar fascia thereby provides an indirect attachment for the transversus abdominis to the lumbar spinous processes. The mechanical significance of these three morphologic features is described below (see Functions).

ACTIONS

The possible actions of the individual back muscles are a function of their orientation and disposition with respect to the vertebral column. To determine thoroughly all the possible actions of a muscle, the orientation of each of its fascicles needs to be analyzed in each of three dimensions. In either lateral or anteroposterior views, the line of action of individual fascicles can be described in terms of two vectors, and the relative size of the vectors reflects the proportion of the contraction force of each fascicle exerted in either direction. It is important to realize that although the description of the action of a muscle can be subdivided into two parts, a muscle with two vectors of action cannot use these vectors independently. If the muscle contracts, then both vectors are exerted simultaneously.

In this section the terms *flexion* and *extension* are not used in the way they are commonly applied to the vertebral column. As described in Chapter 2, the movement of flexion consists of two components: a major rocking movement of the lumbar vertebrae, which strictly is described as anterior sagittal rotation; and a small amplitude sagittal translation. Extension involves a similar but converse combination of movements.

Every back muscle does not contribute to the same extent in controlling or executing the sagittal rotations and the translations that occur in flexion and extension, and so the term *extensor* cannot be universally or indiscriminantly applied. Therefore, in analyzing the actions of the lumbar back muscles, we have specified, where appropriate, how different fascicles contribute to different extents to each of the two components of extension. Thus, certain muscles will be seen to contribute principally, and sometimes exclusively, to posterior sagittal rotation but have less effect or none at all on forward translation. Conversely, others will have a greater effect on translation and less on sagittal rotation.

Interspinales and Intertransversarii

Situated between the spinous processes, the interspinales can act synergistically with the multifidus to produce posterior sagittal rotation of their motion segment, and the spinous processes endow the muscles with powerful levers for this action.

The attachments of the intertransversarii laterales place these muscles in an advantageous position to act as lateral flexors of individual motion segments. The length of the transverse processes provides these muscles with substantial levers to execute this action and act synergistically with other lateral flexors. However, the actions and functions of the intertransversarii mediales are not that readily explained.

The intertransversarii mediales lie lateral to the axis of lateral flexion and behind the axis of sagittal rotation. However, they are very small muscles and their position is very close to these axes. Therefore, it is questionable whether they would contribute any appreciable force in either lateral flexion or posterior sagittal rotation, even if they acted only synergistically. It might be argued that larger muscles provide the bulk of the power to move vertebrae, and the intertransversarii act to fine tune the movement. However, this suggestion is highly speculative, if not fanciful.

A tantalizing alternative suggestion is that the intertransversarii act as large, proprioceptive transducers. Their value lies not in the force they can exert, but in the muscle spindles they contain. Placed close to the lumbar vertebral column, the intertransversarii could monitor the movements of the column and provide feedback that might control the action of the surrounding muscles. Such a role has been suggested for the cervical intertransversarii, which have been found to contain a high density of muscle spindles.[21-23] However, apart from the preceding comments, a similar role has not been formally suggested for the lumbar intertransversarii.

Multifidus

In a posterior view the fascicles of multifidus are seen to have an oblique, caudolateral orientation. Their line of action, therefore, can be resolved into two vectors: a large vertical; and a considerably smaller horizontal vector (Fig. 4-9).

The small horizontal vector suggests that the multifidus could pull the spinous processes sideways, and therefore produce horizontal rotation. However, horizontal rotation of lumbar vertebrae is impeded by the impaction of the contralateral zygapophyseal joints. Horizontal rotation occurs after impaction of the joints only if an appropriate shear force is applied to the intervertebral discs, but the horizontal vector of multifidus is so small that it is unlikely that multifidus would be capable of exerting such a shear force on the disc by acting on the spinous process. Indeed, electromyographic studies reveal that multifidus is inconsistently active in derotation and that paradoxically it is active in both ipsilateral and contralateral rotation.[24] Rotation, therefore, cannot be inferred to be a primary action of multifidus. In this context, multifidus has been said to act only as a "stabilizer" in rotation,[17,24,25] but the aberrant movements that it is supposed to stabilize have not been specified.

The principal action of multifidus is expressed by its vertical vector and further insight is gained when this vector is viewed in a lateral projection. Each fascicle of multifidus, at every level, acts virtually at right angles to its spinous process of origin. Thus, using the spinous process as a lever, every fascicle is ideally disposed to produce posterior sagittal rotation of it vertebra. The right-angle orientation, however, precludes any action as a posterior horizontal translator. Therefore the multifidus can exert or control only the "rocking," or rotatory, component of extension of the lumbar spine, and can control this component during flexion.

Having established that multifidus is primarily a posterior sagittal rotator of the lumbar spine, it is possible to resolve the paradox about its activity

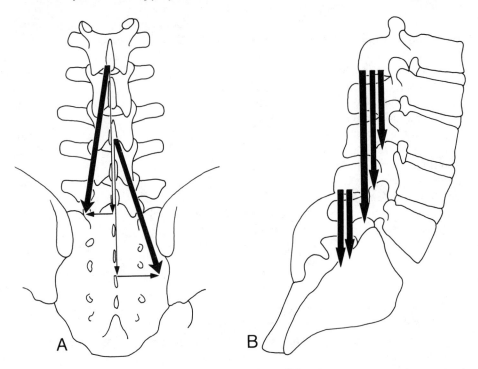

Fig. 4-9.   The action of multifidus. The action of multifidus (**bold** arrow) can be resolved into a small horizontal vector and a large vertical vector. (A) Posterior view. (B) Lateral view.

during horizontal rotation of the trunk.[9] In the first instance, it should be realized that rotation of the lumbar spine is an indirect action. Active rotation of the lumbar spine occurs only if the thorax is first rotated, and is therefore secondary to thoracic rotation. Secondly, it must be realized that a muscle with two vectors of action cannot use these vectors independently. If the muscle contracts, then both vectors are exerted. Thus, multifidus cannot exert axial rotation without simultaneously exerting a much larger posterior sagittal rotation.

The principal muscles that produce rotation of the thorax are the oblique abdominal muscles. The horizontal component of their orientation is able to turn the thoracic cage in the horizontal plane and thereby impart axial rotation to the lumbar spine. However, the oblique abdominal muscles also have a vertical component to their orientation. Therefore, if they contract to produce rotation they will also simultaneously cause flexion of the trunk, and therefore, of the lumbar spine. To counteract this flexion, and maintain pure axial rotation, extensors of the lumbar spine must be recruited, and this is how multifidus becomes involved in rotation.

The role of multifidus in rotation is not to produce rotation, but to oppose the flexion effect of the abdominal muscles as *they* produce rotation. The aberrant motion "stabilized" by multifidus during rotation is, therefore, the unwanted flexion unavoidably produced by the abdominal muscles.[9]

Apart from its action on individual lumbar vertebrae, the multifidus, because of its polysegmental nature, can also exert indirect effects on any interposed vertebrae. Since the line of action of any long fascicle of multifidus lies behind the lordotic curve of the lumbar spine, such fascicles can act like bowstrings on those segments of the curve that intervene between the attachments of the fascicle. The bowstring effect would tend to accentuate the lumbar lordosis, resulting in compression of intervertebral discs posteriorly and strain of the discs and longitudinal ligament anteriorly. Thus, a secondary effect of the action of multifidus is to increase the lumbar lordosis and the compressive and tensile loads on any vertebrae and intervertebral discs interposed between its attachments.

Lumbar Longissimus

Each fascicle of the lumbar longissimus has both a dorsoventral and a rostrocaudal orientation. Therefore, the action of each fascicle can be resolved into a vertical vector and a horizontal vector, the relative sizes of which differ from L1–5 (Fig. 4-10). Consequently, the relative actions of longissimus differ at each segmental level. Furthermore, the action of longissimus, as a whole, will differ according to whether the muscle contracts unilaterally or bilaterally.

The large vertical vector of each fascicle lies lateral to the axis of lateral flexion and behind the axis of sagittal rotation of each vertebra. Thus, contracting unilaterally the longissimus can laterally flex the vertebral column, but acting bilaterally the various fascicles can act, like multifidus, to produce posterior sagittal rotation of their vertebra of origin. However, their attachments to the accessory and transverse processes lie close to the axes of sagittal rotation and, therefore, their capacity to produce posterior sagittal rotation is less efficient than that of multifidus, which acts through the long levers of the spinous processes.

The horizontal vectors of the longissimus are directed backward. Therefore, when contracting bilaterally the longissimus is capable of drawing the lumbar vertebrae backward. This action of posterior translation can restore the anterior translation of the lumbar vertebrae that occurs during flexion of the lumbar column. The capacity for posterior translation is greatest at lower lumbar levels where the fascicles of longissimus assume a greater dorsoventral orientation.

Reviewing the horizontal and vertical actions of longissimus together, it can be seen that longissimus expresses a continuum of combined actions across the lumbar vertebral column. From below upward its capacity as a posterior sagittal rotator increases while reciprocally, from above downward, the fascicles are better designed to resist or restore anterior translation.

It might be deduced that the horizontal component of longissimus, if acting unilaterally, could draw the accessory and transverse processes backward and

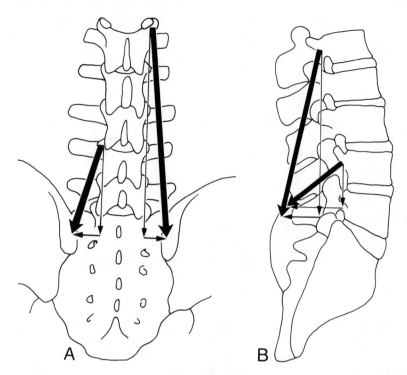

Fig. 4-10. The action of the lumbar longissimus. The action of longissimus (bold arrow) can be resolved into a small horizontal vector and a large vertical vector. (A) Posterior view. (B) Lateral view.

therefore produce horizontal rotation. However, in this regard, the fascicles of longissimus are orientated almost directly towards the axis of horizontal rotation and so are at a marked mechanical disadvantage of produce horizontal rotation.

Lumbar Iliocostalis

The disposition of the lumbar fascicles of iliocostalis is similar to that of the lumbar longissimus, except that the fascicles are situated more laterally. Like that of the lumbar longissimus, their action can be resolved into horizontal and vertical vectors (Fig. 4-11).

The vertical vector is still predominant, and therefore, the lumbar fascicles of iliocostalis contracting bilaterally can act as posterior sagittal rotators, but because of the horizontal vector, a posterior translation will be exerted simultaneously, principally at lower lumbar levels where the fascicles of iliocostalis have a greater forward orientation. Contracting unilaterally, the lumbar fascicles of iliocostalis can act as lateral flexors of the lumbar vertebrae for which action the transverse processors provide very substantial levers.

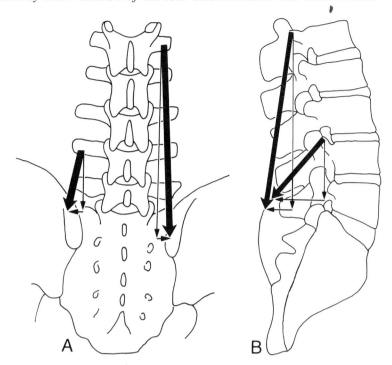

Fig. 4-11. The action of the lumbar iliocostalis. The action of the lumbar fascicles of iliocostalis (**bold** arrow) can be resolved into a small horizontal vector, and a large vertical vector. (A) Posterior view. (B) Lateral view.

Contracting unilaterally, the fibers of iliocostalis are better suited to exert axial rotation than the fascicles of lumbar longissimus, for their attachment to the tips of the transverse processes displaces them from the axis of horizontal rotation and provides them with substantial levers for this action. Because of this leverage, the lower fascicles of iliocostalis are the only intrinsic muscles of the lumbar spine reasonably disposed to produce horizontal rotation. Their effectiveness as rotators, however, is dwarfed by the oblique abdominal muscles that act on the ribs and produce lumbar rotation indirectly by rotating the thoracic cage. However, because iliocostalis cannot exert axial rotation without simultaneously exerting posterior sagittal rotation, the muscle is well suited to cooperate with multifidus to oppose the flexion effect of the abdominal muscles when they act to rotate the trunk.

Thoracic Longissimus

The thoracic longissimus is designed to act on thoracic vertebrae and ribs. Nonetheless, when contracting bilaterally it acts indirectly on the lumbar vertebral column, and uses the erector spinae aponeurosis to produce an increase in the lumbar lordosis. However, not all of the fascicles of longissimus thoracis span the entire lumbar vertebral column. Those from the second rib and T2 reach only as far as L3, and only those fascicles arising from T6-7 to T12 actually span the entire lumbar region. Consequently, only a portion of the whole thoracic longissimus acts on all the lumbar vertebrae.

The oblique orientation of the thoracic longissimus also permits it to laterally flex the thoracic vertebral column and thereby indirectly flex the lumbar vertebral column laterally.

Thoracic Iliocostalis

The thoracic fascicles of iliocostalis have no attachment to lumbar vertebrae, but attach to the iliac crest and thereby span the lumbar vertebral column. Consequently, by acting bilaterally, it is possible for them to exert an indirect "bowstring" effect on the vertebral column creating an increased lordotic curvature of the lumbar spine. Acting unilaterally, the thoracic iliocostalis can use the leverage afforded by the ribs to laterally flex the thoracic cage and thereby, indirectly, the lumbar vertebral column. The distance between the ribs does not shorten greatly during ipsilateral rotation of the trunk and therefore the thoracic iliocostalis can have little action as a horizontal rotator. However, the contralateral rotation greatly increases this distance and the thoracic iliocostalis can serve to derotate the thoracic cage and, therefore, the lumbar spine.

FUNCTIONS

Geometric analysis reveals that each of the lumbar back muscles is capable of several possible actions. No action is unique to a muscle and no muscle has a single action. Instead, the back muscles provide a pool of possible actions that may be recruited to suit the needs of the vertebral column. Therefore, the functions of the back muscles need to be considered in terms of the observed movements of the vertebral column. In this regard, three types of movements can be addressed: (1) minor active movements of the vertebral column; (2) postural movements; and (3) major movements in forward bending and lifting. In this context, postural movements refers to movements, usually subconscious, that occur to adjust and maintain a desired posture when this is disturbed, usually by the influence of gravity.

Minor Active Movements

In the upright position, the lumbar back muscles play a minor or inactive role in executing movement, for gravity provides the necessary force. During extension, the back muscles contribute to the initial tilt, drawing the line of gravity backward,[25,26] but are unnecessary for further extension. Muscle activity is recruited when the movement is forced or resisted,[27] but is restricted to muscles acting on the thorax. The lumbar multifidus, for example, shows little or no involvement.[28]

The lateral flexors can bend the lumbar spine sideways, but once the center of gravity of the trunk is displaced, lateral flexion can continue under the influence of gravity. However, the ipsilateral lateral flexors are used to direct the movement, and the contralateral muscles are required to balance the action of gravity and control the rate and extent of movement. Consequently, lateral flexion is accompanied by bilateral activity of the lumbar back muscles, but the contralateral muscles are relatively more active for it is they that must balance the load of the laterally flexing spine.[25,26,29–32] If a weight is held in the hand on the side to which the spine is laterally flexed, a greater load is applied to the spine, and the contralateral back muscles show greater activity to balance this load.[31,32]

Maintenance of Posture

The upright vertebral column is well stabilized by its joints and ligaments. Nonetheless, it is still liable to displacement by gravity or when subject to weight bearing, and the back muscles serve to correct such displacements. As the upright vertebral column sways slightly, intermittent activity occurs in the appropriate muscles to correct that sway.[25,27,28,30,34,35] Unilateral weight bearing displaces the center of gravity and tends to cause lateral flexion. To preserve the upright position, the contralateral lateral flexors (longissimus and iliocostalis) contract.[25,34]

During sitting, the activity of the back muscles is similar to that during standing.[35,36] But in supported sitting, as with the elbows resting on the knees[25,30] or resting on a desk,[35,36] there is no activity in the lumbar back muscles. In reclined sitting the back rest supports the weight of the thorax lessening the need for muscular postural support. Consequently, increasing the reclination of the back rest of a seat decreases lumbar back muscle activity.[35–38]

Major Active Movements

Forward flexion and extension of the spine from the flexed position are movements during which the back muscles exert their most important function. As the spine bends forward there is an increase in the activity of the back muscles.[24–30,32,33,39,40] The movement of forward flexion is produced by gravity, but the extent and the rate at which it proceeds is controlled by the eccentric contraction of the back muscles. The descent of the thorax is controlled by the long thoracic fibers of longissimus and iliocostalis. The long tendons of insertion allow these muscles to act around the convexity of the increasing thoracic kyphosis and anchor the thorax to the ilium and sacrum. In the lumbar region, the multifidus and the lumbar fascicles of longissimus and iliocostalis act to control the anterior sagittal rotation of the lumbar vertebrae. At the same time the lumbar fascicles of longissimus and iliocostalis also act to resist the associated anterior translation of the lumbar vertebrae.

At a certain point during forward flexion the activity in the back muscles ceases, and the vertebral column is braced by the locking of the zygopophyseal joints and tension in its posterior ligaments.[41] This phenomenon is known as *critical point*.[26,33,42,43] However, critical point does not occur in all individuals, or in all muscles.[14,24,25,30]

Extension of the trunk from the flexed position is characterized by high levels of back muscle activity.[24–26,33,40] In the thoracic region, the iliocostalis and longissimus, acting around the thoracic kyphosis, lift the thorax by rotating it backward. The lumbar vertebrae are rotated backward principally by the lumbar multifidus, causing their superior surfaces to be progressively tilted upward to support the rising thorax. The contraction of the lumbar multifidus and the thoracic longissimus and iliocostalis would tend to increase the lumbar lordosis because of their bowstring effect. However, this action is balanced by the simultaneous horizontal component of the action of both the lumbar longissimus and iliocostalis, which draw the lumbar vertebrae posteriorly, preventing the development of an excessive lumbar lordosis.

Because of the downward direction of their action as the back muscles contract, they exert a longitudinal compression of the lumbar vertebral column. This compression raises the pressure in the lumbar intervertebral discs. Any activity that involves the back muscles, therefore, is associated with a rise in nuclear pressure. As measured in the L3-4 intervertebral disc, the nuclear pressure correlates with the degree of myoelectric activity in the back muscles.[31,32,38,44,45] As muscle activity increases, disc pressure rises.

Disc pressure and myoelectric activity of the back muscles have been used extensively to quantify the stresses applied to the lumbar spine in various postures and by various activities.[35,37,38,46–52] From the standing position, forward bending causes the greatest increase in disc pressure. Lifting a weight in this position raises disc pressure even further, and the pressure is greatly increased if a load is lifted with the lumbar spine both flexed and rotated. Throughout these various maneuvers back muscle activity increases in proportion to the load lifted and the disc pressure sustained.

One of the prime revelations of combined discometric and electromyographic studies of the lumbar spine during lifting relates to the comparative stresses applied to the lumbar spine by different lifting tactics. In essence, it has been shown that, on the basis of changes in disc pressure and back muscle activity, there are no differences between using a *stoop* lift or a *leg* lift (i.e., lifting a weight with a bent back versus lifting with a straight back).[32,37,38,53] The critical factor is the distance of the load from the body. The further the load is from the chest the greater the stresses on the lumbar spine, and the greater the disc pressure and back muscle activity.[53]

Although electromyographic studies show that the back muscles are markedly active during forward flexion and lifting, electromyography alone does not prove that the muscles are responsible for executing the movement. It shows only that they are active during the movement. In this respect, lifting involves more than just the action of the back muscles, and the mechanism of lifting warrants a more detailed description.

Lifting

The force exerted on the spine by a weight is proportional not only to the weight itself but also on its distance from the body (see Kippers and Parker[43] for a review). The force exerted on any lumbar vertebrae is the product of the mass of the weight to be lifted and its horizontal distance from the vertebra, and is known as the *moment*. Moments can be increased by increasing the weight to be lifted, or by increasing the distance of a constant weight from the body. reciprocally, moments can be decreased by decreasing the mass, or by shortening the distance from the body.

In simple movements of the trunk when large weights are not being lifted, the moments involved are not large. They are the product of the weight of the upper trunk and the distance the trunk bends in front of the lumbar spine. The back muscles are quite capable of balancing these moments, and therefore, are quite capable of controlling flexion and then restoring the upright position. However, in weight lifting a different set of forces prevail. In the early phases of a weight lift, the lumbar spine is subject to a massive moment because the large mass to be lifted lies substantially in front of the body. Calculations reveal that even with maximal contraction, the back muscles cannot generate enough force to balance the large moment, and therefore, lift the weight.[54]

It should also be remembered that lifting involves not only extension of the spine but also extension of the hip. Much of the forward movement seen in forward flexion occurs at the hip joints,[42] and during extension and lifting this movement is reversed. The muscles producing hip extension are the gluteus maximus and medius and the hamstrings. These muscles in combination are massive and are quite capable of balancing the moments generated by large weights and hence of lifting the weights.[55] However, the mechanical problem that occurs is the need to transmit the effort of the hip extensors to the thorax. The forces involved are beyond the capacity of the back muscles, and they alone cannot be responsible for the transmission. They must be assisted by additional factors.

Two theories have been elaborated, which describe mechanisms that provide the additional forces needed to execute a heavy lift. One relates to the balloon effect of intraabdominal pressure, and the other relates to the role of the posterior ligamentous system. While each of these theories has its staunch advocates, neither has been fully confirmed experimentally, nor has either been totally refuted. Therefore, it is still unclear whether either theory alone, a combination of both, or neither is the explanation for the mechanism of lifting.

The intraabdominal pressure theory[56] maintains that during weight lifting, the abdominal muscles contract to raise intraabdominal pressure. This pressure then acts upwards on the diaphragm like a balloon, and serves to lift or support the thorax, thereby assisting the back muscles in raising the trunk. While endorsed by some authorities,[26,57–61] this theory has not been formally tested experimentally. Such data as is available from related experiments show that although intraabdominal pressure does rise during lifting, the correlation between intraabdominal pressure and disc pressure, back muscle activity, and the load on the lumbar spine is irregular and poor.[45,62]

The abdominal balloon theory has also been challenged on theoretical grounds. It has been calculated that in order to provide the required upward force on the thorax, intraabdominal pressure must exceed systolic aortic blood pressure.[63] Consequently, lest the circulation to the lower limbs be compromised, such pressures could not be sustained for longer than a brief moment. Moreover, it has been calculated that the force of contraction of the abdominal muscles necessary to generate this pressure exceeds the maximum possible hoop tension of these muscles.[63–65] Furthermore, in contracting to raise pressure, the abdominal muscles must also impart a flexion moment on the thoracic cage,[54,55] which would counteract any antiflexion effect of the raised pressure.[64]

These theoretical deductions and the lack of experimental verification of the balloon mechanism have led to the conclusion among some authorities that whatever effect abdominal pressure has in lifting, it cannot be the major factor assisting the back muscles in extension.[45,55,63,64] In turn, these reservations have led to the development of an alternative theory, which involves a crucial role of the posterior ligaments and thoracolumbar fascia in lifting.[20,55,64]

This theory maintains that a lift can be performed provided that the power of the hip extensors can be transmitted through the lumbar spine to the trunk and upper limbs, which are lifting the weight. The muscles of the lumbar spine are not strong enough to transmit the necessary force but can be assisted by the capsules of the zygapophyseal joints, the posterior ligaments, notably the interspinous and supraspinous ligaments, and the posterior layer of thoracolumbar fascia. Collectively these structures form what has been called the *posterior ligamentous system*.[20,55,64]

The posterior ligamentous system is said to be able to transmit forces through the lumbar spine in two ways, which can act cooperatively to assist the back muscles in executing a lift. A passive mechanism is exerted by the posterior ligaments and the zygapophyseal-joint capsules, while a more dynamic mechanism is exerted by the thoracolumbar fascia.

When tensed, the posterior ligaments and joint capsules are strong enough to sustain very large forces. Therefore, if the lumbar spine remains flexed, it can be used passively to raise large weights. With the spine flexed, and the ligaments taut, the hip can be extended and the pelvis rotated backward. This posterior sagittal rotation of the pelvis can then be transmitted to the lumbar spine through the lumbosacral joints, the L5-S1 interspinous ligament, the iliolumbar ligaments, and the alar ligaments of the thoracolumbar fascia. It is subsequently transmitted through the lumbar spine to the thorax along the posterior ligaments and, as a result, the thorax can be rotated posteriorly, achieving a lift.

For the ligaments to transmit the force of the hip extensors, they must remain taut, and therefore, the lumbar spine must remain flexed. Activity of the back muscles would cause extension, and thereby would defeat this requirement. Therefore, in terms of this theory, back muscle activity, in the initial phases of lifting, is not only superfluous, but is outrightly disadvantageous. It is therefore, natural that no activity should occur during the initial phases of a lift.

Flexion of the lumbar spine can be maintained passively by the resistance of the weight to be lifted, and actively by the contraction of the abdominal muscles.[55] Consequently, the purpose of the abdominal muscle activity during lifting is not to raise abdominal pressure, but to flex the lumbar spine and maintain ligamentous tension. In this regard, intraabdominal pressure is more a side effect of this activity, rather than its primary purpose.

Once the weight has been raised, and is progressively brought closer to the trunk, the moment it exerts is reduced. The size of the moment decreases until it is within the capacity of the trunk muscles, and gradually the back muscles can be recruited to take over the load. Thus, once the moment is small enough, the back muscles can balance it and relieve the ligaments, and under the action of the muscles, the lumbar spine extends, i.e., "deflexes."

The essence of this theory is that the power of lifting stems from the hip extensors. The back muscles do not provide the power. They are relatively too small to lift large weights. During lifting, the lumbar spine acts passively, and is kept flexed to allow the power of the hip extensors to be transmitted through its posterior ligaments. As the spine approaches the upright position, the moment exerted by the lifted weight is reduced, and the back muscles are capable, at last, of continuing the lift.

A limitation to the passive role of the posterior ligamentous system is that the lumbar spine must remain in a flexed position for the ligaments to remain taut and be able to transmit tension. The moment the spine extends, the ligaments relax and can no longer transmit forces from the hip to the thorax. This observation suggests that, at some stage in the lift, there must be an abrupt transition from ligamentous to muscular support of the flexed lumbar spine. However, the posterior ligamentous theory provides for an additional mechanism superimposed on the passive role of the posterior ligaments that is largely independent of the angle of flexion. This mechanism is provided by the posterior layer of thoracolumbar fascia.

The posterior layer of thoracolumbar fascia can function in three ways to stabilize the flexed lumbar spine and to aid in lifting. The most overt mechanism is the passive ligamentous role of the deep lamina. The L4 and L5 spinous processes are directly connected to the ilium by fibers of the deep lamina (Fig. 4-8). These connections would be tensed in the flexed lumbar spine, and would provide a route of transmission to the lumbar spine of the posterior sagittal rotation of the pelvis, complementing the role of the interspinous and iliolumbar

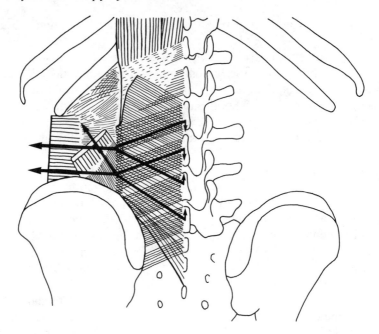

Fig. 4-12. The combined action of the deep and superficial laminae of the posterior layer of thoracolumbar fascia. (Bogduk N, Macintosh JE: The applied anatomy of the thoracolumbar fascia. Spine 9:164, 1984.)

ligaments in this regard. The actual extent to which these structures contribute to the transmission of force is still unknown, but it is being investigated.

The second function of the thoracolumbar fascia stems from the bilaminar structure of the posterior layer and its connections, through the lateral raphe, with the transversus abdominis (Fig. 4-12). These connections allow the transversus abdominis to exert an "antiflexion" effect on the lumbar spine. Both the superficial and deep laminae of the posterior layer fuse with the lateral raphe. Therefore, from any point in the lateral raphe a fiber from the superficial lamina extends caudomedially to the midline, and a fiber from the deep lamina extends rostromedially. Consequently, the posterior layer can be perceived as consisting of a series of overlapping triangles of fibers, each with its apex in the lateral raphe and its basal corners at the midline.[7] The divergence of the fibers is such that the base of each triangle is about two segments long (Fig. 4-13).

The effect of this arrangement is that when lateral tension is applied to the apex of a triangle, tension develops along its two sides. The upper corner of the triangle is thereby subjected to a downward and outward tension, while the lower corner is subjected to an upward and outward tension. Because of the mutually opposed downward and upward tension exerted on the corners, they tend to approximate,[7,64] and it can be shown mathematically that in the upright position the size of this approximating force is about 57 percent of the

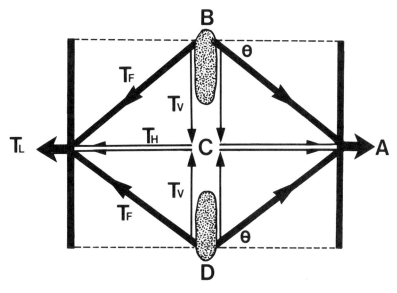

Fig. 4-13. Diagram representing the force transmission through the posterior layer of thoracolumbar fascia.

force applied to the lateral raphe (see the Appendix). This increase has been described as the *gain* of the thoracolumbar fascia.[64]

Relating this to the transversus abdominis, it can be seen that from the lateral raphe where the transversus abdominis attaches fibers of the posterior layer radiate to subtend two pairs of vertebrae: L2, L4 and L3, L5. Therefore, through the triangular network in the posterior layer, contraction of the transversus abdominis results in a vertical midline tension that tends to approximate the spinous process of L2 to L4, and L3 to L5. Because of this tension, contraction of the transversus abdominis will resist separation of these spinous processes, and therefore, flexion of these vertebrae. Thus, the second function of the thoracolumbar fascia is to provide a mechanism whereby transversus abdominis can act to "brace" the lumbar spine by resisting flexion of its lower vertebrae.

This bracing action is independent and additional to any effect that abdominal contraction may have in raising intraabdominal pressure and exerting a balloon effect on the thorax. Moreover, it is conceivable that this direct action of the transversus abdominis may be the cardinal role of the abdominal muscles in lifting.

The third function of the posterior layer of thoracolumbar fascia stems from its retinacular structure. As the lumbar back muscles contract, they shorten and expand, evidenced clinically by the enhanced prominence of their contour. The posterior layer of thoracolumbar fascia will resist this expansion, and tension will develop in it as the back muscles contract. This tension will be additional to any tension already developed either by the passive ligamentous action of the deep lamina or by the contraction of the transversus abdominis. By increasing the tension in the posterior layer, contraction of the lumbar back muscles enhances the antiflexion functions of the thoracolumbar fascia. This phenomenon has been called the *hydraulic amplifier mechanism*.[66]

The hydraulic amplifier mechanism and the contraction of the transversus abdominis enable tension in the thoracolumbar fascia to be sustained throughout a lift. Thus, even when the other components of the posterior ligamentous system are relaxed by the onset of spinal extension, the thoracolumbar fascia can continue to exert an antiflexion action that can act synergistically with the back muscles to brace the extending, though still partially flexed, lumbar spine.

The posterior ligamentous theory is consistent with the known anatomy of the lumbar spine, and is consistent with the tensile properties and capacities of its ligaments and fasciae. Mathematically, the theory does account for the missing forces required to execute a heavy lift. However, to date, the theory has not been evaluated experimentally or clinically, and this remains its major liability. On paper and in computer models, the posterior ligamentous theory seems to explain the mechanism of lifting better that the intraabdominal balloon mechanism, but the critical experiments to ratify or refute either theory have yet to be performed.

APPENDIX

The authors are indebted to Dr. Serge Gracovetsky for his assistance in formulating the following mathematical description of the posterior layer of thoracolumbar fascia.

The lateral tension (T_T) applied to the lateral raphe is exerted on the midline through fibers of the posterior layer of thoracolumbar fascia (T_F), which are oriented at 0 degrees to the horizontal axis. This oblique tension (T_F) can be resolved into a horizontal tension (T_H) and a vertical tension (T_V) (Fig. 4-13):

$$T_H = T_F \cos\theta \tag{1}$$

$$T_V = T_F \sin\theta \tag{2}$$

T_L must equal the sums of the horizontal tensions in the triangles ABC and ADC, i.e., $T_L = 2 T_H$

Therefore, from (1)

$$T_L = 2T_F \times \cos\theta$$
$$T_F = \frac{T_L}{2\cos\theta} \tag{3}$$

From (2), (3)

$$T_v = \frac{T_I \cdot \sin\theta}{2\cos\theta}$$

$$= \frac{T_L}{2} \cdot \tan\theta$$

The force approximating B and D will be the sum of the vertical forces generated in the triangles ABC and ADC, i.e.,

$$F = 2T_V$$

$$= 2 \cdot \frac{T_L \tan\theta}{2}$$

$$= T_L \tan\theta$$

Since

$$\theta = 30°$$

then

$$F = 0.577 \, T_L$$

REFERENCES

1. Basmajian JV: Grant's Method of Anatomy. 10th Ed. Williams & Wilkins, Baltimore, 1980
2. Hollinshead WH, Jenkins DB: Functional Anatomy of the Limbs and Back. 5th Ed. Saunders, Philadelphia, 1981
3. Snell RS: Clinical Anatomy for Medical Students. 2nd Ed. Little, Brown, Boston, 1981
4. Warwick R, Williams PL (eds): Gray's Anatomy. 35th Ed. Longman, London, 1973
5. Bogduk N: A reappraisal of the anatomy of the human lumbar erector spinae. J Anat 131:525, 1980
6. Bogduk N: The myotomes of the human multifidus. J Anat 136:148, 1983
7. Bogduk N. Macintosh JE: The applied anatomy of the thoracolumbar fascia. Spine 9:164, 1984
8. Macintosh JE, Bogduk N: The qualitative biomechanics of the lumbar back muscles. J Anat 142:218, 1985
9. Macintosh JE, Bogduk N: The detailed biomechanics of the lumbar multifidus. Clin Biomech 1:196, 1986

10. Macintosh JE, Bogduk N: Biomechanics of the thoracolumbar fascia. Clin Biomech 1:196, 1986
11. Macintosh JE, Bogduk N: The anatomy and biomechanics of the lumbar erector spinae. Spine (submitted)
12. Macintosh JE, Valencia F, Bogduk N, Munro RR: The morphology of the human lumbar multifidus. Clin Biomech 1:205, 1986
13. Valencia F, Munro RR: Electromyography of lumbar multifidus in man. J Anat 142:218, 1985
14. Valencia F, Munro RR: An electromyographic study of the lumbar multifidus in man. Electromyogr Clin Neurophysiol 25:205, 1985
15. Bogduk N, Wilson AS, Tynan W: The human lumbar dorsal rami. J Anat 134:383, 1982
16. Cave AJE: The innervation and morphology of the cervical intertransverse muscles. J Anat 71:497, 1937
17. Lewin T, Moffet B, Viidik A: The morphology of the lumbar synovial intervertebral joints. Acta morphol Neerl Scand 4:299, 1962
18. Leong JCY, Luk KDK, Ho HC: The iliolumbar ligament—Its anatomy, development and clinical significance. Paper presented at the twelfth annual meeting of the International Society for the Study of the Lumbar Spine. Sydney, Australia, 1985
19. Fairbanks JCT, O'Brien JP: The abdominal cavity and thoracolumbar fascia as stabilizers of the lumbar spine in patients with low back pain. p. 83. In Engineering Aspects of the Spine. Vol 2. Mechanical Engineering Publications, London, 1980
20. Gracovetsky S, Farfan HF, Lamy C: The mechanism of the lumbar spine. Spine 6:249, 1972
21. Abrahams VC: The physiology of neck muscles; their role in head movement and maintenance of posture. Can J Physiol Pharmacol, 55:332, 1977
22. Abrahams VC: Sensory and motor specialization in some muscles of the neck. TINS 4:24, 1981
23. Cooper S, Danial PM: Muscles spindles in man, their morphology in the lumbricals and the deep muscles of the neck. Brain 86:563, 1963
24. Donisch EW, Basmajian JV: Electromyography of deep back muscles in man. Am J Anat 133:25, 1972
25. Floyd WF, Silver PHS: The function of the erectores spinae muscles in certain movements and postures in man. J Physiol 129:184, 1955
26. Morris JM, Benner G, Lucas DB: An electromyographic study of the intrinsic muscles of the back in man. J Anat 96:509, 1962
27. Ortengren R, Andersson GBJ: Electromyographic studies of trunk muscles with special reference to the functional anatomy of the lumbar spine. Spine 2:44, 1977
28. Morris JM, Lucas DB, Bresler B: Role of the trunk in stability of the spine. J Bone Joint Surg (Am) 43A:327, 1961
29. Carlsoo S: The static muscle load in different work positions: an electromyographic study. Ergonomics 4:193, 1961
30. Portnoy H, Morin F: Electromyographic study of the postural muscles in various positions and movements. Am J Physiol 186:122, 1956
31. Ortengren R, Andersson G, Nachemson A: Lumbar loads in fixed working postures during flexion and rotation. p. 159 In Asmussen E, Jorgensen K (eds): Biomechanics VIB, International Series on Biomechanics. Vol. 2B. Human Kinetics, Champaign, Illinois, 1978
32. Andersson GBJ, Ortengren R, Nachemson A: 1978 Intradiskal pressure, intra-abdominal pressure and myoelectric back muscle activity related to posture and loading. Clin Orthop 129:156, 1977

33. Floyd WF, Silver PHS: Function of erectores spinae in flexion of the trunk. Lancet 1:133, 1951
34. Jonsson B: The functions of the individual muscles in the lumbar part of the spinae muscle. Electromyography 10:5, 1970
35. Andersson BJG, Ortengren R: Myoelectric activity during sitting. Scand J Rehab Med (suppl)3:73, 1974
36. Andersson BJG, Jonsson B, Ortengren R: Myoelectric activity in individual lumbar erector spinae muscles in sitting: a study with surface and wire electrodes. Scand J Rehab Med (suppl)3:91, 1974
37. Nachemson AL: The lumbar spine. An orthopaedic challenge. Spine 1:59, 1976
38. Nachemson A: Lumbar intradiscal pressure. p. 341. In Jayson MIV (ed): The Lumbar Spine and Backache. 2nd Ed. Pitman, London, 1980
39. Okada M: Electromyographic assessment of the muscular load in forward bending postures. J Fac Sci Univ Tokyo 8:311, 1970
40. Pauly JE: An electromyographic analysis of certain movements and exercises. I. Some deep muscles of the back. Anat Rec 155:223, 1966
41. Twomey LT, Taylor JR: Sagittal movements of the human lumbar vertebral column: A quantitative study of the role of the posterior vertebral elements. Arch Phys Med Rehabil 64:322, 1983
42. Kippers V, Parker AW: Posture related to myoelectric silence or erectores spinae during trunk flexion. Spine 7:740, 1984
43. Kippers V, Parker AW: Electromyographic studies of erectores spinae: symmetrical postures and sagittal trunk motion. Aust J Physiother 31:95, 1985
44. Ortengren R, Andersson GBJ, Nachemson AL: Studies of relationships between lumbar disc pressure, myoelectric back muscle activity, and intra-abdominal (intragastric) pressure. Spine 6:98, 1981
45. Andersson GBJ: Loads on the lumbar spine: in vivo measurements and biomechanical analyses. p. 32. In Winter DA, Norman RW, Wells RP, Hayes KC, Patla AE (eds): Biomechanics IXB, International Series on Biomechanics. Human Kinetics, Champaign, Illinois, 1983
46. Nachemson A: The load on lumbar disks in different positions of the body. Clin Orthop 45:107, 1966
47. Nachemson AL, Elfstrom G: Intravital dynamic pressure measurements in lumbar discs. A study of common movements, maneuvers and exercises. Scand J Rehabil Med 2(suppl)1:1, 1970
48. Nachemson A, Morris JM: In vivo measurements of intradiscal pressure. J Bone Joint Surg (Am) 46A:1077, 1964
49. Andersson BJG, Ortengren R, Nachemson A, Elfstrom G: Lumbar disc pressure and myoelectric activity during sitting. I. Studies on an experimental chair. Scand J Rehabil Med 6:104, 1974
50. Andersson BJG, Ortengren R, Nachemson AL, Elfstrom G: Lumbar disc pressure and myoelectric back muscle activity during sitting. IV > Studies on an a car driver's seat. Scand J Rehabil Med 6:128, 1974
51. Andersson BJG, Ortengren R, Nachemson AL, Elfstrom G, Broman H: The sitting posture: an electromyographic and discometric study. Orthop Clin North Am 6:105, 1975
52. Andersson GBJ, Ortengren R, Nachemson A: Quantitative studies of the back in different working postures. Scand J Rehabil Med (suppl)6:173, 1978
53. Andersson GBJ, Ortengren R, Nachemson A: Quantitative studies of back loads in lifting. Spine 1:178, 1976

54. Farfan HF: The biomechanical advantage of lordosis and hip extension for upright activity. Man as compared with other anthropoids. Spine 3:336, 1978
55. Farfan HF: Muscular mechanism of the lumbar spine and the position of power and efficiency. Orthop Clin North Am 6:135, 1975
56. Bartelink DL: The role of abdominal pressure in relieving the pressure on the lumbar intervertebral discs. J Bone Joint Surg (Br) 39B:718, 1957
57. Troup JDG: Relation of lumbar spine disorders to heavy manual work and lifting. Lancet 1:857, 1965
58. Troup JDG: Dynamic factors in the analysis of stoop and crouch lifting methods: a methodological approach to the development of safe materials handling standards. Orthop Clin North Am 8:201, 1977
59. Troup JDG: Biomechanics of the vertebral column. Physiotherapy 65:238, 1979
60. Davis PR: Posture of the trunk during the lifting of weights. Br Med J 1:87, 1959
61. Davis PR, Troup JDG: Pressures in the trunk cavities when pulling, pushing and lifting. Ergonomics 7:465, 1964
62. Leskinen TPJ, Stalhammar HR, Kuorinka IAA, Troup J DG: Hip torque, Lumbosacral compression, and intraabdominal pressure in lifting and lowering tasks. p. 55. In Winter DA, Norman RW, Wells RP, Hayes KC, Patla AE (eds): Biomechanics IXB, International Series of Biomechanics. Human Kinetics, Champaign, Illinois, 1983
63. Farfan HF, Gracovetsky S: The abdominal mechanism. Paper presented at meeting of the International Society for the Study of the Lumbar Spine, Paris, 1981
64. Gracovetsky S, Farfan HF, Helleur C: The abdominal mechanism. Spine 10:317, 1985
65. Farfan HF, Gracovetsky S, Helleur C: The role of mathematical models in the assessment of task in the workplace. p. 38. In Winter DA, Norman RW, Wells RP, Hayes KC, Patla AE (eds): Biomechanics IXB, International Series on Biomechanics. Human Kinetics, Champaign, Illinois, 1983
66. Gracovetsky S, Farfan HF, Lamy C: A mathematical model of the lumbar spine using an optimized system to control muscles and ligaments. Orthop Clin North Am 8:135, 1977

5 The Maitland Concept: Assessment, Examination, and Treatment by Passive Movement

Geoffrey D. Maitland

It would be difficult for me as an individual who has been involved in the practice of manipulative physical therapy in Australia for the past three decades to objectively assess my particular contribution to the discipline. I therefore begin this chapter, by way of explanation and justification, with a relevant and pertinent quotation from Lance Twomey, who asked me to write it.

> In my view, the Maitland approach to treatment differs from others, not in the mechanics of the technique, but rather in its approach to the patient and his particular problem. Your attention to detail in examination, treatment and response is unique in Physical Therapy, and I believe is worth spelling out in some detail:
> — the development of your concepts of assessment and treatment;
> — your insistence on sound foundations of basic biological knowledge;
> — the necessity for high levels of skill;
> — the evolution of the concepts. It did not "come" to you fully developed, but is a living thing, developing and extending;
> — the necessity for detailed examination and for the examination/treatment/re-examination approach.

(This area is well worth very considerable attention because, to me, it is the essence of "Maitland")

Although the text of this chapter deals with "passive movement," it must be very clearly understood that the author does not believe that passive movement is the only form of treatment that will alleviate musculoskeletal disorders. What the chapter *does* set out to do is to provide a conceptual framework for treatment, which is considered by many to be unique. Thus, for want of a better expression, the particular approach to assessment, examination, and treatment outlined in this paper is described as "the Maitland concept," and referred to hereafter as "the concept."

To portray all aspects of "the concept" by the written word alone is difficult since so much of it depends upon a particular clinical pattern of reasoning. The approach is not only methodical, but also involved, and therefore, difficult to describe adequately without clinical demonstration. *The Maitland concept requires open-mindedness, mental agility, and mental discipline linked with a logical and methodical process of assessing cause and effect. The central theme demands a positive personal commitment (empathy) to understand what the person (patient) is enduring.* The key issues of "the concept" that require explanation are personal commitment, mode of thinking, techniques, examination, and assessment.

A PERSONAL COMMITMENT TO THE PATIENT

All clinicians would claim that they have a high level of personal commitment to every patient. True as that may be, many areas of physical therapy require that a deeper commitment to certain therapeutic concepts be developed than is usual. Thus, the therapist must have a personal commitment to care, reassure, communicate, listen and inspire confidence.

All therapists must make a conscious effort (particularly during the first consultation), to gain the patient's confidence, trust, and relaxed comfort in what may be at first an anxious experience. The achievement of this trusting relationship requires many skills, but it is essential if proper *care* is to be provided.

Within the first few minutes, the clinician must make the patient believe that he wants to know what the patient feels; not what his doctor or anyone else feels, but what the patient himself feels is the main issue. This approach immediately puts the patient at ease by showing that we are concerned about his symptoms and the effect they are having.

We must use the patient's terminology in our discussions: we must adapt our language (and jargon) to fit his; we must make our *concern* for his symptoms show in a way that matches the patient's feelings about the symptoms. In other words, we should adapt our approach to match the patient's mode of expression, not make or expect the patient to adapt to our personality and our knowledge. The patient also needs to be *reassured* of the belief and understanding of the therapist.

Communication is another skill that clinicians must learn to use effectively and appropriately. As far as personal commitment is concerned, this involves understanding the nonverbal as well as the verbal aspects of communication so that use can be made of it to further enhance the relationship between patient and clinician. Some people find that this is a very difficult skill to acquire, but however much effort is required to learn it, it must be learned and used.

Listening to the patient must be done in an open-minded and nonjudgmental manner.

It is most important to accept the story the patient weaves, while at the same time being prepared to question him closely about it. Accepting and listening are very demanding skills, requiring a high level of objectivity.

It is a very sad thing to hear patients say that their doctor or physical therapist does not listen to them carefully enough or with enough sympathy, sensitivity, or attention to detail. The following quotation from *The Age*,[1] an Australian daily newspaper, sets out the demands of "listening" very clearly:

> Listening is itself, of course, an art: that is where it differs from merely hearing. Hearing is passive; listening is active. Hearing is involuntary; listening demands attention. Hearing is natural; listening is an acquired discipline."

Acceptance of the patient and his story is essential if trust between patient and clinician is to be established. We must accept and note the subtleties of his comments about his disorder even if they may sound peculiar. Expressed in another way, he and his symptoms are "innocent until proven guilty" (that is, his report is true and reliable until found to be unreliable, biased, or false). In this context, he needs to be guided to understand that his body can tell him things about his disorder and its behavior that we (the clinicians) cannot know unless he expresses them. This relationship should *inspire confidence* and build-up trust between both parties.

This central core of the concept of total commitment must begin at the outset of the first consultation and carry through to the end of the total treatment period.

Other important aspects of communication will be discussed later under Examination and Assessment.

A MODE OF THINKING: THE PRIMACY OF CLINICAL EVIDENCE

As qualified physical therapists, we have absorbed much scientific information and gained a great deal of clinical experience, both of which are essential for providing effective treatment. The "science" of our discipline enables us to make diagnoses and apply the appropriate "art" of our physical skill. However, the accepted theoretical basis of our profession is continually developing and changing. The gospel of yesterday becomes the heresy of tomorrow. It is essential that we remain open to new knowledge and open-minded in areas of uncertainty, so that inflexibility and tunnel vision do not result in a misapplication of our "art." Even with properly attested science applied in its right context, with precise information concerning the patient's symptoms and signs, a correct diagnosis is often difficult. Matching of the clinical findings to particular theories of anatomic, biomechanical, and pathologic knowledge, so as to attach a particular "label" to the patient's condition, may not always be appropriate. Therapists must remain open-minded so that as treatment progresses, the patient is reassessed in relation to the evolution of the condition and the responses to treatment.

In summary, the scientific basis underlying the current range of diagnoses of disorders of the spine is incompletely understood. It is also changing rapidly with advances in knowledge and will continue to do so. In this context, the therapist may be sure of the clinical evidence from the patient's history and clinical signs, but should beware of the temptation to "fit the diagnosis" to the inflexible and incomplete list of options currently available. The physical therapist must remain open-minded, not only at the initial consultation, but also as noting the changing responses of the patient during assessment and treatment. When the therapist is working in a relatively "uncharted area" like human spinal disorders, one should not be influenced too much by the unreliable mass of inadequately understood biomechanics, symptomatology, and pathology.

As a consequence of the above, a list of practical steps to follow has been drawn up. In the early era of its evolution, "the Maitland concept" had as its basis the following stages within a treatment:

1. Having assessed the effect of a patient's disorder, to perform a single treatment technique
2. To take careful note of what happens during the performance of the technique
3. Having completed the technique, to assess the effect of the technique on the patient's symptoms including movements
4. Having assessed steps 2 and 3, and taken into account the available theoretical knowledge, to plan the next treatment approach and repeat the cycle from step 1 again

It becomes obvious that this sequence can only be useful and informative if both the clinical history taking and objective examinations have been accurate.

The actual pattern of the concept requires us to keep our thoughts in two separate but interdependent compartments: the *theoretical* framework; and the *clinical* assessment. An example may help to clarify these concepts. We know that a lumbar intervertebral disc can herniate and cause pain, which can be referred into the leg. However, there are many presentations that can result from such a herniation (Table 5-1).

Table 5-1. One Diagnosis With Many Presentations

Theory	Clinical
Diagnosis: disc herniation	H_1(history); Sy_1 (symptoms); S_1 (signs)
	H_2 Sy_2 S_2
	H_3 Sy_3 S_3
	etc.

The reverse is also true—a patient may have one set of symptoms for which more than one diagnostic title can be applied[2] (Table 5-2).

Table 5-2. Different Diagnoses for One Set of Symptoms and Signs*

Theory	Clinical
Diagnosis 1	
Diagnosis 2	$H; Sy; S$
Diagnosis 3	
Diagnosis 4	

* (H = history; Sy = symptoms; S = signs)

Because of the circumstances shown in Tables 5-1 and 5-2, it is obvious that it is not always possible to have a precise diagnosis for every patient treated. The more accurate and complete our theoretical framework, the more appropriate will be our treatment. If the theoretical framework is faulty or deficient (as most are admitted to be), a full and accurate understanding of the patient's disorder may be impossible. The therapist's humility and open-mindedness are therefore essential, and inappropriate diagnostic labels must not be attached to a patient prematurely. The theoretical and clinical components must, however, influence one another. With this in mind, I have developed an approach separating theoretical knowledge from clinical information by what I have called the *symbolic, permeable brick wall* (Table 5-3). This serves to separate theory and practice, and to allow each to occupy (although not exclusively) its own compartment. That is, information from one side is able to filter through to the other side. In this way, theoretical concepts influence examination and treatment, while examination and treatment lead one back to a reconsideration of theoretical premises.

Using this mode of thinking, the brick-wall concept frees the clinician's mind from prejudice, allowing the therapist to ponder the possible reasons for a patient's disorder; to speculate, consider a hypothesis, and discuss with others

Table 5-3. Symbolic, Permeable Brick Wall (H = history, Sy = symptoms, S = signs)

THEORY	B R I C K	W A L L	CLINICAL
Diagnosis			$H; Sy; S$

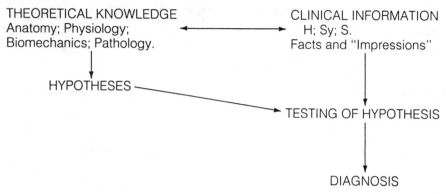

THEORETICAL KNOWLEDGE   CLINICAL INFORMATION
Anatomy; Physiology;   ◄────────►   H; Sy; S.
Biomechanics; Pathology.   Facts and "Impressions"

            HYPOTHESES

                                      TESTING OF HYPOTHESIS

                                              DIAGNOSIS

Fig. 5-1.   Flowchart demonstrating relationships and contexts for theoretical and clinical knowledge with related hypotheses. (H = history; Sy = symptoms; S = signs)

the possibilities regarding other diagnoses without anyone really knowing all the answers, yet all having a clear understanding of the patient's symptoms and related signs (Fig. 5-1).

This mode of thinking requires the use of accurate language, whereas inaccurate use of words betrays faulty logic. The way in which an individual makes a statement provides the listener with an idea both of the way that person is thinking and of the frame of reference for the statement.

A simple example may help to make this point clear. Imagine a clinician presenting a patient at a clinical seminar, and on request the patient demonstrates his area of pain. During the ensuing discussion, the clinician may refer to the patient's pain as "sacroiliac pain." This is a wrong choice of words. To be true to "the concept" we have outlined, of keeping clinical information and theoretical interpretations separate, one should describe the pain simply as a "pain in the sacroiliac area." It would be an unjustified assumption to suggest that pathology in the sacroiliac joint was the source of pain, but the former description above could be interpreted in this way. On the other hand, describing the pain as "in the sacroiliac area" indicates that we are considering other possible sites of origin for the pain besides the sacroiliac joints, thereby keeping our diagnostic options open until we have more evidence. This is an essential element to "the concept." Some readers may believe that attention to this kind of detail is unnecessary and pedantic. Quite the opposite is true. The correct and careful choice of words indicates a discipline of mind and an absence of prejudice, which influence all our diagnostic procedures including the whole process of examination, treatment, and interpretation of the patient's response.

A clinician's written record of a patient's examination and treatment findings also show clearly whether the therapist's thinking processes are right or wrong. A genuine scientific approach involves logical thinking, vertical and lateral thinking, and inductive and deductive reasoning. It requires a mind that is uncluttered by confused and unproven theory, which is at the same time able to use proven facts, and has the critical ability to distinguish between well-attested facts and unsubstantiated opinions. It requires a mind that is honest, methodical, and self-critical. It also requires a mind that has the widest possible scope in the areas of improvization and innovation.

TECHNIQUES

Many physical therapy clinicians are continually seeking new techniques of joint mobilization. When they hear a new name or when a new author has written a book on manipulation, they attempt to acquire the "new" technical skills, and immediately apply them. In reality, the techniques are of secondary importance. Of course, if they are poorly performed or misapplied, treatment may fail and the therapist may lose confidence in the techniques. However, in my view there are many acceptable techniques each of which can be modified to suit a patient's disorder and the clinician's style and physique. Accordingly, I consider that there is no absolute set of techniques that can belong or be attributed to any one person. There should be no limit to the selection of technique: the biomechanically-based techniques of Kaltenborn; the "shift" techniques of McKenzie; the combined-movements technique of Edwards; the osteopathic and chiropractic technique; the Cyriax techniques; the Stoddard technique; the bonesetters' techniques; the Maigne techniques; and the Mennell techniques. All of these techniques are of the present era. Every experienced practitioner must feel totally free to make use of any of them. The most important consideration is that the technique chosen be appropriate to the particular patient or situation, and that its effect should be carefully and continually assessed.

Techniques of Management

Within the broad concept of this chapter, there are certain techniques of management that are continually used, but are not described by other authors. These techniques are as follows.

When treating very painful disorders passive-treatment movements can be used in an oscillatory fashion ("surface stirring" as described by Maitland[3]) but with two important provisos:

1. The oscillatory movement is performed without the patient experiencing any pain whatsoever, nor even any discomfort.
2. The movement is performed only in that part of the range of movement where there is no resistance, i.e., where there is no stiffness or muscle spasm restricting the oscillations.

One may question how a painfree oscillatory movement, which avoids every attempt to stretch structures, can produce any improvement in a patient's symptoms. A scientific answer to this question has been suggested [3] but there is a far more important clinical conclusion. It has been repeatedly shown clinically that such a technique does consistently produce a measurable improvement in range of movement with reduction in pain and disability and no demonstrable harmful effects. This demonstrates that the treatment is clinically, and therefore "scientifically," correct even though an adequate theoretical explanation for its effectiveness may not yet be available. Reliable and repeated demonstration of effectiveness must validate a treatment method. To know how the method achieves the result is a theoretical problem for science to solve. The "scientific" examination must match the primary clinical observation, the latter being the aspect of which we can be sure.

This example demonstrates once more how this mode of thinking so essential to "the concept" is so necessary for the further development of treatment methods. Without this mode of thinking we would never have found that passive-movement treatment procedures can successfully promote union in nonuniting fractures.[4,5]

Oscillatory movements as an important component of passive movement are referred to above in relation to the treatment of pain. There is another treatment procedure that requires oscillatory movement to be effective. This is related to the intermittent stretching of ligamentous and capsular structures. There are clearly defined areas of application for this treatment, which are described elsewhere.[3]

There are occasions when a passive treatment movement needs to be performed with the opposing joint surfaces compressed together.[6] Without the compression component, the technique would fail to produce any improvement in the patient's symptoms.

Utilizing the movements and positions by which a patient is able to reproduce his symptoms as an initial mandatory test is essential to "the concept." This tactic, like the formalized examination of combined movements (the original contribution in cooperation with Edwards[7]) is very special to "the concept."

Although it is frequently recognized that straight-leg raising can be used as a treatment technique for low lumbar disorders, it is not widely appreciated that the technique may be made more effective by using straight-leg raising in the "Slump test" position.[8] In the same slumped position, the neck flexion component of the position may be effectively utilized when such movement reproduces a patient's low back pain.

"Accessory" movements produced by applying alternating pressure on palpable parts of the vertebrae are also very important in terms of techniques and "the Maitland concept." Any treatment concept that does not include such techniques is missing a critical link essential to a full understanding of the effects of manipulation on patients with low lumbar disorders.

It is important to remember that there is no dogma or clear set of rules that can be applied to the selection and use of passive-movement techniques; the choice is open ended. A technique is the brainchild of ingenuity. "The achievements are limited to the extent of one's lateral and logical thinking."[9]

EXAMINATION

The care, precision, and scope of examination required by those using this "concept" are greater and more demanding than other clinical methods I have observed. "The concept's" demands differ from those of other methods in many respects.

The history taking and examination demand a total commitment to understanding what the patient is suffering and the effects of the pain and disability on the patient. Naturally, one is also continually attempting to understand the cause of the disorder (the theoretical compartment of "the concept").

Examination must include a sensitive elucidation of the person's symptoms in relation to:

1. Precise area(s) indicated on the surface of the body.
2. The depth at which symptoms are experienced.
3. Whether there is more than one site of pain, or whether multiple sites overlap or are separate.
4. Changes in the symptoms in response to movements or differences in joint positions in different regions of the body.

The next important and unique part of the examination is for the patient to reenact the movement that best reveals his disorder or, if applicable, to reenact the movement that produced the injury. The function or movement is then analyzed by breaking it into components in order to make clinical sense of particular joint-movement pain responses, which are applicable to his complaint.

The routine examination of physiologic movements performed with a degree of precision rarely utilized by other practitioners. If the person's disorder is an "end-of-range" type of problem, the details of the movement examination required are:

1. At what point in the range are the symptoms first experienced; how do they vary with continuation of the movement; and in what manner do the symptoms behave during the symptomatic range?
2. In the same way and with the same degree of precision, how does muscle spasm or resistance vary during the symptomatic range?
3. Finally, what is the relationship of the symptoms (a) to the resistance or spasm; and (b) during that same movement? There may be no relationship whatsoever, in which case, for example, the stiffness is relatively unimportant. However, if the behavior of the symptoms matches the behavior of the stiffness, both should improve in parallel during treatment.

An effective method of recording the findings of all components of a movement disorder is to depict them in a "movement diagram." These also are an innovative part of "the concept." The use of movement diagrams facilitates demonstration of changes in the patient's condition in a more precise and objective manner. They are discussed at length in the fifth edition of "Vertebral Manipulation."[10]

If the patient's disorder is a "pain through range" type of problem, the details of the movement examination required are:

1. At what point in the range does discomfort or pain first increase?
2. How do the symptoms behave if movement is taken a short distance beyond the onset of discomfort? Does intensity markedly increase or is the area of referred pain extended?
3. Is the movement a normal physiological movement in the available range or is it protected by muscle spasm or stiffness? Opposing the abnormal movement and noting any change in the symptomatic response compared with entry 2 is performed to assess its relevance to the course of treatment.

Palpatory Techniques

The accessory movements are tested by palpation techniques and seek the same amount and type of information as described above. They are tested in a variety of different joint positions. The three main positions are:

1. The neutral mid-range position for each available movement i.e., midway between flexion/extension, rotation left and right, lateral flexion left and right, and distraction/compression.
2. The joint is in a "loose-packed position,"[11] at the particular position where the person's symptoms begin, or begin to increase.
3. Position is at the limits of the available range.

These palpatory techniques of examination and treatment have been peculiar to this "concept" from its beginnings. As well as seeking symptomatic responses to the movement as described above, the palpation is also used to assess positional anomalies and soft-tissue abnormalities, which are at least as critical to "the concept" as the movement tests.

The testing of physiologic and accessory movement can be combined in a variety of ways in an endeavor to find the comparable movement sign most closely related to the person's disorder. Edwards[12] originally described a formal method of investigating symptomatic responses and treating appropriate patients using "combined movement" techniques. In addition, joint surfaces may be compressed, both as a prolonged, sustained firm pressure, and as an adjunct to physiologic and accessory movement. These are two further examples of examination developed as part of "the Maitland concept."

Differentiation tests are perfect examples of physical examination procedures that demonstrate the mode of thinking so basic to "the Maitland concept." When any group of movements reproduces symptoms, "the concept" requires a logical and thoughtful analysis to establish which movement of which joint is affected. The simplest example of this is passive supination of the hand

and forearm, which when held in a stretched position, reproduces the patient's symptoms. The stages of this test are as follows:

1. Hold the fully supinated hand/forearm in the position that is known to reproduce the pain.
2. Hold the hand stationary and pronate the distal radio-ulnar joint 2 or 3 degrees.
3. If the pain arises from the wrist, the pain will increase because in pronating the distal radio-ulnar joint, added supination stress is applied at the radiocarpal and midcarpal joints.
4. While in the position listed in entry 1, again hold the hand stationary, but this time increase supination of the distal radioulnar joint. This decreases the supination stretch at the wrist joints and will reduce any pain arising from the wrist. However, if the distal radio-ulnar joint is the source of pain, the increased supination stretch will cause the pain to increase.

All types of differentiation tests require the same logically ordered procedure. These objective tests follow the same logic as the subjective modes of assessment described at the beginning of this chapter, and provide additional evidence leading to accurate diagnosis.

ASSESSMENT

In the last few years it would appear that physical therapists have discovered a new "skill," with the lofty title of "problem solving." This is, and always should be, the key part of all physical therapy treatment. Being able to solve the diagnostic and therapeutic problems and thus relieve the patient of his complaint is just what physical therapists are trained to do. For many years, manipulative physical therapy has been rightly classed as empirical treatment. However, since manipulative physical therapists began to be more strongly involved in problem-solving skills, treatment has become less empirical and more logical. On the basis that the pathology remains unknown in the majority of cases and the effects of the treatment on the tissues (as opposed to symptoms) is unknown, the treatment remains empirical in form. This is true with almost all of the medical science. Nevertheless, the approach to the patient and to physical treatment has become more logical and scientific within "the Maitland concept."

Minds existed before computers were developed, and manipulative therapists are trained to sort out and access "input" so that appropriate and logical "output" can be produced. Appropriate problem-solving logic will relate clinical findings to pathology and mechanical disorders. This process of "sorting out" we have called *assessment,* and assessment is the key to successful, appropriate, manipulative treatment, which, because of the reliability of its careful and logical approach, should lead to better and better treatment for our patients.

Assessment is used in six different situations:

1. Analytical assessment at a first consultation
2. Pretreatment assessment
3. Reassessment during every treatment session proving the efficacy of a technique at a particular stage of treatment
4. Progressive assessment
5. Retrospective assessment
6. Final analytical assessment

Analytical Assessment

A first consultation requires skills in many areas, but the goals require decisions and judgments from the following five areas:

1. The diagnosis
2. The phase of the disorder
3. The degree of stability of the disorder at the time of treatment
4. The presenting symptoms and signs
5. The characteristics of the person

Without communication and an atmosphere of trust, the answers to the different assessment procedures (1–5) cannot be reliably determined. By using one's own frame of reference, and endeavoring to understand the patient's frame of reference, the characteristics of the patient can be judged. By making use of nonverbal skills, picking out key words or phrases, knowing what type of information to listen for, and recognizing and using "immediate-automatic-response" questions (all described later), accurate information can be gained at this first consultation. The objective examination is discussed under the heading, Examination.

Pretreatment Assessment

As the beginning of each treatment session a specific kind of assessment is made of the effect of the previous session on the patient's disorder, its the symptoms and changes in movement. Since the first consultation includes both examination of movements and treatment of movements, the assessment at the second treatment session will not be as useful for therapy as it will be at the following treatment sessions.

When the patient attends subsequent treatment sessions, it is necessary to make both subjective and objective assessments, i.e., subjective in terms of how they feel; objective in terms of what changes can be found in quality and range of movement, and in related pain response. When dealing with the subjective side of assessment, it is important to seek spontaneous comments. It is wrong to ask, "How did it feel this morning when you got out of bed, compared with how it used to feel?" The start should be "How have you been?'' or some such general question, allowing the patient to provide some information that seems most important to him. This information may be more valuable because of its spontaneous nature.

Another important aspect of the subjective assessment is that statements of fact made by a patient must always be converted to comparisons to previous statements. Having made the subjective assessment, the comparative statement should be the first item recorded on the patient's case notes. And it must be recorded as a *comparison-quotation* of his opinion of the effect of treatment. (The second record in the case notes is the comparative changes determined by the objective movement tests.) To attain this subjective assessment, communication skills are of paramount importance. There are many components that make up the skill, but two are of particular importance:

1. *Key words or key phrases.* Having asked the question, "How has it been?" a patient may respond in a very general and uninformative way. However, during his statements he may include, for example, the word "Monday." Latch on to Monday, because Monday meant something to him. Find out what it was and use it. "What is it that happened on Monday? Why did you say Monday?"

2. A patient frequently says things that demand an immediate-automatic-response question. As a response to the opening question given above, the patient may respond by saying, "I'm feeling better." The immediate-automatic-response to that statement, even before he has had a chance to take breath and say anything else, is, "better than what?" or "better than when?" It may be that after treatment he was worse and that he is better than he was then but that he is not better than he was before the treatment.

One aspect of the previous treatment is that it (often intentionally) provokes a degree of discomfort. This will produce soreness, but if the patient says he has more pain, the clinician needs to determine if is it treatment-soreness or disorder-soreness? For example, a patient may have pain radiating across his lower back and treatment involves pushing on his lumbar spine. He is asked to stand up and is asked, "How do you feel now compared with before I was pushing on your back?" He may say, "it feels pretty sore." He is then asked, "Where does it feel sore?" If he answers, "it's sore in the center," the clinician may consider that it is likely to be treatment soreness. But if he answers, "it's sore across my back," then the clinician may conclude that it is disorder soreness. If it were treatment soreness it would only be felt where the pressure had been applied. If the soreness spreads across his back, the treatment technique must have disturbed the disorder.

In making subjective assessments, a process is included of educating the patient in how to reflect. If a patient is a very good witness, the answers to questions are very clear, but if the patient is not a good witness, then subjective assessment becomes difficult. Patients should learn to understand what the clinician needs to know. At the end of the first consultation, patients need to be instructed in how important it is for them to take notice of any changes in their symptoms. They should report all changes, even ones they believe are trivial. The clinician should explain, "Nothing is too trivial. You can't tell me too much; if you leave out observations, which you believe to be unimportant, this may cause me to make wrong treatment judgments." People need to be reassured that they are not complaining, they are informing. Under circumstances when a patient will not be seen for some days or if full and apparently trivial detail is needed, they should be asked to write down the details. The criticism that is made of asking patients to write things down is that they become hypochondriacs. This is a wrong assessment in my experience, as the exercise provides information that might otherwise never be obtained.

There are four specific times when changes in the patient's symptoms can indicate the effect of treatment. They are as follows:

1. *Immediately after treatment.* The question can be asked, "How did you feel when you walked out of here last time compared with when you walked in?" A patient can feel much improved immediately after treatment yet experience exacerbation of symptoms one or two hours later. Any improvement that does not last longer than one hour indicates that the effect of the treatment was only palliative. Improvement that lasts more than four hours indicates a change related to treatment.

2. *Four hours after treatment.* The time interval of four hours is an arbitrary time and could be any time from three to six hours. It is a "threshold" time interval beyond which any improvement or examination can be taken to indicate the success or failure of the treatment. Similarly, if a patient's syndrome is exacerbated by treatment, the patient will be aware of it at about this time.

3. *The evening of the treatment.* The evening of the day of treatment provides information in regard to how well any improvement from treatment has been sustained. Similarly, an exacerbation immediately following treatment may have further increased by evening. This is unfavorable. Conversely, if the exacerbation has decreased, it is then necessary to know whether it decreased to its pretreatment level or decreased to a level that was better than before that day's treatment. This would be a very favorable response, clearly showing that the treatment had alleviated the original disorder.

4. *On rising the next morning.* This is probably the most informative time of all for signalling a general improvement. A patient may have no noticeable change in his symptoms on the day or night of the treatment session, but may notice that on getting out of bed the next morning his usual lower back stiffness and pain are less, or that they may pass off more quickly than usual. Even at this time span, any changes can be attributed to treatment. However, changes that are noticed *during* the day after treatment, or on getting out of bed the second morning after treatment, are far less likely to be as a result of treatment. Nevertheless, the patient should be questioned in depth to ascertain what reasons exist, other than treatment, to which the changes might be attributed.

Because accurate assessment is so vitally and closely related to treatment response, each treatment session must be organized in such a way that the assessments are not confused by changes in the treatment. For example, if a patient has a disorder that is proving very difficult to help, and at the eighth treatment session he reports that he feels there may have been some slight favorable change from the last treatment, the clinician has no alternative in planning the eighth treatment session. In the eighth treatment, that which was done at the seventh must be repeated in exactly the same manner in every respect. To do otherwise could render the assessment at the ninth treatment confusing. If the seventh treatment is repeated at the eighth session, there is nothing that the patient can say or demonstrate that can confuse the effect attributable to that treatment. If there was an improvement between the seventh and the eighth treatment (and the eighth treatment was an identical repetition of the seventh treatment), yet no improvement between the eighth treatment and the ninth treatment time, the improvement between treatments seven and eight could not have been due to treatment.

There is another instance when the clinician must recognize that there can be no choice as to what the eighth treatment must be. If there had been no improvement with the first six treatments, and at the seventh treatment session a totally new technique was used, the patient may report at the eighth session that there had been a surprisingly marked improvement in symptoms. It may be that this unexpected improvement was due to treatment or it may have been due to some other unknown reason. There is only one way that the answer can be found—the treatment session should consist of no treatment techniques at all. Objective assessment may be made but no treatment techniques should be performed. At the ninth session, if the patient's symptoms have worsened considerably, the treatment cannot be implicated in the cause because none had been administered. The clinician can then repeat the seventh treatment and see if the dramatic improvement is achieved again. If it is, then the improvement is highly likely to have been due to that treatment.

Whatever is done at one treatment session is done in such a way that when the patient comes back the next time, the assessment cannot be confusing.

Another example of a different kind is that a patient may say at each treatment session that he is "the same," yet assessment of his movement signs indicates that they are improving in a satisfactory manner, and therefore that one would expect an improvement in his symptoms. To clarify this discrepancy, specific questions must be asked. It may be that he considers he is "the same" because his back is still just as stiff and painful on first getting out of bed in the morning as it was at the outset of treatment. The specific questioning may divulge that he now has no problems with sitting, and that he can now walk up and down the stairs at work without pain. Although his sitting, climbing, and descending stairs have improved, his symptoms on getting out of bed are the same, and this explains his statement of being "the same." The objective movement tests will have improved in parallel with his sitting the stair-climbing improvements.

Assessment during Every Treatment Session

Proving the value or failure of a technique applied through a treatment session is imperative. Assessment (problem solving) should be part of all aspects of physical therapy. In this chapter it is related to passive movement. There are four kinds of assessment, and probably the one that most people think of first is the one in which the clinician is trying to prove the value of a technique that is being performed on a patient.

Proving the Value of a Technique

Before even choosing the technique to be used it is necessary to know what symptoms the patient has and how his movements are affected in terms of both range and the pain response during the movement. Selection of a treatment technique depends partly on knowing what that technique should achieve while it is being performed. In other words, is it the aim to provoke discomfort and, if so, how much "hurt" is permissible? It is also necessary to have an expectation of what the technique should achieve after it has been performed.

With these considerations in mind, it is necessary to keep modifying the treatment technique until it achieves the expected goal during its performance. Assuming that this is achieved and that the technique has been performed for the necessary length of time, the patient is then asked to stand, during which time he is watched to see if there are any nuances that may provide a clue as to how his back is feeling. The first thing is to then ask him is, "How do you feel now compared with when you were standing there before the technique?" It is then necessary to clarify any doubts concerning the interpretation of what he says he is feeling. It is important to understand what the patient means to say if the subjective effect of the technique is to be determined usefully.

Having subjectively assessed the effect of the technique, it is then necessary to reexamine the major movements that were faulty, to compare them with their state before the technique. An important aspect of checking and rechecking the movements is that there may be more than one component to the patient's problem. For example, a man may have back pain, hip pain, and vertebral-canal pain. Each of these may contribute to the symptoms in his lower leg. On reassessing him after a technique, it is necessary to assess at least *one* separate movement for *each* of the components, so it can be determined what the technique has achieved for each component. It is still necessary to check all of the components even if it is expected that a change will only be effected in one of the components. Having completed all of these comparison assessments, the effect of that technique at that particular stage of the disorder is now recorded in detail.

Progressive Assessment

At each treatment session the symptoms and signs are assessed for changes for their relation to the previous treatment session and to "extracurricular" activities. At about each fourth treatment session a subjective assessment is made, comparing how the patient feels today with how he felt four treatments previously. The purpose of this progressive assessment is to clarify and confirm the treatment by assessment of the treatment response. One is often surprised by the patient's reply to a question, "How do you feel now compared with ten days (i.e., four treatments) ago?" The goal is to keep the treatment-by-treatments assessment in the right perspective in relation to the patient's original disorder.

Retrospective Assessment

The first kind of retrospective assessment is that made routinely at each group of three or four treatment sessions when the patient's symptoms and signs are compared with before treatment began, as described above.

A second kind of retrospective assessment is made toward the end of treatment when the considerations relate to a final assessment. This means that the clinician is determining:

1. Whether treatment should be continued
2. Whether spontaneous recovery is occurring
3. Whether other medical treatments or investigations are required
4. Whether medical components of the disorder are preventing full recovery
5. What the patient's future in terms of prognosis is likely to be

A third kind of retrospective assessment is made when the patient's disorder has not continued to improve over the last few treatment sessions. Under these circumstances, it is the subjective assessment that requires the greatest skill, and its findings are far more important than the assessment of the objective-movement tests. The clinician needs to know what specific information to look for. This is not a facetious remark, since it is the most common area where mistakes are made, thereby ruining any value in the assessment. The kinds of question the clinician should ask are as follows:

"During the whole time of treatment, is there anything I have done that has made you worse?"

"Of the things I have done to you, is there any one particular thing (or more) that you feel has helped you?"

"Does your body tell you anything about what it would like to have done to it to make it start improving?"

"My record of your treatment indicates that after the lumbar-traction treatment last Friday, you had a bad day Saturday, but that by Monday the pain had subsided and you thought you might have been better than you were before the traction. Looking back to that weekend now, do you feel that the traction did help you? Do you feel that if the traction had been gentler and of shorter duration that you might not have had the recurrence of symptoms, and that you might then have been more sure of the treatment's effect?''

"Do your symptoms tell you that it might be a good plan to stop treatment for, say, two weeks after which a further assessment and decision could be made?"

And so the probing interrogation continues until two or three positive answers emerge, which will guide the further measures that should be taken. The questions are the kind that involve the patient in making decisions, and that guide the clinician in making a final decision regarding treatment.

There is a fourth kind of retrospective assessment. If treatment is still producing improvement but its rate is less than anticipated, a good plan is to stop treatment for two weeks and to then reassess the situation. If the patient has improved over the two week period, it is necessary to know whether the improvement has been a day-by-day affair thus indicating a degree of spontaneous improvement. If the improvement only occurred for the first two days after the last treatment, then it would seem that the last treatment session was of value and that a further three or four treatments should be given followed by another two week break and reassessment.

Final Analytical Assessment

When treatment has achieved all it can, the clinician needs to make an assessment in relation to the possibility of recurrence, the effectiveness of any prophylactic measures, the suggestion of any medical measures that can be carried out, and finally an assessment of the percentage of remaining disability. The answers to these matters are to be found by analyzing all the information derived from:

1. The initial examination
2. The behavior of the disorder throughout treatment
3. The details derived from retrospective assessments
4. The state of affairs at the end of treatment, taking into account the subjective and objective changes

This final analytical assessment is made easier as each year a clinician's work builds up experience. It is necessary for this experience to be based on a self-critical approach and on analysis of the results, with the reasons for these results.

CONCLUSION

The question has often been asked, "How did this method of treatment evolve?" The attributes necessary to succeed in this treatment method are an analytical, self-critical mind and a talent for improvisation.

   With this as a basis, the next step is to learn to understand how a patient's disorder affects him. Coupled with this is the need to have sound reasons for trying a particular technique and then the patience to assess its effect. In "the Maitland concept," over the years this has developed into a complex inter-related series of assessments as described in the body of this text.

Q: Why are painless techniques used to relieve pain?

A: Experience with patients who have had manipulative treatment elsewhere, allows us to inquire as to which kind of technique was used and to observe its effect. When patients emphasize the extreme gentleness of some suc-cessful clinicians, one is forced to the conclusion that there must be ways of moving a joint extremely gently and thus improving patients' symptoms. Having accepted this fact (and that is not always easy) the obvious next step is to reproduce these techniques. For example, a technique one patient may describe can then be used on other patients who fit into the same kind of category. The clinician can learn what its possibilities are via the assessment process.

Q: Why conversely, are some of the techniques quite vigorous and painful?

A: When treatment reaches a stage when nothing seems to help, a useful axiom is, "Find the thing that hurts them, and hurt them." This should not be interpreted as being cruel to a patient, or that one is "out to hurt them," come what may. The hurting is a controlled progressive process with a strong emphasis on assessment. From using this kind of treatment on appropriate patients, it has become obvious how firmly some disorders need to be pushed to the point of eliciting pain in order to aid recovery. This approach may be seriously questioned by some practitioners, but it can be a most useful technique in appropriate circumstances.

Q: How did treating joints using strong compression of the joint surfaces come about?

A: If, for example, a patient has shoulder symptoms only when lying on it, and if normal examination methods reveal very little, then the thought processes go something like this:

   "I believe him when he says he has a shoulder problem."

   "There is nothing to indicate any serious or sinister disorder."

   "He hasn't responded to other treatments."

   "So it *must* be possible to find something on examination that relates to his problem."

   "How can I find that something? What lead is there?"

      "He says, 'I can't lie on it.'"

   "So I will ask him to lie on it and then move it around and see what happens."

By thus experimenting with techniques (improvisation) until the patient's pain can be reproduced, having found the thing that hurts him, treatment should then aim to hurt him in this *controlled* manner, as stated above.

A quandary then arises:

   "As the patient doesn't move his shoulder around when he's asleep and lying on it, why is my examination using compression only, without movement, *not* painful."

One would expect it to be painful!

"However, he has to lie on it for half an hour before pain forces him to change his position, so try compression again but make it stronger and sustain it longer."

After half a minute or so of sustained maximum compression without movement his pain will certainly appear.

Q: How about the Slump test and treatment, how did this evolve?

A: Some patients who have low back pain complain about difficulty getting into a car. By reenacting the action and analyzing it, it is found that it was not the flexing of the lumbar spine that made getting into the car difficult; i.e., was the head/neck flexion that provoked the low back symptoms. Examination using standard movement tests for structures between the head and the sacrum do not reveal anything; so reenact the particular movements and remember that the only structure connecting both areas must be in the vertebral column, most likely within the vertebral canal. To put these structures on stretch was the only method that *reproduced* the complaint. The maximum stretch position is the position now referred to as the slump position.

Q: We now read of using mobilizing techniques to make a nonuniting fracture unite. How did this come about?

A: In the past, traditional methods used to stimulate union have been: (1) Remove all support for the fracture site and allow the patient to take weight through the fracture; and (2) Surgically explore the area and make both ends of the fracture site bleed, and then splint them in apposition again. If such things can promote union then why not try passively moving the fracture site? Based on this reasoning, and linking it with our axiom "find the thing that hurts and hurt them," it was found that it was possible to cause "fracture-site pain." This characteristic pain was found to have two other characteristics: (1) Pain stopped *immediately* when the treating movement was stopped; and (2) No side effects were provoked. This then meant that the treatment could be repeated, and in fact pain became harder to provoke: union took place.

REFERENCES

1. The Age. 21 August 1982
2. MacNab I: Negative disc exploration: An analysis of the causes of nerve root involvement in 68 patients. J Bone Joint Surg 53A:891, 1971
3. Maitland GD: Passive movement techniques for intra-articular and periarticular disorders. Aust J Physiother 31:3, 1985
4. McNair JFS: Non-uniting fractures management by manual passive mobilization. Proceedings Manipulative Therapists' Association of Australia, 88, Brisbane, 1985
5. McNair JFS, Maitland GD: The role of passive mobilization in the treatment of a non-uniting fracture site—A case study. International Conference on Manipulative Therapy, Perth, 1983

6. Maitland GD: The hypothesis of adding compression when examining and treating synovial joints. Orthop Sports Phys Ther 2:7, 1980
7. Edwards BC: Combined movements of the lumbar spine: Examination and clinical significance. Aust J Physiother 25:147, 1979
8. Maitland GD: Negative disc exploration: Positive canal signs. Aust J Physiother 25:6, 1979
9. Hunkin K: Unpublished publication. 1985
10. Maitland GD: Vertebral manipulation. 5th ed. Butterworth, London, 1986
11. MacConaill MA, Basmajian SV: Muscles and Movements. Waverley Press, Baltimore, 1969
12. Edwards BC: Movement patterns. International Conference on Manipulative Therapy, Manipulative Therapists' Association of Australia, Perth, 1983

6 | Mechanical Diagnosis and Therapy for Low Back Pain: Toward a Better Understanding

Robin A. McKenzie

This chapter is an attempt to persuade those interested in the topic that a more organized and rational approach to the mechanical treatment of spinal pain is desirable. It proposes that simple modifications to our present diverse and complex therapeutic approaches would result in both short- and long-term improvement in patient care. This goal is well within the reach of the physical therapy profession, providing it organizes and coordinates energies, which at the moment can be seen to be fragmented, if not divisive.

Having now had the opportunity and pleasure to visit and demonstrate my methods in over 20 countries, I have come to realize that physical therapy means different things in different places. Legislation may impose limits on the profession so that physical therapists in some countries may be more constrained than in others. Ethical considerations and sheer conservatism within the medical community may also inhibit the healthy growth of the profession. But, sadly, in many countries where high levels of development exist throughout the profession in general and where manipulative skills abound, the problems lie more in seeking prestige and in the maintenance of status. It is sometimes hard to know which will cause the most harm in the long term.

My own belief is that this profession of ours is at a crossroads and must recognize the historical lessons of the past in order to avoid the mistakes made by chiropractors and osteopaths.

Over the next few years, physical therapy will have the opportunity to become the key profession within medicine responsible for the delivery of conservative care for mechanical disorders of the spine. If the appropriate steps are not taken now, we may never again have another such opportunity.

In attempting this persuasion, I am aware that many will feel an affront and some will ridicule the necessity for change. I rely on the future members of the profession to judge the sense of my proposals.

In order to understand our present predicament, it is necessary to review some aspects of pathology, responsibility for conservative spinal care, the treatments delivered, and the philosophies of various approaches.

PATHOLOGY

The pathology or the micromechanical disorders that give rise to low back pain are still rather obscure, just as they were when Hippocrates first described his methods of treatment for "hyboma" or acute lumbar kyphosis.[1] Hippocrates believed the cause to be a dislocation backward of one vertebra onto another. Today, although our understanding has improved immensely especially in the past 20 years, with the exception of the sequestrated disc,[2] we are still unable to identify with certainty or precision the offending structure causing pain in many particular instances.

Since the search for exact causes of low back pain began, every structure in the lower back has been considered suspect at one time or another. The reasons proposed for onset of pain have been innumerable, but they have ranged from the witch's curse inflaming the nerves to the proverbial chill in the kidneys acquired by sitting in a draft.

Modern medicine has advanced with such rapidity that it can be fairly stated that man has learned more of the precise nature of the causes of spinal pain in the past 20 years than he has in all of previous recorded history, and the search has narrowed to two structures likely to be involved in the production of most mechanical back pain.[2]

The intervertebral disc with its strong anulus fibrosus, retaining the gel-like nucleus, probably attracts the most attention. Over the past 10 years, the journal *Spine* has published the results of many studies aimed at the examination of intervertebral disc structure, function, pathology, and treatment. The other mobile structures to capture the attention of those investigating back pain are the zygapophyseal joints. These are also probable sources of pain, but the precise pathology causing the pain is frequently difficult to identify.

The pathologic changes occurring between birth and death are now well described[3,19,20,22] but disagreement remains about certain fundamental aspects of that pathology. Recently, for instance, quite contrary to material that has appeared before, evidence is accumulating stating that the intervertebral disc actually thickens rather than thins with the aging process.[3] This must inevitably lead to reappraisal of the hypothetical basis of some of our therapies. Indeed, until more precise technology provides an answer, our conceptualization regarding the reasons for treatment effectiveness must continue to remain flexible and open to change.

Although so much regarding the causes of low back pain remains to be discovered, many physical therapists either remain unaware or choose to ignore certain established findings within orthopedics. Disorders of the sacroiliac joint occur without doubt, but most are inflammatory in origin. That true mechanical lesions occur is also recognized. They are, however, uncommon and usually only occur following pregnancy.[4] Physical therapists, especially in the United States,[31] or wherever therapists are receiving instruction from osteopaths, are "discovering" sacroiliac pathology in many of their patients. It is likely that either the proponents are wrong or the literature is in error.

The historical obsession of physical therapists with the musculature as the main source of backache has already been exposed.[5] Although orthopedic opinion does not support the proposal,[6] muscle imbalance as well as muscle strain are still considered by some physical therapists to be common causes of persistent back pain and account for the degree of lordosis present.

It appears now to be generally accepted within medicine that many low back problems are mechanical in origin, probably arising in the intervertebral disc early in life and in the apophyseal joints much later in life.[3,19,20,22] The treatment for these particular problems, therefore, should in the main be mechanical. This fact has been recognized through 2,500 years of recorded history[7] and most treatments today given for the alleviation of back pain contain mechanical components.

The problem remains, however, and is likely to remain for the forseeable future that, even with the most sophisticated and detailed investigations, the precise pathology responsible for the pain remains a mystery.

There is a danger that physical therapists will develop (as occurred with the chiropractors and osteopaths) a system of "pathology" quite separate and contrary to that which exists within medicine as a whole, and orthopedics in particular. Medicine has always been able to exert control over and put pressure on its wayward practitioners in order to protect the public from outrageous claims and methods of treatment.

Is it not time to adopt those controls within physical therapy, especially when we see such fringe concepts as craniosacral technique and myofascial release techniques being taught without the slightest scientific evidence to support their consideration as tools for the treatment of spinal disorders? If we fail to curb the development of unscientific cultism, we deserve to lose what should be our rightful place within the medical team.

RESPONSIBILITY

In years past little was known about the likely causes of low back problems and every health related specialty attempted to obtain for themselves the role of responsibility for care of the back by administering the skills of their particular specialty. This situation persists today to a lesser degree.

Thus, we see some physicians proposing that the answer to most back pain problems lies in the dispensing of medicines, pills, and embrocations, despite evidence to support the view that most back problems are mechanical in nature. Surgeons attempt to provide solutions by removing, replacing, or modifying various parts of the spinal column, and osteopaths and chiropractors have for almost 100 years applied manipulative procedures to the painful back albeit for different reasons.

Physical therapists have in the past traditionally applied heat, massage, and exercises, as well as various forms of electrotherapy, and these methods are still used in some clinics today. Only in the past 40 years have physical therapists regularly adopted manipulative procedures for spinal therapy.

The mechanical therapies in most common use today are spinal manipulative therapy (SMT), mobilization, traction, massage, and exercises. At the present time, there are three main groups dispensing mechanical therapies, competing with each other to become the profession responsible for the conservative management of low back pain. In this chapter I will confine myself to discussing only those groups involved in the provision of mechanical therapies.

Physical therapists, chiropractors, and osteopaths all apply what must appear to the uninitiated as a bewildering array of mechanical procedures and all uphold basic concepts as diverse as can be imagined. All groups claim great benefit to the patient as a result of dispensing various forms of mobilization, manipulation, or traction, with its untold variations, or massage and exercises, which also contain mechanical elements.

Up until the present time, no treatment has been found to provide a reliable long-term benefit for people with low back pain. The responsibility for the conservative care of people with low back pain will ultimately be decided by the public and the system chosen will be that which provides a long-term benefit.

DIAGNOSIS

It is frustrating indeed to have to accept that so often we do not have a complete or even partial diagnosis when commencing our various therapies. But as physical therapists we have one important advantage over our colleagues in the medical profession. By the nature of their training as well as the expectations of the public, physicians and surgeons are predisposed to prescribe drugs for inflamed or painful joints, to surgically immobilize or even remove severely painful joints and to replace them with metal implants. The surgical procedures require a high degree of accuracy in execution if success is to follow. A successful outcome of treatment is dependent therefore on positive identification of the site of the lesion and as is well known the surgical procedures are fraught with hazard. On the other hand, since physical therapists are not engaged in delivering invasive therapies, precise identification of the structure affected and location of the offending lesion are less critical.

It has always been my own feeling that the patient in the first instance should be screened by the family medical practitioner. Thus we will receive into our clinics patients who have been appropriately screened, who are judged to have mechanical disorders, and in whom serious pathologies have been eliminated. We are then in a position to attempt the definition of the mechanical problem.

Mechanical Diagnosis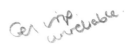

There are many differing views regarding the best method of establishing a mechanical diagnosis. It is agreed almost universally that it is necessary to obtain detailed information from the patient by way of history but confusion reigns about the relevance of various questions and answers.

Some therapists attach much more importance to one particular response, others will disregard that aspect as irrelevant. Some clinicians obtain large amounts of detailed information, which is admirable. However, in the long run the final decision as to the mechanical approach to be adopted is decided by the patient's response to the mechanical forces applied. The clinician has a simple choice. If he wishes to obtain a large range of detailed information he must realize that much of it will be irrelevant or unreliable.[24] If he is prepared to limit the information then he will increase its reliability and relevance.

There are those, mainly osteopathically oriented, who decide the nature of the mechanical problem principally by palpatory means; some even claim to be able to determine by palpation alone the levels of existing pathology. While it is the experience of many that rather gross losses of movement are detectable by palpation, there is only one study[8] of which I am aware that indicates palpation to be reliable, and unfortunately it is seriously flawed by having no objective and independent assessors involved in the outcomes. On the contrary, intertherapist reliability has generally been extremely poor.[9,10] Matyas and Bach[32] have shown poor intertest and intertherapist reliability for passive intervertebral testing.[32] A recent study comparing intertester reliability in examination of sacroiliac dysfunction has also shown extremely poor correlation; in 11 of 13 tests, agreement was 50 percent or less. Palpatory skills were fundamental to 10 of the 13 cases. All the therapists involved were experienced and trained in orthopedic manual therapy.[31]

Chiropractors rely on a combination of diagnostic criteria, but mainly on information obtained from radiologic and palpatory findings. These have always been their main tools of diagnosis and remain so today. Their treatments, however, have expanded significantly as they have embraced more and more of orthodox medicine in recent years.

Physical therapists in different parts of the world exhibit differing attitudes to the problem of mechanical diagnosis. This has come about because of the influence of three people in particular. Some, especially in Europe and countries influenced by the Norwegian system, have opted to follow the osteopathic concepts and their modifications developed by Kaltenborn, while others, mainly in Commonwealth countries, have adopted a more orthopedically oriented approach probably because of the influence of James Cyriax. In Australia, Geoffrey Maitland has developed a blend of the orthopedic together with his own system of palpatory examination and treatment. So there are in so many places differing mechanical approaches to the treatment of the same mechanical disorders.

Those familiar with my own approach to patient selection will realize that serious pathologies should already have been eliminated from the patient population by virtue of medical screening; that radiologic information eliminates most serious disorders and exposes architectural faults unsuitable for the mechanical approach; and that palpatory diagnosis is rejected on two counts:

1. The widespread incidence of tropism[33,34] causes palpatory findings to be unreliable, constantly suspect, and open to misinterpretation.
2. Our inability to demonstrate intertherapist reliability casts serious doubts on our findings.[32]

My conclusion on completion of the evaluation process is based almost entirely on the effects produced on the patients' symptoms by repeating well-defined movements performed in the standing and lying positions. Following the performance of these movements a subdivision of patients within the non-specific spectrum of back pain is possible, allowing us to classify them into categories entitled postural syndrome, dysfunction syndrome, and derangement syndrome. Patients in the derangement group are by far the most frequently encountered and are further subdivided into seven clinically identifiable entities.[11] The precise means of identification and the concepts and methods of treatment of these syndromes is described in detail elsewhere.[11]

My approach to the treatment of low back pain and a description of the three identifiable syndromes is given in Chapter 9 and described in detail elsewhere,[11] while a brief summary is provided below.

Postural Syndrome

Patients with this syndrome are usually under 30 years of age, have sedentary occupations, and frequently do not engage in regular exercise. They develop pain that appears locally, usually adjacent to the midline of the spinal column. The pain is provoked by mechanical deformation of soft tissues, which occurs only when spinal segments are subjected to prolonged static loading with joints at end range. This occurs most commonly when poor sitting or standing postures are adopted.

They frequently complain of pain felt either separately or simultaneously in the cervical, thoracic, and lumbar areas.

Pain from the postural syndrome is never induced by movement, never referred, and never constant. There is no pathology, no loss of movement, and there are no signs in this syndrome. There is nothing to see.

Movements are normal and patients with this syndrome are sometimes described as being hypermobile. The only objective information appears on examination of posture at the time of onset of pain when the patient will be seen to adopt poor postures and will be seen to "hang" at the end of range of movement.

Pain from the postural syndrome can arise from any part of the mobile segment or from the adjacent soft tissues. It is probably ligamentous or peri-articular in origin in the zygapophyseal joints. Described simply, postural pain appears eventually by prolonged over stretching of normal tissue.

Dysfunction Syndrome

Patients with this syndrome are usually over 30 years of age except where trauma can be identified as the original cause of their problem. They commonly exhibit poor posture and are frequently under exercised.

Their pain develops insidiously, appearing locally, adjacent to the midline of the spinal column. The pain is provoked on attempting full movement, by mechanically deforming shortened soft tissues in segments that have reduced elasticity and movement. The pain is always felt at end range and never felt during the movement. With the exception of a patient with an adherent nerve root, pain from dysfunction is never referred.

The loss of movement evident in the dysfunction syndrome arises from two common causes. The first and most common cause of reduced spinal mobility is poor postural habits maintained during the first few decades of life. This is especially so when the individual does not exercise regularly. Poor postural habits allow adaptive shortening of certain structures. The result is a gradual reduction of mobility with aging. The movements reduced are usually those extension movements essential for the maintenance of the very erect posture. The second cause of reduced spinal mobility is contracture of fibrous scar tissue developed during repair following trauma. Thus, an inextensible scar can form within or adjacent to otherwise health structures, and will cause reduced mobility. The pain resulting from stretching of this inextensible scar appears only on attempting full end range movement. The pain does not occur during the movement or before the structure is placed under tension. Surrounding healthy structures would be capable of further extensibility but are now restricted by the scar.

It is not possible to identify the structure causing the pain of dysfunction, but any of the soft tissues adjacent to the vertebral column may adaptively shorten or may be damaged. Thus the pain may result from adaptive shortening or injury to any of the ligamentous structures in the segment, from the intervertebral disc, the zygapophyseal joints, or the superficial or deep muscles or their attachements. The pain may also result from adherence of the spinal nerve root or dura following severe intervertebral disc bulging but this is more easily identified. Described simply, the pain of dysfunction is produced immediately by over stretching of shortened tissues.

Derangement Syndrome

Patients with the derangement syndrome are usually between 20 and 55 years of age. They invariably have poor sitting posture, which may be a postural or a structural problem.

They develop pain, usually of sudden onset; that is, in a matter of a few hours or over a day or two they change from completely normal to significantly disabled beings. Very often this syndrome appears for no apparent reason. The symptoms may be felt locally, adjacent to the midline of the spinal column and may radiate and be referred distally in the form of pain, parasthesia or numbness. The symptoms are produced, abolished, increased, or reduced and made better or worse by performance of certain movements or the maintenance of certain positions.

Pain from the derangement syndrome may alter and change both in regard to the site of the pain, or the extent of the area affected, which may increase or decrease. Pain from the derangement syndrome may cross the midline, for example, move from the right of the low back to the left.

Discogenic pathology must always be suspected when the patient describes his pain as changing position and radiating when he changes position or performs different movements. When the referred pain changes its distribution, shape, or position, this may mean that there has been nuclear displacement through incomplete anular cracks or tears within the intervertebral disc as the disc changes its shape or position during movement or sustained postures.

Pain from the derangement syndrome is frequently constant in nature. There may be no position in which the patient can find relief. The pain therefore may be present whether movement is performed or not and this pain is usually described as an ache. That ache is then made worse by movement in certain directions and reduced by movement in other directions.

In the derangement syndrome, especially in severe cases, gross loss of movement may occur. Also in severe cases, postural deformities, such as kyphosis and scoliosis are seen frequently. Sudden loss of spinal mobility and the sudden appearance of postural deformity in acute low-back and neck pain may be likened to the sudden locking that may occur in the knee joint where internal derangement of the meniscus is common.

The mechanism of internal derangement of the intervertebral disc is not fully understood. That the nucleus pulposus can be displaced towards and escape through a damaged anular wall is inarguable.[28,29] It is highly likely that this will follow as a consequence of sudden or violent movement, or with sustained postures in younger patients. Older patients have a stiffer, less fluid nucleus (Ch. 1), which is less likely to be displaced from within its anular envelope.[27–29] It is also hypothesized that prior to a frank anular lesion with nuclear herniation, there exists incomplete tears into which nuclear material may be displaced. This alters the joint biomechanics and may be responsible for the temporary postural deformities (e.g., localized scoliosis) observed.

Creep of the fluid nucleus/anulus complex will disturb the normal alignment of adjacent vertebrae[30] and change the resting shape of the disc.[27] This change of shape will also affect the ability of the joint surface to move in normal pathway[30] and deviation to the right or left of the saggital plane result on attempting flexion or extension.

Described simply, the pain of derangement occurs as a consequence of a change in disc shape with related malalignment of the mobile segment and its associated abnormal stresses.

Identification of the different syndromes is based on the effects that movements have on the initiation of the pain: the point in the movement pathway where pain is first perceived; the site of the pain and subsequent change of location of the pain; the increasing or decreasing intensity of the pain; and finally abolition of the pain. Mechanical pain can arise only from a limited number of events or combination of events causing force to be applied to innervated soft tissues. Those soft tissues may be in a normal state, a contracted state, or in an anatomically altered state with a change in the shape of the disc. Any of these events can be identified by the response of the patient's pain to the deliberate application of certain mechanical stresses.

Patients with inflammatory disorders, with spondylolisthesis or other undetected minor fracture and with pathologies unsuited to mechanical therapies will not respond in a predictable fashion, and will be quickly exposed and recognized when tested in the manner I have described.

MECHANICAL TREATMENTS

Spinal Manipulative Therapy

All over the world enthusiastic physical therapists frustrated by years of domination by medicine or disillusioned by the use of ineffective methods of physical therapy are rediscovering mobilization and manipulation, and are providing it as the treatment of choice for many patients with spinal pain. No one who is experienced in the use of such therapy has failed to be excited on the many occasions when a spectacular improvement is obtained. There is no doubt that many patients benefit from spinal manipulative therapy (SMT). Several studies support the view that there is a short term benefit from SMT.[12,35,37-39]

From within the ranks of the physical therapists and especially from chiropractors and osteopaths, from time to time there emerge claims expounding the advantages of one form of manipulative therapy in preference to another. While one cannot with any hope of resolution enter the arguments for or against the concepts attached to the various systems it is comparatively simple to cut through the mystique of the procedures utilized to achieve the same end result. As far as I am aware, no study demonstrates that any one particular form of manipulative therapy is superior to another. In one study at least, it has been established that osteopathic manipulation at the end of four weeks was no better than a placebo (detuned short wave diathermy).[13] Schiotz and Cyriax[7] describe these situations well, "It is not the elegance or alleged specificity of some maneuver that matters, it is its therapeutic effectiveness."

Physical therapists should not allow history to repeat itself, as already within the ranks of our profession there is a tendency for those schooled in one particular method of mobilization to denigrate other systems. Already we can see Kaltenborn followers, Maitland, Cyriax, and Paris devotees all enthusiastically supporting their particular guru and unfortunately failing to recognize that each group is probably dispensing the same mechanical maneuver using a different title, philosophy, and technique.

Once familiar with the various techniques of SMT, it becomes clear that the basic maneuvers in common usage today, by whichever profession, are essentially the same. Although differences may exist in the manner of delivery, as yet these differences have not been shown to affect the final outcome. I am sure this statement will be strenuously challenged by the purists. This is the way it should be, of course, and we shall eagerly await the definitive study that demonstrates the superiority of one form of SMT over another.

There are several problems and concerns arising from the current wave of enthusiasm for SMT and its related techniques. These problems exist because in many parts of the world manipulation by physical therapists is only now being developed and the initial enthusiasm, although understandable, must be tempered and brought into perspective. Inexperienced physical therapists see manipulation as the answer to the back problem and a panacea for whatever ails the patient. There is a danger that many in our profession will in essence become chiropractors in another guise. The world does not deserve or require a third profession whose sole means of treating the spine is by the application of manipulative therapy.

Those in the profession who have longer experience of the benefits and limitations of SMT must make the benefit of that experience available to moderate the enthusiasm of those entering the field. Until we have learned to distinguish between when a patient is responsive to treatment as opposed to a natural resolution of symptoms with the passage of time our credibility is at risk. When our patients improve over a period of three to four months, can we seriously attribute their recovery to our manipulative or mechanical prowess delivered over this period?

In order to dispense manipulative therapy, it has always been necessary for the therapist to do something to the patient. Thus, irrespective of whether the patient's improvement is due to the passage of time or to the techniques of therapy, the patient, rightly or wrongly, attributes his recovery to what was done to him. He becomes dependent on whatever therapy was received and in the event of recurrence hurries back to the therapist of whatever calling. In his own mind and often in the mind of the therapist, he must receive more of the same in order to recover.

It has been demonstrated that SMT provides a short term benefit. There are no known long term benefits.[36] If physical therapy is to become the profession responsible for the treatment and management of people with mechanical spinal problems, we must also find treatments that have the potential to provide long term benefits. Is it ethical to confine our practice to treatments that contain only a short term benefit potential?

Spinal manipulation by physical therapists was introduced to New Zealand when Dr. Cyriax's physical therapist, Jennifer Hickling, toured the country in 1952.

The new found tool was used with enthusiasm on anyone with a pain in the back, and at that time I must confess to a certain guilt in this regard. It was so satisfying to feel the *click*. It is not until much later that one realizes that all the normal joints click.

We have used manipulative and mobilizing procedures in New Zealand extensively since that date, and we have been told by many outside groups whose visiting lecturers have advised us that we should do it, "my way." From time to time we adopted the advice but today in New Zealand it would be very hard to find a member of the New Zealand Manipulative Therapists Association who used only one method of mobilization or manipulation. We have adopted all those procedures that have been demonstrated effective, irrespective of origin. Although the process is incomplete, we have discarded most of the hocus pocus that surfaces from time to time and have strenuously resisted the temptation to adopt the current fringe procedures of cranial suture mobilization, or the craniosacral and myofascial release techniques so popular in areas where osteopathic concepts are embraced.

Thus, when visiting clinics in New Zealand, the observer will see a fine mixture of the philosphies and techniques of Cyriax, Maitland, Stoddard, and Kaltenborn, all of whom have added to the quality of manual procedures.

During her tour in New Zealand, Hickling demonstrated that there was a benefit to be obtained from SMT. In 1955 and 1956, it was my good fortune to chance upon a series of clinical events that immediately attracted my attention and, which suggested that a potential exists to impart a long term benefit to low back pain patients. With the available knowledge of the day, the only explanation I could accept was found in the techniques or the philosophy and practice of Cyriax.[14]

The observations were simple, very definite, and almost immediate. One patient, in pain for three weeks, lay inadvertently in a certain position on my treatment table. After about ten minutes he arose completely relieved of leg pain. He returned the following day almost totally symptom free. Another patient after a change of position experienced a complete reversal of his pain from the right to the left side; another patient with a neck problem abolished all symptoms by repeatedly combing his hair with the head laterally flexed to one side. The pain did not return. These and other clinical observations allowed me to develop several rather different avenues of diagnosis and therapy.[11] The main points emanating from these observations were:

1. That patients, without therapist assistance, could significantly affect the course of their own disorder.
2. That persons performing certain movements or adopting certain positions, which were productive of persisting pain could, if properly instructed, reverse the situation.
3. That without our special skills and magic fingers, certain mechanical

disorders were rapidly reversible using the patient's own movement and positions.

4. That most of the benefits obtained from mobilization or manipulation could be achieved more safely, efficiently, quickly, less expensively, and with lasting benefit to the patient without therapist intervention.

5. All that is required in order to apply this information is to determine the direction in which the appropriate movements must be made.

The time to apply our special techniques of mobilization and manipulation arrives when the patient, having exhausted all possibilities of self treatment, requires an increase in the degree of pressure in the appropriate direction; that direction has already been determined and mobilizing procedures should be commenced. Failing improvement with the use of mobilization, then and only then is manipulation indicated. Maitland and Kaltenborn have both expressed similar opinions regarding the application of pressures from without. Thus, the gradual development of increasing force to bring about change is a logical and safe method of applying mechanical therapies, assuming that vertebral and vascular pathology are excluded. The ultimate weapon we have is the manipulative thrust technique. Why use that weapon on day one when it may well be that the patient without being approached by the therapist is capable of causing the change himself (and learning an important self-management lesson)?

I have, therefore, proposed since that time that we should postpone or avoid mobilization and manipulation until we have determined that resolution of the problem is impossible utilizing the patient's own positions and movements. This concept offers up to 70 percent of people referred to physical therapists with mechanical low back pain the opportunity to treat and manage their own problem and thus become independent of therapists.[15]

The remaining 30 percent including patients categorized by myself as having derangement (4 or 6)[11] and therefore unable to apply self-treatment procedures with lasting benefit will always require the special skills of the manipulative therapist for correction of any lumbar or sciatic list.[16] Others will require techniques in the form of mobilization and some of those will additionally require manipulative thrust procedures.

I am not proposing that mobilization and manipulation are no longer required in our armamentarium. Spinal manipulative therapy has a particular and important part to play in the treatment of mechanical spinal pain but its dispensation is greatly misused. I am proposing that the time has come when we must rationalize the use of such methods. We are now able to determine within at least 48 hours from commencement of assessment whether manipulative therapy will be necessary at all. It should no longer be ethical to apply the technique in order to find out retrospectively if the procedure was indicated. Spinal mobilization and manipulation should not be dispensed to the entire population with back pain in order to ensure that the very few who really need it actually receive it. That philosophy is abhorrent. To add further controversy to the subject, I would wish to propose that in the not too distant future we may well arrive at the point where, apart from four or five obvious exceptions, the unlocking mechanism applicable to mechanical spinal disorders will be so well understood that few problems affecting the spinal segments will require manipulation at all; that our understanding will be so much improved that most patients will be able to self-treat most mechanical disorders.

Traction

As with studies into the efficacy of SMT,[12] most of the studies investigating clinical efficacy of traction are flawed. However, some evidence remains to suggest it is premature to discard the treatment as ineffectual. The most recent addition to the various themes of traction is the autotraction devised by Lind.[17]

Originally designed for the treatment of major disc herniation causing sciatic syndromes, it is recently in the United States being recommended by some as a panacea for back pain in general and its worth may be misjudged accordingly. No such claims were made by its inventor and hopefully it will be further investigated properly by appropriate independent assessors, although one recent study indicated that the response to autotraction was no different from the response to manual traction at two weeks and three months.[26] One study already completed[23] indicates that during autotraction pressures within the disc increased considerably. Passive traction levels remain unaffected. No negative pressures were recorded.

Gravity traction and inversion traction are other methods of treatment currently in vogue in the United States. No reliable data or objective assessments are yet forthcoming as far as I am aware. As with other therapies, so it is with traction; improvement must be seen to be as a result of the treatment and not the result of the passage of three or four weeks of time as the natural history of the condition runs its course.

It has been my own experience that patients other than those I have classified as having derangement 6[11] will benefit more rapidly using self-treatment procedures than from the use of traction. Patients with derangement 6 seem to resolve with the passage of time rather than from traction itself, but the advent of autotraction may alter this view.

Massage

Massage is still used for the treatment of low back pain and it can certainly have a mechanical effect on superficial structures.

When applied with sufficient pressure, there must also be a mechanical effect on the articulations of the spine. Under certain circumstances, it is likely that firm massage is as beneficial as gentle mobilization.

Exercise

Exercise has been the mainstay of the physical therapy profession, especially after the development of Swedish Remedial Exercises.[25] in the early part of this century. In the treatment of spinal disorders there has always been a conflict between those who have advocated flexion exercises based on the rationale proposed by Williams[21] and those who advocated the use of extension to treat low back pain. Williams' philosophy was most strongly established in the United States and Canada where almost anyone with low back pain or sciatica would routinely receive the standard exercises prescribed orriginally by Williams.

Extension, on the other hand, having been graphically described by Hippocrates,[1] has been in use throughout the rest of the world it seems since the earliest records were kept.[7]

Of course, it is not possible to take the whole spectrum of mechanical disorders of the low back and arbitrarily decide that all must flex or all must extend. Utilizing the repeated movement system I have described,[11] it is possible to determine the direction in which any particular patient must be moved in order to bring about resolution of their particular problem.

It is now clear that some patients must flex in a particular way in order to abolish pain; others must extend in a particular way to achieve that state. There are others who must flex and then extend in order to become symptom free.

SUMMARY

Pathology

With one exception,[18] we are not yet in a position to positively identify precisely the structures involved in the production of common low back problems.

Responsibility

Physical therapists, by virtue of their training, their relationship with the medical profession, and their now improved public esteem are without doubt the profession most appropriately situated to assume responsibility to dispense conservative spinal therapy for mechanical disorders.

We must ensure, however, that this opportunity is not lost by allowing some of our less particular colleagues to perpetuate hocus pocus type treatments. Ridding ourselves of outmoded therapies is an urgent priority. It is appropriate, at this point to quote directly from Nachemson[18]:

> In the therapeutic field today, it is virtually impossible to introduce a
> new drug without clinical and laboratory tests to prove its effectiveness

and we are increasingly alert to and critical of different types of pharmacological side effects.

The same approach should be used for the different forms of treatment of low back pain and we should critically re-assess our present methods.

Mechanical Diagnosis and Treatment

Three clinically identifiable syndromes exist in the nonspecific spectrum of low back pain.[11] Identification of these does not depend on naming the involved structure. Soft tissues are affected by mechanical forces that will result in the production of pain only in three particular conditions. These conditions can be (a) normal; (b) shortened; and (c) anatomically disrupted and displaced.

Postural Syndrome

Normal tissues can become painful in everyday life by the application of prolonged stresses commonly appearing during static postural loading conditions, such as prolonged sitting, standing, or bending.

Treatment.   Correction of faulty postural habit removes causative stresses. No other treatment is required. SMT mobilization and traction are of no use. In order to remove the cause of pain, the therapist must help the patient to correct position.

Dysfunction Syndrome

Shortened structures cause limited movement and simultaneously cause pain when the shortened structure is stretched.

Treatment.   Lengthen short structures by the regular application of stretching exercises. Dysfunction is not rapidly reversible; weeks are required to remodel and lengthen. SMT is of no use. Structures that have adaptively shortened over weeks and months cannot suddenly lengthen by the application of high velocity thrusts without incurring damage. Mobilization must, however, be considered as the most likely therapy to influence shortened structures. Traction is unlikely to remodel.

Derangement Syndrome

An example of this syndrome is frank tears of the anulus fibrosus with nuclear displacement or anular bulging. The patient experiences aching without movement, increased pain with movement in certain directions as displacement increases, and reduced pain in other directions as displacement decreases.

Treatment. This syndrome is subject to mostly rapid reversal. Reduce derangement by applying appropriate movements; maintain reduction by correcting posture and avoiding wrong positions; restore function before adaptive changes are established; and teach prevention of recurrence and self treatment. Mobilization and SMT now become important and may be required if self treatment applies insufficient reductive pressures.

Mechanical forces used to treat mechanical disorders of the low back should be applied in a graduated form, firstly, utilizing patient self-treatment repeated movements, progressing through mobilization and, finally, the application of manipulative procedures.

With no resolution of symptoms, exploration of other mechanical devices, such as traction, should follow. The only patients to receive modalities should be patients failing to respond to the mechanical approach. Modalities, such as TENS, Interferential Therapy, Microwave, and others should only be used to modulate pain when mechanical methods have failed. The physical therapy profession, however, must ask itself whether modulating pain by using expensive physical therapy is better for the patient and society as a whole than dispensation of rather inexpensive medications.

REFERENCES

1. Hippocrates: Corpus Hippocrateum. Peri arthron. Ch. 47. 400 BC (Cited by Cyriax, 1980)
2. Nachemson A: A critical look at conservative treatment of low back pain. In Jayson (ed): The Lumbar Spine and Back Pain. Pitman Medical, Tunbridge Wells, 1980
3. Twomey L, Taylor J: Age changes in the lumbar intervertebral discs. Acta Orthop Scand 56:6, 496, 1985
4. Dixon A: Diagnosis of low back pain. In Jayson M (ed): The Lumbar Spine and Back Pain. Pitman Medical, Tunbridge Wells, 1980
5. Cyriax J: Textbook of Orthopaedic Medicine. Vol. 1. 5th Ed. Baillière Tindall, London, 1980
6. Suzuki N, Seiichi E: A quantitative study of trunk muscle strength and fatigability in the low back pain syndrome. Spine 8:1, 1983
7. Schiotz EH, Cyriax J: Manipulation past and present. Heinmann, London, 1975
8. Jull G: The reliability of manual palpation. Proceedings of a Low Back Pain Conference. Man Ther Assn Conf Aust Melbourne, 1984, (in press)
9. Nachemson A: Lumbar spine instability. Spine 10:3, 1985
10. Gonnella C, Paris S, Kutner M: Reliability in evaluating passive intervertebral motion. Phys. Ther 62:437, 1982
11. McKenzie RA: The Lumbar Spine. Spinal Publications, Waikanae, New Zealand, 1980
12. Brunarski DJ: Clinical trials of spinal manipulation. J Manip Physiol Ther 7:4, 1984
13. Gibson T, Blagrave P, Harkness J et al: Low back pain treated by an osteopath. Br J Rheumatol 24:92, 1985
14. Cyriax J: Textbook of Orthopaedic Medicine. Vol. 1. Baillière Tindall, London, 1954
15. McKenzie RA: Prophylaxis in recurrent low back pain. NZ Med J 89:627, 1979

16. McKenzie RA: Manual correction of sciatic scoliosis. NZ Med J 76:484, 1972
17. Larsson U, Chöler U, Lidström A et al: Auto traction for treatment of lumbago-sciatica. Acta Orthop Scand 51:791, 1980
18. Nachemson A: Conservative treatment of low back pain. 2nd Ed. Jayson M (ed): In The Lumbar Spine and Back Pain. Pitman Medical, Tunbridge Wells, 453, 1980
19. Coventry MB, Ghormley, RK, Kernohan JW: The intervertebral disc: Part II. Changes in the intervertebral disc concomitant with age. J Bone Joint Surg 27:233, 1945
20. Coventry, MB, Ghormley, RK, Kernohan, JW: The intervertebral disc: Part III. Pathological changes in the intervertebral disc. J Bone Joint Surg 27:460, 1945
21. Williams CP: The lumbosacral spine. McGraw-Hill, New York, 1965
22. Vernon-Roberts B: The pathology and interrelation of intervertebral disc lesions. In Jayson M (ed): The Lumbar Spine and Back Pain. 2nd Ed., 1980
23. Andersson BJG, Schultz AB, Nachemson A: Intervertebral disc pressures during traction. J Rehabil Med suppl 9:88, 1983
24. Nelson MA, Allen P, Clamp S et al: Reliability and reproducibility of clinical findings in low-back pain. Spine 4:2, 1979
25. Prosser E: Manual of massage and movements. Faber & Faber, London, 1945
26. Ljunggren AE, Webber H, Larson S: Auto traction v. manual traction in patients with prolapsed lumbar intervertebral discs. Scan J Rehab Med 16:117, 1984
27. Farfan HF: Mechanical Disorders of the Low Back. Lea & Febiger, Philadelphia, 1973
28. Adams MA, Hutton WC: Prolapsed intervertebral disc: a hyperflexion injury. Spine 7:3, 1982
29. Adams MA, Hutton WC: Gradual disc prolapse. Spine 10:6, 1985
30. Panjabi M, Krag MH, Chung TQ: Effects of disc injury on mechanical behaviour of the human spine. Spine 9:7, 1984
31. Potter NA, Rothstein JM: Intertester reliability for selected clinical tests of the sacroiliac joint. Phys Ther 65:1671, 1985
32. Matyas TA, Bach TM: The reliability of selected techniques in clinical arthrometrics. Aust J Physiother 31:175, 1985
33. Cyron BM, Hutton WC: Articular trophism and instability of the lumbar spine. Spine 5:168, 1980
34. Willis TA: The lumbo-sacral anomalies. JBJS 41A:935, 1959
35. Farrell JB, Twomey LT: Acute low back pain. Comparison of two conservative treatment approaches. MTAA Proceedings, Perth, WA, 162, 1983
36. Moritz U: Evaluation of manipulation and other manual therapy. Criteria for measuring the effect of treatment. Scand J Rehab Med 11:173, 1979
37. Doran ML, Newell DJ: Manipulation in treatment of low back pain: A multicentre study. Br Med J 2:161, 1975
38. Hoehler FK, Tobis JS, Buerger AA: Spinal manipulation for low back pain. JAMA 245:1835, 1981
39. Sims-Williams H, Jayson MIV, Young SMS et al: Controlled trial of mobilisation and manipulation for patients with low back pain in general practise. Br Med J 2:1338, 1978

7 | Clinical Assessment: The Use of Combined Movements in Assessment and Treatment

Brian C. Edwards

The physical examination of the lumbar spine requires a high degree of skill combined with a thorough knowledge of structure and function, particularly when the treatment to be prescribed is manipulative therapy. This is because very close attention needs to be paid to the way in which the patient's signs and symptoms react to relatively small changes in posture and movement. If movement is the preferred method of treatment, the more precise the information on the reaction of signs and symptoms to movement, the more specific and effective the passive movement (manipulative procedure) will be.

However, it is important to expand the usual orthopedic examination by including movements that will highlight signs and symptoms that might normally be masked. This involves combining movements, which will increase or decrease the stretch and compressive effects on structures associated with the joint (e.g., the capsule, ligaments, and muscle attachments). This enables the therapist to establish movement patterns, which assist not only in the choice of the movement techniques to be used, but also in the prognosis.

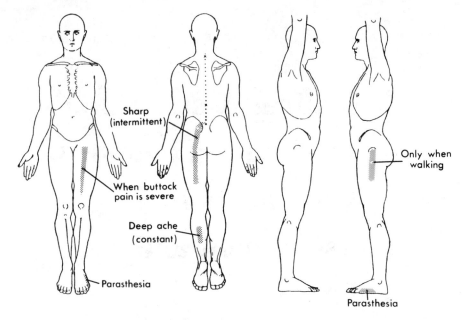

Fig. 7-1. A body chart used to show distribution of symptoms in a patient.

HISTORY TAKING AND SUBJECTIVE EXAMINATION

A standard orthopedic examination of the lumbar spine initially involves history taking. At the outset, an accurate account of the symptoms and their distribution must be obtained. This can be achieved in a number of ways. The patient can be given a simple body chart (Fig. 7-1) and asked to draw in the areas of pain or discomfort. However, such a method usually requires the therapist to repeat the examination in more detail, which can be very time consuming. A useful compromise is to ask the patient to map out on the body chart using one finger the areas of paresthesia and anesthesia, including a description of the type and depth of pain. In the case of the lumbar spine particularly, specific questions need to be asked related to perineal anesthesia or paresthesia alteration in micturition or bowel habit (particularly if associated with severe pain), and the responses require careful assessment. Care must be taken at this point to explain to the patient that it is important and necessary to describe the symptoms experienced at the time of assessment. If the distribution of symptoms has changed, the change can be superimposed on the same diagram or a separate diagram may be used. This is an important aspect of the examination since a clear understanding of those symptoms that are currently experienced as compared to those originally experienced can have an important bearing on both the diagnosis of the condition and selection of the treatment techniques.

Once descriptions of the symptoms and their distribution have been established, the patient should be questioned about how symptoms in different areas are related to each other (e.g., has there been an increase in pain in one area with a corresponding change in another area? In what sequence did the symptoms originally appear?). Such questioning is often omitted in history taking. However the answers provided by the patient highlight and implicate the anatomical structures likely to be affected, which may be the cause of the patient's symptoms.

The constancy of a patient's symptoms or the variability in the intensity of pain are also important aspects of the history taking and must be established. Following this, activities that cause any change in symptoms should be noted (i.e., the ease with which symptoms are aggravated; the activities that cause this aggravation; the relation between the type of activity and the duration and intensity of the symptoms produced, sometimes called irritability). These are often a useful guide to the amount of physical examination or treatment that may be carried out on the first day.

Activities that aggravate, relieve, or do not affect the symptoms need to be carefully described and analyzed in relation to the anatomy and biomechanics of the vertebral column, and to the distribution of the patient's symptoms. The simple activity of digging in the garden may be performed quite differently by two patients. If sitting, standing, or lying positions aggravate or relieve the symptoms this should be carefully noted. Particular attention should be paid to the positions adopted by the patient at the time of examination and treatment.

The history of present and past attacks of low back pain in terms of the type of activity responsible (if any) and the mode of onset of the symptoms needs to be clearly described by the patient and noted by the physical therapist. The onset of the symptoms is frequently related to and may have resulted from a particular incident or activity. However, it is not unusual for patients to have difficulty in remembering the particular incident, as they may regard it as trivial or it may have occurred some time before the onset of the symptoms.

The need for accurate questioning and skill in the interpretation of answers cannot be overemphasized. It is essential to have this information as a sound base before proceeding to the next step of the objective examination. The interpretation of the subjective examination also requires considerable patience and skill on the part of the therapist.

OBJECTIVE EXAMINATION OF LUMBAR SPINE

General

The term *objective examination* is something of a misnomer. Objectivity in its pure form is difficult to achieve when the physical therapist includes in such examination not only movements but also the patient's description of the symptoms reproduced by the movements.

The objective examination therefore contains some elements that are subjective in the sense that patient response requires interpretation by the therapist. It is important that reference is constantly made to the specific areas of pain and the symptoms for which the patient has come seeking treatment. It cannot be overemphasized that attention to (a) small details of a patient's answers, and (b) individual movements, is essential if the objective examination is to help identify particular structures as a likely sources of the patient's symptoms.

The principal aim of the objective examination is to establish the effect of movement of the lumbar spine on those symptoms that have already been described by the patient. In doing this the identification of the muscles, joints, and ligaments involved by the patient's disorder is of primary importance. Careful observation of the way the vertebral column moves, areas of hyper- and hypomobility, and areas of relative muscle hypertrophy or atrophy are assessed.

Observation

The first part of the examination consists of observation. Three important aspects of observation are general movement, posture and shape of joints, and gait.

General Movement

Observation of the care with which a patient moves while adopting the sitting position or moves out of such a position, of how the patient moves while disrobing, with any changes in facial expression, assists the interpretation of the patient's symptoms. A pertinent question to be asked when a particular posture produces pain is, "Is it "the" pain or is it different from the pain for which you are seeking treatment?" Such observations may suggest to the therapist the movements that are likely to reproduce the symptoms.

Posture and Shape of Joints

Alterations in posture and joint outline may be of recent or long standing duration and indeed many so-called postural deformities may well be perfectly normal for a particular individual. It should be emphasized that some fairly obvious deformities, for example, marked kyphosis, lordosis, or scoliosis may be of no significance in the patient's current problem.

Gait

Obvious gait alterations can be observed initially. Changes such as altered weight distribution and lack of mobility in hips, knees, or ankles, or a positive Trendelenburg sign may be noted. With the exception of the latter, lack of mobility may be inhibition of movement due to pain originating in the lumbar spine, or due to a previous unrelated peripheral joint involvement.

SPECIFIC MOVEMENT AND OBSERVATION

The patient needs to be undressed sufficiently to observe the whole of the spine as well as the lower limbs.

Observation from Behind

When observing from behind the following may be observed and variation noted:

1. Altered leg length
2. Altered shoulder height
3. Position of head on neck and neck on shoulders
4. Kyphosis or lordosis (exaggerated or diminished)
5. Position of scapulae
6. Valgus or varus deformity of knees and feet
7. Scoliosis (postural or structural)
8. Position of sacrum and iliac crests
9. Prominence or depression of vertebral spinous processes
10. Skin contour and color

Observation from in Front

When observing from the front, a clinician should take note of the following features:

1. Height or level of iliac crests
2. Position or level of the knees
3. Shape of trunk
4. Relative positions of shoulders, head, and feet
5. Skin contour

Observation from the Side

When observing from the side, a clinician should be aware of:

1. Position of head

2. Shape of cervical, thoracic, and lumbar spinal curves (any increased or decreased kyphosis or lordosis)
3. Skin contour.

Movements

The lumbar spine is most easily examined from behind.

Flexion

When suitably undressed the patient is asked first to describe exactly where the symptoms are at present. The patient is then asked to bend forward to where there is any increase in any part of the symptom complex. This flexion range is usually recorded by measuring the distance from the outstretched finger tips to the floor or in relation to position the fingertips on legs (e.g., patella, midthigh etc.). The patient is then asked to move in a controlled manner further into the painful range (Fig. 7-2). This range and any alteration in the symptoms are noted.

Assessment during Flexion. Not only is the full range of movement noted, considerable attention is paid to the way in which the individual vertebrae move during flexion. Areas of hyper- and hypomobility are recorded as well as any deviation from the median sagittal plane. Surface contour should be carefully considered, particularly noting areas of prominence or depression.

At this time it is important to compare those symptoms and signs produced on flexion to those answers given to the related subjective questions. Thus, any links may be established between the symptoms described by the patient and those elicited by the movement.

The distribution of the symptoms and the range of movement needs to be very carefully recorded. In one patient buttock pain may be produced during the first 10 degrees of flexion, but the patient may also be able to continue to full range without any alteration in the distribution of the pain. In another patient buttock pain may be produced in the first 10 degrees of flexion but on continuing the movement toward full range the pain may progress to the calf. *Both patients have the same range of forward flexion but they produce quite different symptoms, which need to be treated quite differently.*

The effect of a controlled amount of overpressure (i.e., gentle passive forcing of the movement from the patient's end range further into range) is also necessary under certain circumstances, not only to observe the way the symptoms react, but also to test the *end feel* of the physiologic movement. The end feel of a movement is the relationship between the pain experienced and the resistance to movement. Such resistance may be due to intrinsic muscle spasm or tightness of the ligaments and capsule of the joint.

The end feel of the physiologic movement, mentioned above, may be different to the end feel with llocalized passive movement procedures (described

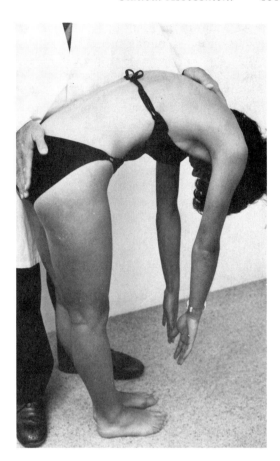

Fig. 7-2. Part 1 of the general examination: Flexion.

later). However, quite distinct solid, springy, soft, or hard end feelings may be distinguished. The end feel needs to be noted because if there is a difference between what is found with localized procedures compared to the more general movement procedures, then an attempt needs to be made to define those differences and the possible reasons for them.

On occasion it is important to hold the full range position of flexion for a period of time. This becomes a necessary part of the examination especially if during the subjective examination an activity involving sustained flexion is reported by the patient as a position where symptoms are eased. Such a procedure is valuable because if the symptoms are not eased more detailed questioning and examination is necessary.

The return from the flexed to the upright position is also an important movement to monitor, both in terms of the way the vertebral column moves and the production of symptoms. A postural scoliosis or tilt may be seen on adoption of the erect position, which is not evident on bending forward. Another important aspect of assessment of flexion and the return to the upright position is the reproduction of a painful arc; that is, pain that is produced through a part of the range and then is eased as the movement continues. This can happen either during the flexion movement or during the return to the upright position. The range within which such symptoms are produced, as well as the distribution of the symptoms, should be carefully recorded and related if possible to the subjective findings. Often those patients with painful arcs are slower to respond to treatment, particularly if the painful arc is variable in its position in the range.

On occasion, symptoms may be produced some time after the movement has been completed (i.e., latent pain). This latent pain possibly may have a large chemical component in its production or etiology. Occasionally repeated flexion movements or varying the speed of the movement may be necessary to reproduce this symptom.

As well as the general observation of changes in signs and symptoms on full range flexion, particular consideration needs to be given to the way in which motion segments are moving. On flexion there is a cephalad movement of the inferior zygapophyseal facets at one level in relation to the superior facets of the level below. This is accompanied by a stretching of the soft tissues of the posterior elements of the motion segment, including the posterior parts of the disc and the canal structures, as well as the posterior ligaments, capsules, and muscles. There is an accompanying compression of the anterior parts of the disc (nucleus and anterior anulus including the anterior longitudinal ligament).

Lateral Flexion

The patient stands in the same position as for flexion and is asked to slide his or her hand down the lateral aspect of the leg. Measurement is usually taken of the distance from the finger tips to the head of the fibula. Areas of hypo- and hypermobility can be observed at segmental levels by closely matching the movement behavior of the vertebrae. As with flexion, the use of over-pressure and repeated and sustained movements may be necessary in addition to the observance of deformity and presence or absence of a painful arc.

The effect of lateral flexion on that part of the motion segment on the contralateral, extended side (away from that which the movement is performed on) is similar to that observed with sagittal plane flexion. There is a cephalad movement of the inferior zygapophyseal facet of the superior vertebra on the superior zygapophyseal facet of the vertebra below. This stretches the soft-tissue structures (discs, joint capsules, etc.) on the side opposite the direction of lateral flexion. On the side toward which the lateral flexion is performed, these structures are compressed (Fig. 7-3).

Extension

The therapist stands behind the patient who is asked to bend backwards. Measurement can be made of the distance the finger tips pass down the posterior aspect of the thigh. Areas of hypo- and hypermobility are observed, as

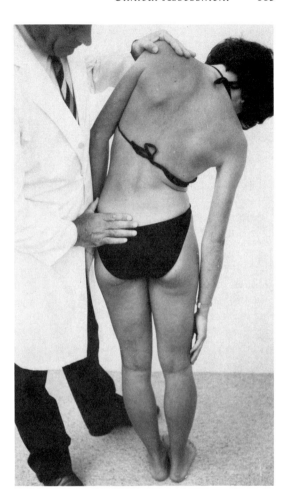

Fig. 7-3. Part 2 of the general examination: Right lateral flexion.

well as the distribution of symptoms at the end of range and through range. The use of overpressure and repeated and sustained movements are used as necessary.

The effect of extension on the motion segment is such that there is a caudal movement of the inferior zygapophyseal facets of a vertebra on the facets of the vertebra below. There is also a compression of the posterior parts and a stretching of the anterior parts of the intervertebral disc (Fig. 7-4).

Axial Rotation

Rotation as a testing procedure in the lumbar spine is not a movement that often produces significant alteration in signs and symptoms. Strangely enough, it is a movement often preferred as a passive movement treatment technique by therapists. One method of testing rotation is for the therapist to stand on

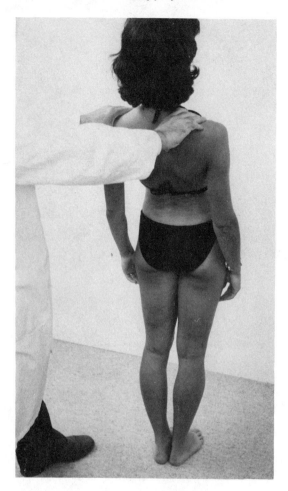

Fig. 7-4. Part 3 of the general examination: Thoracolumbar extension.

the left side of the patient and take hold of the patient's right ileum with the right hand and the patient's right shoulder with the left. The patient's pelvis is then rotated to the right while applying counter resistance to the shoulder (Fig. 7-5).

General Assessment of Standard Active Physiologic Movements.   In addition to recording the ranges of movements that are available and the way in which the vertebral segments move, detailed attention must also be given to (a) the distribution of the symptoms, and (b) the type of symptoms involved with each movement. The importance of the patient's descriptions of these symptoms cannot be overemphasized. Comparison needs to be made between the way the patient describes the symptoms produced with various activities as elicited during the subjective questioning, to those produced and observed in the objective testing of lumbar movements, mentioned above. Similar descriptions of type of symptoms, as well as distribution are important (i.e., the pain may be described as diffuse, lancinating, or referred to a limb, etc.). At this stage, the therapist should look for similarities between the movements of general

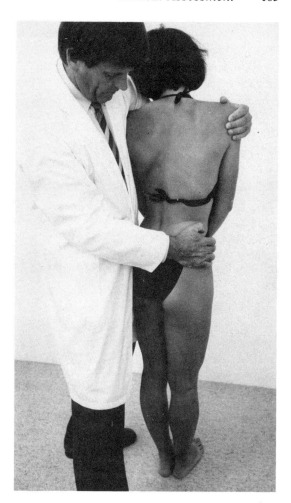

Fig. 7-5. Part 4 of the general examination: Lumbar rotation to the left.

daily activities that bring on the symptoms and the active movements that elicit the pain. For example, a patient may report that bending activity in the garden for about one hour brings on back pain, while on subsequent examination one repetition of forward flexion is shown to produce the same pain. Careful questioning is required to define the type and distribution of the symptoms as sustained flexion (if that is the movement he adopts while gardening) is unlikely to produce the same quality and quantity of pain as would be produced by one movement of flexion. Such careful questioning can help both in diagnosis as well as the selection of a treatment technique.

Combined Movements

Habitually, movements of the vertebral column occur in combination across planes rather than as pure movements in one plane only. Many aspects of this phenomenon have been investigated.[4,8,12,14] Gregson and Lucas[5] found

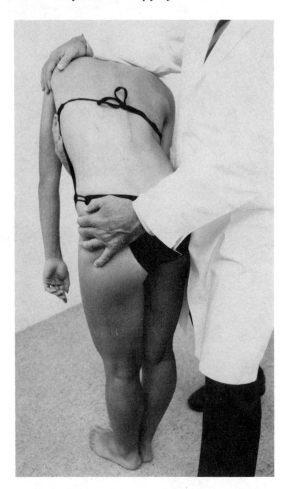

Fig. 7-6. Part 1 of the combined movements examination: Lateral flexion in flexion.

that axial rotation of the lumbar spine to the left accompanied lateral flexion to the left, and rotation to the right accompanied lateral flexion to the right. However, in one case they found the reverse combination occurred. Stoddard[13] stated that the direction of this conjoined rotation varied depending on whether the lateral flexion was performed with the lumbar spine in flexion or extension. He suggested that the conjoined rotation is to the same side when the movement of lateral flexion is performed in flexion, and to the opposite side when the movement of lateral flexion is performed in extension. Kapandji[7] also states that lateral rotation occurs in conjunction with lateral flexion. Personal laboratory observation on fresh human cadaveric specimens seems to indicate that the direction of axial rotation is in the opposite direction to that to which the lumbar spine is laterally flexed, regardless of whether the spine is in flexion or extension. The presence of degenerative processes within the disc or zygapophyseal joints affects the amount of rotation, and occasionally there is an unexplained apparent reversal of the axial rotation.

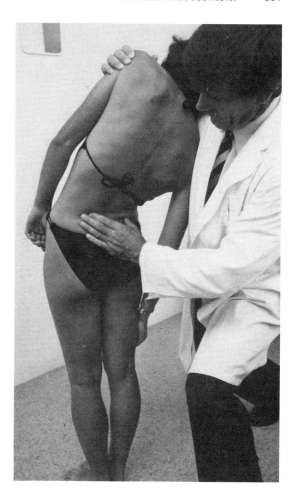

Fig. 7-7. Part 2 of the combined movements examination: Lateral flexion in extension.

Because of this, the usual objective examination of the lumbar spine should be expanded to incorporate combined movements. This is because symptoms and signs produced by lateral flexion, flexion, extension, and rotation as pure movements may alter when these movements are performed in a combined manner.[2]

Lateral Flexion in Flexion

The therapist stands on the right-hand side of the patient so that the therapist's right anterosuperior iliac spine is in contact with the lateral aspect of the patient's right hip. The therapist's right hand is placed over the posterior aspect of the patient's left shoulder. The therapist's left hand grips the patient's left ilium. The patient is asked to bend forward; the range at which the symptoms are reproduced is noted, and while this position is maintained, lateral flexion to the right is included as part of the total pattern (Fig. 7-6).

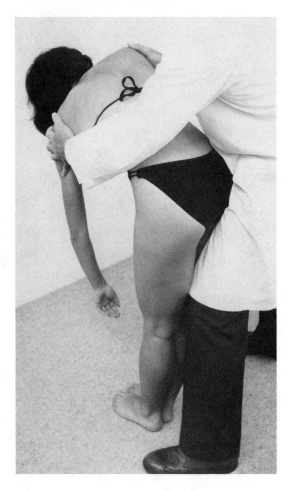

Fig. 7-8. Part 3 of the combined movements examination: Flexion and rotation.

Lateral Flexion in Extension

The therapist stands on the right-hand side of the patient, with the right arm placed around the patient's chest so that the therapist's right hand grips the patient's left shoulder. The thumbs and index finger of the therapist's left hand are placed over the transverse process of the vertebral level to be examined. The patient is then bent backward and laterally flexed to the right (Fig. 7-7).

Flexion and Rotation

The therapist stands on the right-hand side of the patient and places his hands posteriorly on the patient's shoulder. The patient then bends forward and rotates to the right (Fig. 7-8).

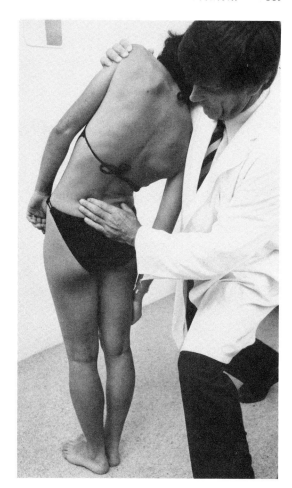

Fig. 7-9. Part 4 of the combined movements examination: Extension and rotation.

Extension and Rotation

The same hand positions are adopted as with extension and lateral flexion. The patient's lumbar spine is extended and rotated to the right, as well (Fig. 7-9).

Passive Accessory Movements in Combined Positions

The usual accessory movements of transverse, central, and unilateral pressure[10] may also be carried out in combined positions. The lumbar spine is placed in the combined positions described above and the appropriate accessory movements are performed.

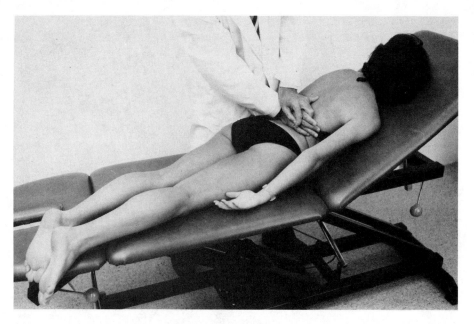

Fig. 7-10. Passive accessory movements in part 1 of the combined positions examination: Central vertebral pressure in extension and right lateral flexion.

Central Vertebral Pressure in Extension and Right Lateral Flexion

The patient lies prone in a position of extension and right lateral flexion. Central vertebral pressure is applied over the spinous process. Then the pressure is directed caudad on the spinous process of L4, the compressive effect particularly on the right-hand side will be increased on the right between L4-5 but decreased between L3-4 (Fig. 7-10).

Transverse Pressure to the Left in Flexion and Left Lateral Flexion

With the patient prone and in a position of flexion and left lateral flexion, transverse pressure over the right side of the spinous process is applied. This will tend to increase the stretching effect on the right (Fig. 7-11).

Unilateral Pressure on the Right in Flexion and Left Lateral Flexion

With the patient positioned in flexion and right lateral flexion, unilateral pressure on the right over the transverse process of the vertebrae is applied. If this pressure is directed cephalad on the transverse process of L4 there will be an increase in the stretching effect on the right between L4-5 and a decrease between L3-4 (Fig. 7-12).

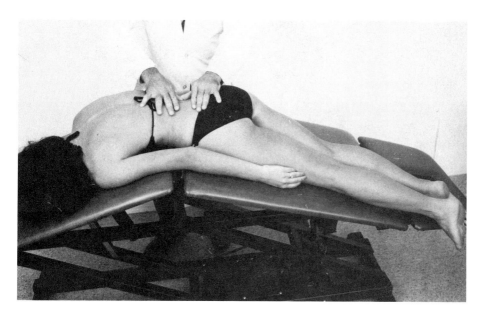

Fig. 7-11. Passive accessory movements in part 2 of the combined positions examination: Transverse pressure to the left in flexion and left lateral flexion.

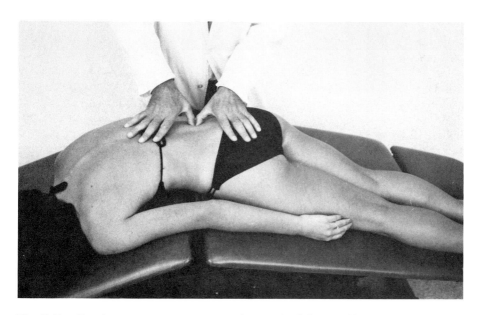

Fig. 7-12. Passive accessory movements in part 3 of the combined positions examination: Unilateral pressure on the right in flexion and left lateral flexion.

Passive Testing of Physiologic Movements

Standard passive physiologic tests of the movements of flexion, extension, lateral flexion, and axial rotation can also be carried out, and are a useful adjunct to the examination procedures.

Assessment of Combined Movements

The movements of flexion, extension, lateral flexion, and rotation performed in the neutral position, are termed *primary movements*. On the initial examination it is usual for one of these *primary movements* to reproduce part or all of the symptoms of which the patient is complaining. It is to this primary movement that the other movements are added. It is essential when performing the primary movement that the movement is taken to the point where the symptoms begin, and then taken in a controlled manner further into the painful range of the movement. At this stage, the movement of lateral flexion or rotation or both is added.

Care must be taken when adding other movements that the starting position into the range of the primary movement is not altered. The basic principle is to combine movements that have similar mechanical effects on the motion segment and to observe if symptoms are increased or decreased by such maneuvers. On flexion there is a cephalad movement of the inferior zygapophyseal facet for instance of L4 on the superior zygapophyseal facet of L5. The posterior elements are stretched; the posterior part of the intervertebral disc; the posterior longitudinal ligament; the ligamentum flavum; and capsules of the zygapophyseal joints. The anterior structures are compressed.

With right lateral flexion, for instance, the left inferior zygapophyseal facet of L4 moves upwards on the left superior zygapophyseal facet of L5. This movement produces a stretching of the elements on the left side of the motion segment with compression of the right side of the motion segment. When flexion and right lateral flexion are combined, the stretching effects on the left are increased and slight stretching effects are produced on the right.

With extension there is a downward movement of the inferior zygapophyseal facet (e.g., of the L4 vertebra on the superior zygapophyseal facet of L5). This is accompanied by compression of the posterior elements of the motion segment. When the movement of right lateral flexion is combined with extension there is an increase in the compressive effects on the right and a decrease on the left.

Regular and Irregular Patterns

The combination of these movements can under many circumstances produce recognizable symptom patterns, which may be described as Regular or Irregular.[3] The regular pattern may be divided further as follows:

1. Regular patterns: stretch and compressive
2. Irregular patterns: those that show no recognizable pattern.

An Example of a Regular Compressive Pattern.   Right lateral flexion increases, right buttock pain. This pain is made worse when right lateral flexion is performed in extension, and eased when right lateral flexion is performed in flexion.

An Example of a Regular Stretch Pattern.   Right lateral flexion increases the left buttock pain. This pain is made worse when right lateral flexion is performed in flexion and eased when right lateral flexion is performed in extension.

An Example of an Irregular Pattern.   All of those patients who do not fit into the regular category are classified as irregular. There are many of these (e.g., when right lateral flexion reproduces right buttock pain, which is made worse when right lateral flexion is combined with flexion on the right). (In this movement, the right compression of right lateral flexion is counteracted by the stretching of flexion.) Another example is left lateral flexion producing right buttock pain (a stretching movement). This pain is made worse when the same movement is performed in extension (a compressing movement) and eased when the movement of left lateral flexion is performed in flexion (another stretching movement).

The irregular pattern may indicate that there is more than one component to the joint disorder (e.g., zygapophyseal joint and intervertebral disc, canal and foraminal structures). Generally traumatic injuries (e.g., whiplash and early disc lesions) have irregular patterns, while chronic disc lesions or zygapophyseal joint lesions with no history of trauma leave regular patterns.

Contained within one type of pattern there may be elements of other patterns. These should be recognized, and time provided so as to decide whether any irregular patterns have some recognizable regular components.

The recognition of different patterns can assist in:

1. Choosing the direction of a technique
2. Allowing a combined movement, end of range procedure to be used (CME)
3. Assessing the manner in which the signs and symptoms may improve

When *choosing the direction of the technique* in the case of regular patterns, (either stretch or compressive), the first choice of movement is in the direction that is away from the movement that reproduces the symptom. For example, if right lateral flexion reproduces the right buttock pain and this pain is made worse when the right lateral flexion is performed in extension (that is a regular compressive pattern), the first choice would be to carry out the opposite movement (i.e., left lateral flexion in flexion). As the symptoms improve the technique of left lateral flexion in flexion is changed to right lateral flexion in flexion and progressed to right lateral flexion in extension as symptoms improve further. If the patient presents with a regular stretch pattern (e.g.,

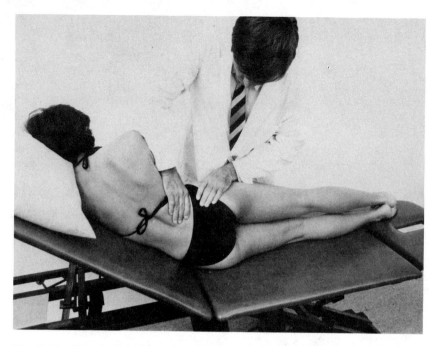

Fig. 7-13.   Part 1 of the technique examination: Right lateral flexion in neutral.

right lateral flexion reproduces left buttock pain and this pain is made worse when right lateral flexion is performed in flexion and eased when right lateral flexion is performed in extension) the first choice technique would be the opposite movement (i.e., left lateral flexion in extension). This technique can then progress to performing right lateral flexion in flexion as the symptoms improve.

Combined movements, end of range procedures (CME) should be used. There is evidence that end of range procedures (i.e., passive movements performed at the limit of a range of movement) are more effective in reducing pain perception and improving the range of movement.[1,6,9,11] By combining movements, it is possible to use end of range movements in a relatively painless way. The most painful movement for the patient can be used as a treatment technique in its least painful combined position. The movement technique can be carried out in a manner that causes the least pain but is performed at the end of the available range. This position is progressed to what was the most painful position for the patient as the symptoms improve.

Assessing the improvement in a patient's condition means recognizing the patterns, regular or irregular, that can help in predicting the way in which the symptoms will improve. In the case of a regular compressive pattern where, for example, right lateral flexion produces right buttock pain and this pain is worse when the movement is performed in extension, then right lateral flexion in neutral will improve before right lateral flexion in extension. With a regular stretch pattern, for example, of right lateral flexion causing left buttock pain,

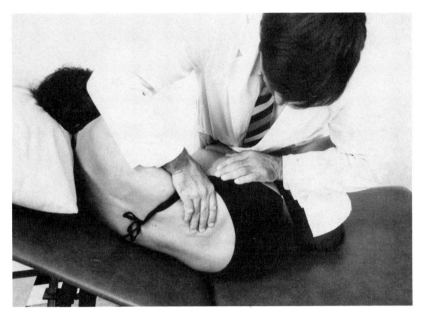

Fig. 7-14. Part 2 of the technique examination: Right lateral flexion in flexion.

this pain being worse when right lateral flexion is performed in flexion, then right lateral flexion in neutral will improve before right lateral flexion in flexion. The response in the case of irregular patterns is not as predictable and the improvement in the signs and symptoms may appear in an apparently random fashion.

Technique

Right Lateral Flexion in Neutral

The treatment table is adjusted so as to have the thoracic spine at the desired position of lateral flexion. This position will correspond to that found on examination. The lumbar spine is placed in a neutral position. The therapist's right hand is placed at the level at which the lateral flexion is to be centered, with the therapist's left hand placed over the patient's right greater trochanter. The movement of lateral flexion is performed by moving the left hand in a cephalad direction so as to laterally flex the pelvis to the right (Fig. 7-13).

Right Lateral Flexion in Flexion

The treatment table is adjusted and the therapist's hands are placed in a manner as described above. The patient's hips and knees are flexed so as to flex the lumbar spine to the required position. The patient's feet are placed

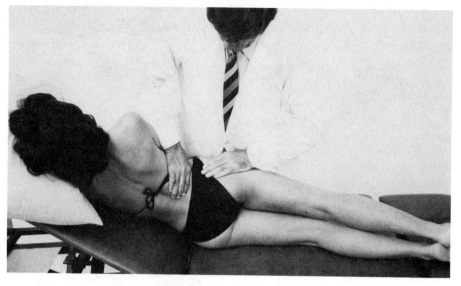

Fig. 7-15.   Part 3 of the technique examination: Right lateral flexion in extension.

over the therapist's flexed left thigh. This maintains the angle of lumbar flexion. The movement of lateral flexion is carried out by moving the left hand cephalad while maintaining the flexion of the lumbar spine (Fig. 7-14).

Right Lateral Flexion in Extension

The table and hand position are placed in a manner as desribed above. The lumbar spine is placed in a position of extension. Lateral flexion is carried out by moving the left hand in a cephalad direction while maintaining the position of extension (Fig. 7-15).

CONCLUSION

The examination of the lumbar spine requires considerable patience and skill. The principle of combining movements provides an addition to the standard examination, and a means by which changes in signs and symptoms can be readily assessed and specific symptom patterns observed. These symptom patterns are of assistance in the selection of passive movement treatment technique, as the ability to be able to predict the likely result enables the therapist to use the end of range combined movement (CME) technique, even in acutely painful conditions. Three techniques of lateral flexion have been described.

ACKNOWLEDGEMENTS

I wish to acknowledge the considerable assistance of David Watkins in the preparation of the photographs used in this chapter.

REFERENCES

1. Baxendale RH, Ferrell WR: The effect of knee joint afferent discharge on transmission in flexion reflex pathways in decerebrate cats. J Physiol 315:231, 1981
2. Edwards BC: Combined movements of the lumbar spine—examination and clinical significance. Aust J Physiother 25:4, 1979
3. Edwards BC: Movement patterns. In Bower K (ed): Proceedings of International Conference on Manipulative Therapy, 1983
4. Farfan HF: Muscular mechanisms of the lumbar spine and the position of power and efficiency. Ortho Clin M Th Amer 6(1):135, 1975
5. Gregerson GC, Lucas DB: An in vivo study of the axial rotation of the human thoraco-lumbar spine. J Bone Joint Surg 49A, 2:247, 1967
6. Grigg P, Greenspan BJ: Response of primate joint afferent neurons to mechanical stimulation of the knee joint. J Neurophys 40:1, 1977
7. Kapandji IA: The Physiology of Joints. Vol. 3. Churchill Livingstone, London, 1974
8. Loebl WY: Regional rotation of the spine. Rheumatol Rehab 12:223, 1973
9. Lundberg A, Malmgren K, Schomburg ED: Role of joint afferents in motor control exemplified by effects on reflex pathways from ib afferents. J Physiol 284:327, 1978
10. Maitland GD: Vertebral Manipulation. Butterworth, London, 1985
11. Nade S, Newbold PJ: Factors determining the level and changes in intra-articular pressure in the knee joint of the dog. J Physiol 338:21, 1983
12. Rolander SD: Motion of the lumbar spine with special reference to the stabilising effect of posterior fusion—an experimental study on autopsy specimens. Acta Orthop Scand suppl 90, 1966
13. Stoddard AC: Manual of Osteopathic Technique. Hutchison, London, 1959
14. Troup JDG, Hood CA, Chapman AE: Measurements of the sagittal mobility of the lumbar spine and hips. Am Phys Med 9, 8:308, 1968

8 | Manipulative Therapy for the Low Lumbar Spine: Technique Selection and Application to Some Syndromes

Patricia H. Trott
Ruth Grant
Geoffrey D. Maitland

Patients referred for manipulative physical therapy can be divided into two groups according to the history: The first group have a *history of injury*, such as a fall, a direct blow, or are referred following surgery. The tissues that are injured depend on the direction and force of the injury, and thus the therapist cannot predict the pattern of the symptoms and signs or the response to treatment. The second group includes patients who have a history of *symptoms occurring spontaneously* or following some trivial incident such as sneezing or bending to pick up a light object. Patients in this group have symptoms, signs, and histories that are easily recognized, and these conditions respond in a predictable way to manipulative physical therapy.

In this chapter the application of manipulative therapy (passive movement) in the treatment of some conditions/syndromes of the low lumbar spine (L4-S1) is presented. Although discussion is restricted to the use of passive movement techniques, the need for a detailed assessment of the soft-tissue components and the muscular control of the spine and pelvis is stressed and these aspects together with ergonomic advice are included in the overall management of low lumbar problems (these aspects are covered in other chapters of this book).

Before describing such lumbar conditions, discussion of the factors that govern the selection of passive movement techniques is necessary.

SELECTION OF TECHNIQUES

Diagnosis

In the clinical setting, reaching a definitive diagnosis is not always possible. This is particularly the case for low lumbar disorders, and relates to the following factors:

1. In many cases the etiology is multifactorial and includes both an inflammatory and a mechanical cause.
2. Pain arising from certain tissues does not follow a specific anatomical pattern.
3. A particular pathologic process can give differing patterns of symptoms and signs.

For example, patients with a diagnosis of disc herniation with nerve root irritation can exhibit differing clinical presentations, that is, the symptoms may be acute and severe or chronic; the distribution of pain may vary, being worse either proximally or distally, with or without neurologic changes. The pattern of limitation of movements may vary from gross restriction of flexion and straight leg raising (SLR) due to pain, to full range and painfree flexion but with marked restriction of extension.

Clearly, a diagnostic label on its own is of limited assistance when choosing physical treatment modalities and in particular when selecting passive movement techniques. Rather, treatment selection is based on the way the condition presents, in terms of the patient's symptoms, abnormalities of movement, and the history of the disorder. Knowing which structures can cause pain and the different patterns of pain response that can occur during test movements is fundamental to the selection of passive movement techniques.

Physical therapists, and in particular manipulative physical therapists, are skilled in diagnosis of mechanical disorders of the neuromusculoskeletal system. They are also trained to recognize when symptoms do not have a mechanical basis and when to suspect an inflammatory component. In many cases radiologic and hematologic tests are required to exclude other pathologies.

Pain-Sensitive Structures and Their Pain Patterns

In the lumbar spine the common structures that cause symptoms are the joints[1,2] and their supportive tissues[2] and the pain-sensitive structures in the vertebral and foraminal canals.[3-7]

The Intervertebral Joints

The Intervertebral Disc. Pain from disorders of the intervertebral disc is commonly deep and illdefined, presenting as a wide area across the low back or as a vague buttock pain. This pain may spread to the upper posterior thigh or lower abdomen, but pain originating in the disc itself is not referred into the lower leg.[8] The pain may be central, to one side, or bilateral (symmetric or asymmetric).

A damaged disc may impinge against the posterior longitudinal ligament or the dura or, as it herniates, disc material can impinge on or irritate the nerve-root sleeve or the nerve root causing referred pain.[2,9]

Discogenic pain behaves differently from pain arising from other structures, in that (a) following a sustained posture, rapid reversal of that posture is both painful and stiff (e.g., to stand up quickly after prolonged sitting), and (b) speed of movement will vary the position in range at which pain is experienced (i.e., with increased speed, pain is experienced earlier in the range). Discogenic pain may be aggravated by either compressive or stretching movements.[10]

The Zygapophyseal Joint. Like other synovial joints, the zygapophyseal joint may present with an intraarticular disorder (which is made worse, i.e., more painful, when the articular surfaces are compressed) or a periarticular disorder (which is worsened by movements that place stress on the capsule).

Commonly, zygapophyseal joint pain is felt locally as a unilateral back pain, which when severe can spread down the entire limb.[2,11] The zygapophyseal joints do not refer pain into the lower limb in a definite pattern and the source of pain must be confirmed by clinical examination. In its chronic form, there may be no local pain over the affected joint, but a distal localized patch of pain. This is a common phenomenon in the thoracolumbar region; similar clinical findings for the lower lumbar area have not been substantiated by research.

Ligamentous and Capsular Structures. Referred pain from specific spinal ligamentous structures follows no known neurologic pattern.[2,12] Based on clinical experience, Maitland[10] reported that ligamentous and capsular pain is felt maximally over the ligament and that the pain may spread into the lower limb. Movements that stretch the ligament/capsule may produce sharp local pain or a stretched sensation at the symptomatic site.

Pain-Sensitive Structures in the Vertebral and Foraminal Canals

The pain-sensitive structures in the vertebral and foraminal canals are the dura anteriorly,[5,6] the nerve-root sleeves, the ventral nerve roots, and the blood vessels of the epidural space.[7,13]

The structures comprising the vertebral canal that are pain sensitive are the posterior longitudinal ligament, posterior portions of the annuli fibrosi, and the anterior aspect of the laminae.[1] The pain sensitive components of the foraminal canals are the posterolateral aspect of the intervertebral discs and the zygapophyseal joints.[1]

Passive-movement tests will implicate a loss of mobility and/or increase in tension of the neuromeningeal tissues.

The Dura and Nerve-Root Sleeve. Dural pain does not have a segmental pattern of reference.[3] However stimulation of the nerve-root sleeve gives rise to symptoms of a similar distribution to those arising from stimulation of that nerve root. The only reported difference is that the nerve root frequently gives rise to symptoms that are more severe distally and the pain is often associated with paresthesia. These phenomena are not seen with irritation of the nerve-root sleeve.[14]

Nerve-Root Pain. Mechanical or chemical irritation of the sensory nerve root causes pain and/or paresthesia to be experienced in the distal part of a dermatome, or if felt throughout a dermatome, these symptoms are often worse distally. Movements that narrow the intervertebral canal and foramen (extension, rotation, and lateral flexion to the affected side) are likely to reproduce or aggravate the nerve-root pain/paresthesia. Clinically, pain can be conclusively attributed to the nerve root only if there are neurologic changes indicating a loss of conduction along that nerve root.

Passive movement tests that specifically test the neuromeningeal structures are Straight Leg Raising (SLR), Prone Knee Flexion (PKF), Passive Neck Flexion (PNF), and the Slump Test. These tests are described in the major textbooks on manipulative therapy.[9,10,15] They are used not only as examination techniques but also in treatment.

Range/Pain Response to Movement

Test movements of the low lumbar intervertebral joints and the neuromeningeal tissues produce common patterns.

Stretching or Compressing Pain

Unilateral back pain may be reproduced by either stretching (e.g., lateral flexion to the other side) or by compressing the faulty tissues (e.g., lateral flexion towards the painful side).

End of Range or Through Range Pain

Pain may be reproduced at the limit of a particular movement (i.e., when the soft-tissue restraints are put on stretch) or during the performance of a movement, increasing near the limit of the movement. Through range pain is common in joints in which there is a constant ache.

Local and Referred Pain

In patients who have referred pain, the pain response to test movements influences the selection of passive movement techniques. For example, test movements even when firmly applied may elicit only local back pain. In these patients the movement may be applied firmly without risk of exacerbation of symptoms. In cases where the test movement has to be sustained at end of range in order to reproduce the referred pain, a treatment technique that is sustained will be required. In contrast to this, test movements that immediately cause distal leg symptoms require very gentle movement in a manner that does not reproduce the distal symptoms. Test movements that cause latent referred pain or that cause the referred pain to linger also indicate caution in treatment.

History

Any history taken should include the onset and progression of the disorder. Conditions that have a spontaneous (nontraumatic) onset have a characteristic progressive history, that is, there is a pattern that is typical of a degenerating disc or of postural ligamentous pain. Knowing the history that is typical for these conditions helps the clinician to recognize the present *stage of the disorder* and to match this with the symptoms and signs to form a syndrome. Typical histories will be presented in Low Lumbar Syndromes.

A detailed history gives information as to the *stability or progressive nature of the disorder*. This will guide the extent and strength of techniques used and may contraindicate certain techniques. This is particularly important in cases of a progressive disc disorder when injudicious treatment may convert a potential disc protrusion into a herniated disc with neurologic changes.

The progression of the disorder allows prediction of the outcome of treatment, the number of treatment sessions needed, and the long term prognosis.

The following case history illustrates these aspects of history taking.

A 25-year-old gardener presented with a 10-year history of low back pain, which started one school vacation when he worked as a builder's laborer. He then remained symptom free until he began work as a gardener seven years ago. Prolonged digging caused low back pain, which initially would be gone by the next morning, but this slowly worsened to the extent that the pain spread to his left buttock and posterior thigh and took longer to settle. In the last six months he has required treatment and two or three treatments of heat and extension exercises have completely relieved his symptoms. Two weeks ago, he tripped over a stone and experienced sharp pain in his left calf and paresthesia of his left fifth toe. This has not responded to heat and exercises, but he has been able to continue his gardening.

This history is typical of a progressive and worsening disc disorder and the patient is now at a stage where he has nerve root irritation. Although a trivial incident provoked this episode, the disorder is relatively stable in that he can continue gardening without worsening his symptoms.

More specific treatment will be required and it can be performed firmly without risk of exacerbation of his symptoms. The expectation of treatment is to make him symptom free while anticipating there may be further episodes due to the progressive nature of his disorder.

Symptoms

The area in which a patient feels his symptoms and the manner in which they vary in relation to posture and movement assist in the recognition of syndromes, and if they match the response to physical examination, can assist in the selection of passive movement techniques. A movement or combination of movements that simulate a position or movement described by the patient as one which causes the pain, can be used as the treatment technique. The following case history illustrates this.

A right-handed tennis player complains of chronic right-side low back pain as he commences serving. In this position his low lumbar spine is extended, laterally flexed, and rotated to the right. Examination confirms that this combined position reproduces his pain and testing of intervertebral movement reveals hypomobility at the L5-S1 joint.

An effective treatment would consist of placing his low lumbar spine into this combined position and then passively stretching one of these movements, carefully localizing the movement to the L5-S1 joint.

Two other important aspects of the patient's symptoms are the severity of the pain and the irritability of the disorder. *Severity* relates to the examiner's interpretation of the severity of the pain based on the patient's description and functional limitations due to the pain. *Irritability* (or touchiness) of the disorder is based on three things:

1. How much activity the patient can perform before being stopped by pain.
2. The degree and distribution of pain provoked by that activity.

3. How long the pain takes to subside to its original level. (This is the most informative part and serves as a guide to the probable response of the symptoms to examination and treatment.)

In the previous example of the tennis player, a nonirritable disorder would be one in which he experiences momentary pain each time he serves (in this case the treatment described previously would be applicable). In contrast to this, an irritable disorder would be one in which his back pain lasts for several minutes after serving a ball and this pain summates to the extent that after 20 serves his back is so painful that he cannot continue to play and has to rest for one hour to ease his pain. In this example, a technique that reproduced his symptoms would not be the initial choice of treatment but rather his lumbar spine would be positioned in the most comfortable position and a technique performed which was pain free.

Signs

Signs refer to physical examination findings. Physical examination tests are used to incriminate or exclude certain structures as the source of a patient's symptoms. In particular, the tests determine the involvement of the intervertebral joints and neuromeningeal tissues and whether conduction of the spinal cord and cauda equina is altered. They help indicate the degree of irritability of the disorder and demonstrate whether symptoms have a stretch or compression component.

The physical examination of movements includes three sections. These are examination of:

1. The gross physiologic movements of the lumbar spine (flexion, extension, lateral flexion, and rotation). It may be necessary to examine these movements in different combinations and in varied sequences, to sustain these positions or to perform them with distraction or compression.

2. Passive physiologic and accessory movements at each intervertebral segment.

3. The neuromeningeal tissues in the vertebral and foraminal canals (using SLR, PNF, PKF, and the Slump test).

Reaching a diagnosis of a mechanical disorder of the neuromusculoskeletal tissues is important, that is, to isolate the structures at fault by knowing the symptom distribution and the response to physical tests. Knowledge of the movements that increase or decrease the symptom response are the main determinants of how to apply passive movement in treatment (not the diagnostic title *per se*).

Selection Based on the Effects of the Technique

Mobilization/Manipulation

Passive movement as a treatment technique can be broadly divided into its use as mobilization (passive oscillatory movements) or manipulation (small amplitude thrust/stretch performed at speed at the limit of a range of movement).

Mobilization is the method of choice for most lumbar conditions because it can be used as a treatment for pain or for restoring movement in a hypomobile joint. It can be adapted to suit the severity of the pain, the irritability of the disorder, and the stages and stability of the pathology.

Manipulation is the treatment of choice when an intervertebral joint is locked. To regain mobility in cases of an irritable joint condition, a single manipulation may be less aggravating than repeated stretching by mobilization.

Position of the Intervertebral (IV) Joint and the Direction of the Movement Technique

Treatment by passive movement involves careful positioning of the particular intervertebral segment and the selection of the most effective direction of movement. These are based on a knowledge of spinal biomechanics and the desired symptom response.

Manipulation. This type of therapeutic technique is applied in the direction of limitation in order to stretch the tissues in that particular direction. For example, using biomechanical principles, the lumbar spine can be positioned (in lateral flexion and contralateral rotation) to isolate movement to the desired intervertebral segment and a rotary thrust applied in the appropriate direction.

Passive Mobilization. When using this technique both the position of the IV joint and the direction of movement are varied according to the desired effect of the technique. Some examples are given below.

In order *to avoid any discomfort or pain*: In cases where the pain is severe or the disorder is irritable, the symptoms should not be provoked or aggravated. The lumbar spine would be positioned so that the painful intervertebral segment was painfree and the movement technique performed must also be painfree.

In order *to cause or to avoid reproduction of referred pain*: Provocation of referred pain is safe when that pain is chronic and nonirritable, and when it is not a nerve-root pain. In these cases it may be necessary to cause some leg pain to gain improvement thus the spine is positioned to either provoke some symptoms or to enable the treatment technique to provoke the referred symptoms. Findings indicating nerve-root pain (i.e., pain worse distally and the presence of neurologic changes) in particular, when the examination of movements reproduces the distal pain, should warn the clinician against using a technique that provoked the referred pain.

In order *to open one side of the intervertebral joint* (i.e., to stretch the disc, distract the zygapophyseal joint, and widen the foraminal canal on one side): This would be the choice in cases of nerve-root irritation/compression or in cases of a progressive unilateral disc disorder. For example, to widen the right side of the L4-5 intervertebral space, the spine would be positioned in the combined position of flexion, lateral flexion, and rotation to the left. Which of these movements would be emphasized as the treatment technique would depend on the pain response.

In order *to stretch tissues that are contracted.* Joints that are both painful and hypomobile can respond differently to passive mobilization depending to a large extent on the irritability. The pain response during the performance of a technique and its effect over a 24-hour period will guide the clinician in the choice of which direction to move the joint and how firmly to stretch the contracted tissues. A favorable response to gentle oscillatory stretches is that the pain experienced during the technique decreases thus allowing the movement to be performed more strongly. A worsening of the pain response indicates that this direction of movement is aggravating the condition.

In order *to move the IV joints or the canal structures.* During the physical examination, if movements of the IV joints and of the neuromeningeal structures in the canal both reproduce the patient's leg pain, a technique directed at altering the IV joint movements should be the first choice of treatment. The effect on the IV joint signs and the canal signs is noted and if the latter are not improving, movement of the neuromeningeal tissues is added or substituted. In cases of only back and/or buttock pain and where the canal tests more effectively reproduce this pain, then the first choice would be to use movement of the canal structures (e.g., passive neck flexion, straight leg raising, prone knee flexion, or the Slump test).

The Manner in Which the Movement Technique Is Performed

Selection of a treatment technique does not merely relate to the direction of movement but also to the manner in which it is applied. The amplitude can be varied from a barely perceptible movement to one that makes use of the total available range. The rhythm can be varied from a smooth evenly applied movement to one that is staccato. Similarly, the speed and the position in range in which the movement is performed can be altered.

Passive movement techniques must be modified according to the intention of the technique and this is based on the symptoms experienced by the patient during the technique, the quality of the movement, the presence of spasm and the end feel. It is not possible to discuss these details in any depth in this chapter, but only to present the two ends of the symptom spectrum that ranges from a constant ache with pain experienced through range to stiffness with mild discomfort felt only at the end of range of certain movements as presented below. For a full description see Maitland.[10]

Constant Aching with Pain through Range. The lumbar spine must be placed in a position of maximal comfort (usually one of slight flexion and mid-position for the other movements). The treatment technique will be of small amplitude, performed slowly and smoothly (so that there is no discomfort produced or where discomfort is constant, no increase in the level of the aching). The movement technique may be a physiologic or an accessory movement, and its performance should result in an immediate lessening of the level of aching. In some patients there may be an immediate effect, but in others the effect should be noted over a 24-hour period.

Stiffness with Mild Discomfort Felt Only at the End of Range of Certain Movements. The lumbar spine is carefully positioned at or near the limit of the stiff directions of movement (i.e., in the position that best reproduces the stiffness and discomfort). The treatment technique will be one that places maximal stretch on the hypomobile IV segment. The technique should be firmly applied, of small amplitude, and either sustained or staccato in rhythm. Should the level of discomfort increase with the firm stretching, large amplitude movements can be interspersed every 40 to 60 seconds.

LOW LUMBAR SYNDROMES

In this section some of the common syndromes with a history of spontaneous onset of symptoms will be presented. Management is restricted to treatment by passive movement. The syndromes are presented as case histories.

Acute Back Pain (Discogenic)

History

A 35-year-old man experienced a mild central low backache after pushing a car one morning. This ache intensified during a 40 minute drive to work, and he was unable to get out of the car unaided due to severe low back pain. He had no previous history of backache and radiographs of his lumbosacral region were reported as being normal. After two days in bed without any improvement in his symptoms, manipulative therapy was requested by his doctor.

Symptoms

There was a constant dull backache centered over the L4-5 region. The patient was unable to move in bed due to sharp jabs of pain. His most comfortable position was supine with his hips and knees flexed over two pillows in crook lying or side lying with his legs (and lumbar spine) flexed.

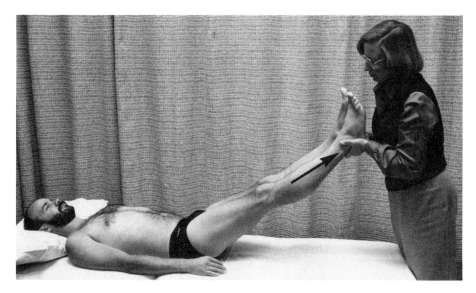

Fig. 8-1. Longitudinal caudad mobilization of the lower lumbar spine is shown, produced by manual traction to the lower limbs.

Physical Signs

The patient was examined supine. SLR was almost full range as was PNF, but both tests slightly increased his back pain. Spreading and compression of the ilia were pain free and there was no abnormality in lower limb reflexes or sensation (testing muscle strength was impossible due to back pain).

Interpretation

The history suggests discogenic pain—pushing a heavy car would raise intradiscal pressure—with pain worsened by sitting followed by inability to extend the spine. The physical examination was too restricted by pain to be helpful in confirming the source of his symptoms.

Treatment

Day 1 (Treatment 1). As SLR was of good range, both legs were comfortably flexed at the hips to 50 degrees and gentle manual traction was applied by pulling on his legs (Fig. 8-1). During traction his backache decreased. A series of four gentle but sharp tugs were applied to his legs. With each tug, a jab of back pain was experienced but there was no increase in his constant backache. On reassessment, PNF was full and painless but SLR remained unchanged. The treatment was repeated resulting in a slight improvement in his SLR on both sides and in his range of lumbar rotations performed in supine.

Day 2 (Treatment 2).   The patient reported greater freedom of movements in bed and had been out of bed twice for a hot shower. Examination of his lumbar mobility in standing showed marked limitation of flexion by pain centered over L5 and there was obvious spasm in his erector spinae. Extension was half range and he had a full range of lateral flexion to each side. Bilateral SLR was full and painless.

Manual traction effected no change in his mobility so he was placed in a prone position with two pillows under his abdomen. From this position of comfort, he was asked to gently passively extend his spine using a modified push-up technique.[16] This technique was repeated 10 times, sustaining the position for 5 seconds. The patient was encouraged to extend his lumbar spine to his comfortable limit. However particular care was taken to avoid development of a backache. On reassessment in standing, flexion had improved so that he could reach finger tips to his patellae and extension was three-quarters of usual range.

The technique was repeated but this time lying over only one pillow. Following two more applications the patient could lie comfortably prone, without a pillow and in weight bearing there was a further slight increase in his ranges of flexion and extension.

The patient was asked to repeat this technique hourly (three lots of 10 push ups at the end of which he allowed his back to sag into sustained extension for 1 minute providing that there was no reproduction of backache). He was allowed out of bed for short periods but was to avoid sitting.

Day 3 (Treatment 3).   The patient was pain free moving in bed and could be ambulant for more than one hour before his ache returned. His range of flexion was such that he was able to reach his fingertips to midshin level (normally he could reach his ankles) and to fully extend his lumbar spine with only a mild ache.

The extension push ups were repeated with the manipulative therapist stabilizing his pelvis flat on the floor. As this was pain free, the patient was asked to sustain the position allowing his lumbar spine to sag fully into extension. In this extended position, gentle posteroanterior pressures were applied to L5 taking care to cause only mild discomfort. On resuming the flat prone position, sharp deep pain was felt over L5 but this quickly subsided with repeated gentle extension.

The above regime was repeated prior to reassessing his mobility in standing. Flexion and extension were now full range. Gentle overpressure to extension reproduced the same deep sharp pain.

Days 4, 6, and 10 (Treatments 4, 5, and 6).   Subsequent treatments were conducted at the manipulative therapist's clinic and consisted of restoration of full pain free range of lumbar extension using posteroanterior pressures on L5 with his lumbar spine in extension. By Day 6 the patient was symptom free, but experienced a deep ache with firm sustained posteroanterior pressure on

L5. When seen four days later, no pain could be elicited by sustained or staccato posteroanterior oscillatory movement.

The patient was discharged with advice regarding lifting and care of his back during sustained postures (especially flexion).

Severe Nerve-Root Pain

History

A 35-year-old young man had suffered from recurrent attacks of low back pain over the last five years. These were associated with lifting strains. This present episode commenced four days ago when he bent to move the garden hose. He experienced only mild aching in his low back but over the next few hours his back pain disappeared and he felt strong pain in his left buttock and calf. His calf pain had worsened in the last 24 hours and spread into his left foot.

Symptoms

The patient had constant severe pain in the lateral aspect of his left calf and foot and numbness of lateral aspect of his left foot. Less severe aching was experienced in his left buttock. Weight bearing and sitting aggravated his back and calf pain, and coughing aggravated his back pain. He could gain some relief of symptoms by lying on his right side with his legs (and lumbar spine) flexed.

Signs

The following movements aggravated his buttock and calf/foot pain: flexion to touch his patellae, left lateral flexion half range, and left SLR limited to 25 degrees. Neurologic examination revealed a reduced left ankle jerk, reduced sensation over the lateral border of foot, and weak toe flexors (unable to test calf power due to pain on weight bearing).

Interpretation of Findings

Evidence of S1 nerve-root compression. The history of a trivial incident causing this episode and the presence of worsening symptoms indicate that the disorder is both unstable and progressive requiring care with treatment so as not to worsen the condition.

Treatment

Day 1 (Treatment 1). In position of ease (i.e., lying on right side with lumbar spine comfortably flexed) the pelvis was gently rotated to the right taking care not to aggravate calf/foot or buttock pain. The technique was performed as far as possible into range without aggravating symptoms; SLR was used as reassessment. After two applications of rotation, flexion was also reassessed. The patient reported easing of his calf symptoms and both flexion and left SLR had minimally improved however extension range remained unaltered.

The patient was advised to rest in bed as much as possible and to avoid sitting.

Day 2 (Treatment 2). Patient reported that his symptoms were unchanged and his physical signs were found to be unaltered.

Rotary mobilization was repeated (as on Day 1) with a similar response.

Day 3 (Treatment 3). No alteration in symptoms or signs.

Lumbar traction was given (15 lb for 10 minutes). During traction his calf/foot pain was eased and afterwards his SLR improved by 10 degrees.

Day 4 (Treatment 4). Definite reduction in calf/foot pain and improvement in all physical signs.

Traction was repeated (15 lb for 20 minutes). At subsequent treatments both the time and the strength of the traction were increased.

Day 10 (Treatment 8). No leg symptoms, but buttock pain was experienced with prolonged sitting. Physical examination revealed full recovery of neurologic function. The extreme range of flexion, with the addition of neck flexion reproduced buttock pain, the other spinal movements were full range and pain free. On passive over pressure, left SLR lacked 20 degrees and also reproduced left buttock pain.

Interpretation of Findings

At this stage, spinal mobility was full and painless but movement of the neuromeningeal tissues was restricted and reproduced the patient's only remaining symptom. A gentle technique to stretch the neuromeningeal tissues should be used but if reproduction of nerve-root symptoms occurred it would contraindicate its use at this stage.

Treatment 8 (continued). A gentle stretch was applied to left SLR causing only buttock pain. Following this, flexion plus neck flexion were pain free.

Day 12 (Treatment 9). The patient was now symptom free, but left SLR still caused buttock pain at 75 degrees.

Interpretation

In view of the progressive disorder, despite an excellent response to treatment, a decision not to stretch his SLR more firmly was taken but to review him in two weeks.

When seen two weeks later he had remained symptom free but his left SLR had not improved. Now that his disorder was stable, his SLR was strongly stretched, restoring full range with no return of symptoms.

Chronic Nerve-Root Aching

This may present as either, (a) residual symptoms from an acute episode of nerve root pain; or (b) chronic aching (not pain) with signs of nerve-root compression.

In both cases, the condition is nonirritable and does not restrict the patients' activities, however as most low-lumbar nerve-root problems are of discogenic origin, sitting causes an increase in leg symptoms. The disorder is stable and permits stronger techniques to be applied safely. The following case history illustrates the second type.

History

A 40-year-old housewife presented with a past history of recurrent low back pain for seven years. One year ago she noticed a dull ache in her left leg. At that time, two or three treatments of passive mobilization completely relieved her symptoms. The current episode began three weeks previously following paving the garden path with bricks. While stooping to lay the bricks she was conscious of aching in her buttock and down the posterior aspect of her left leg. The common treatment of rotary mobilization had not helped.

Symptoms

A constant dull ache spread from her left sacroiliac area, down the posterior aspect of her buttock to the heel, together with paresthesia of the lateral aspect of her foot. The ache in her calf and the paresthesia were worsened if she sustained a flexed posture (vacuuming carpets, etc.) for more than 30 minutes or sat for more than 60 minutes.

Physical Signs

There was a full range of pain-free spinal movements, even when these were sustained. Poor intervertebral movement was noted below L3 on extension and on left lateral flexion. By adding left lateral flexion to the fully extended position, buttock aching was reproduced. The addition of left and right rotation made no change to the symptoms. Testing of intervertebral movement confirmed stiffness at both L4-5 and L5-S1 motion segments and posteroanterior pressure over L5 (performed with her spine in extension/left lateral flexion) caused buttock pain.

Tests for the neuromeningeal tissues revealed full SLR but the left leg had a tighter end feel, and the Slump test was positive (i.e., left knee extension lacked 30 degrees and caused calf pain, which was eased by releasing cervical flexion). She had slight weakness of her left calf, but otherwise showed no neurologic deficit.

Interpretation

The history implicated a disc disorder that was slowly progressing to interfere with nerve-root function. The disorder was stable in that she could continue with her daily activities as a housewife. Treatment to change both her IV joint signs and neuromeningeal signs was necessary, using techniques that temporarily aggravated her leg ache. Treating the IV joint hypomobility first was safer, while observing its effect on both the joint and neuromeningeal signs.

Treatment

Day 1 (Treatment 1). With her low lumbar spine positioned in extension/left lateral flexion, firm posteroanterior pressures were applied to L4 and L5 spinous processes for 60 to 90 seconds causing local pain and a mild increase in left buttock aching (Fig. 8-2). On reassessment, lumbar extension/left lateral flexion no longer reproduced an increase in buttock ache and low lumbar mobility had improved. The Slump test had improved (left knee extension improved by 10 degrees). Treatment was repeated with no further gain in mobility.

Day 3 (Treatment 2). The patient reported no ill effects from treatment, but a lessening of her left leg aching. Physical examination showed that she had maintained the improvement gained on Day 1. Neurologic function was unchanged. The above treatment was repeated even more strongly and sustained to stretch the tightened tissues. The reproduction of only local pain (no referred buttock pain) supported the safety of using a strong stretch. The result of this stretch was that extension/left lateral flexion was painful only when sustained, and in the slump position, knee extension improved by another 10 degrees. Repeating the technique twice gained no further change to the Slump test.

Day 5 (Treatment 3). The patient was delighted with her progress. She no longer had a constant ache down her left leg. The ache returned only if she sat for more than one hour. On examination, her left calf had regained full strength; left SLR was no longer tighter than on the right, however, in the

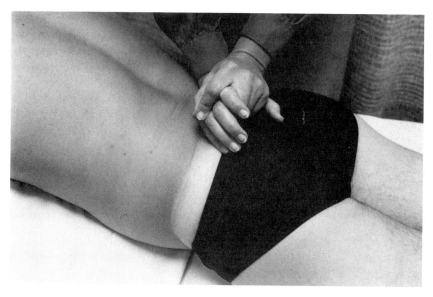

Fig. 8-2.   Posteroanterior pressures on L5 with the lumbar spine positioned in extension/left lateral flexion.

slump position, left knee extension still lacked 10 degrees and caused buttock pain.

Treatment was changed to restore mobility in the neuromeningeal tissues. In the slump position, her left knee was stretched into full extension causing sharp buttock pain (Fig. 8-3). This technique was not repeated until its effect on nerve-root conduction was known. This can only be assessed over 24 to 48 hours.

Day 7 (Treatment 4).   There was no return of symptoms following the last treatment. Her calf strength and ankle reflex were normal. In the slump position, knee extension still reproduced sharp buttock pain. The stretch to the neuromeningeal tissues was increased by stretching the knee into full extension and stretching the ankle into full dorsiflexion in the slump position. This again caused sharp buttock pain. Reassessment of knee extension in the slump position showed it to be full range with minimal buttock pain. The technique was repeated once more. The patient was asked to experiment with activities such as sustained flexion and sitting for long periods during the next week.

Day 14 (Treatment 5).   The patient reported that she experienced no leg symptoms but that her back ached after activities involving sustained flexion for more than 45 minutes and after sitting more than 90 minutes. She considered that this was better than she had been for several years. Examination of the Slump test revealed full mobility, but caused slight buttock pain.

The patient was discharged with a home exercise program to maintain the mobility of both her lower lumbar spine and her neuromeningeal tissues.

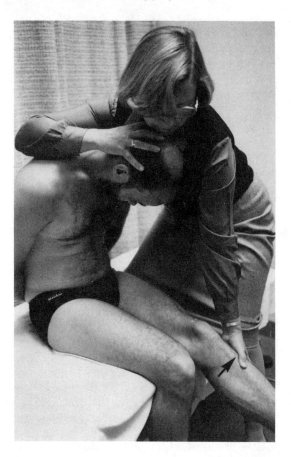

Fig. 8-3. Passive extension of the left knee done while in the slump position.

Mechanical Locking

History

A 20-year-old man complained of a sudden onset of unilateral back pain, which prevented him from standing upright. He had bent forward quickly to catch a ball near his left foot and he was unable to straighten because of sharp back pain. He had no past history of back pain and no spinal radiographs had been taken.

Symptoms

There was no pain when his back was held in slight flexion but on standing upright, pain was experienced to the right of the L5 spinous process.

Physical Signs

He was prevented by pain from extending, laterally flexing, or rotating his low lumbar spine to the right. The other movements were full and painless. Passive testing of intersegmental movement revealed an inability to produce the above painful movements at L4-5 with marked spasm on attempting to do so. Unilateral posteroanterior pressures over the right L4-5 zygapophyseal joint produced marked pain and spasm.

Interpretation

A quick movement in flexion/left lateral flexion gaps the right lumbar zygapophyseal joints following which there is mechanical blocking of the movements that normally appose the articular surfaces (extension, lateral flexion, and rotation of the trunk to the right). The mechanism of mechanical locking is still a contentious issue.[17-19]

A manipulation, localized to the affected intervertebral level, to gap in this case the right L4-5 zygapophyseal joint, will restore normal joint function.

Treatment

A rotary manipulation was performed to gap the right L4-5 zygapophyseal joint. The patient was positioned on his left side with his low lumbar spine flexed and laterally flexed to the right until movement could be palpated at the L4-5 intervertebral level (Fig. 8-4). In this position, with thumb pressure against the right side of the spinous process of L4 (to stabilize L4) a quick left rotary thrust was applied through the pelvis and to L5 by finger pressure against the left side of L5 spinous process (to pull L5 into left rotation).

Immediately afterwards the patient could fully extend, laterally flex, and rotate his trunk to the right with only soreness experienced at the extreme of these movements. This soreness was lessened by gentle large amplitude posteroanterior pressures performed unilaterally over the right L4-5 zygapophyseal joint.

Zygapophyseal Joint Arthropathy (Causing Only Referred Symptoms)

History

A 50-year-old man described a gradual onset, over three days, of aching in the right trochanteric area. This had been present for one month. He could not recall any injury to his back, hip, or leg, and he had not experienced pain in any other area. He had no past history of back or leg symptoms.

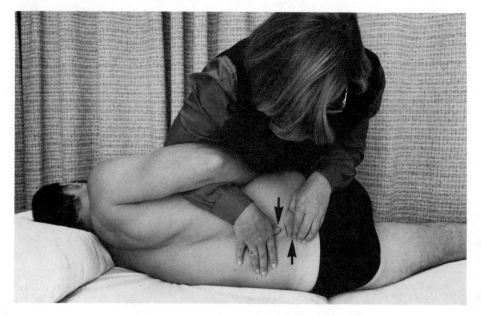

Fig. 8-4.   Rotary manipulation is used to open the right L4-5 zygapophyseal joint.

Radiographs of the lumbar spine and hip were reported to be normal. He was diagnosed by the referring doctor as suffering from trochanteric bursitis.

Symptoms

He experienced a constant deep ache over his right greater trochanter, which was unaltered by posture or activity.

Physical Signs

Lumbar movements were full and pain free with over pressure. Tests for the neuromeningeal tissues, hip, and trochanteric bursitis were negative.

Deep palpation (through the erector spinae) over the right L4-5 zygapophyseal joint revealed stiffness, local spasm, and tenderness and there was an area of thickening at the right side of the interspinous space between L4 and L5. These signs were absent on the left side. Reproduction of referred pain was not possible.

Interpretation

Anatomically, pathology of the L4-5 zygapophyseal joint could give rise to referred pain at the trochanteric area. In the absence of other physical signs, it would be appropriate to mobilize the hypomobile L4-5 zygapophyseal joint and note any effect on his trochanteric aching. An association between the hypomobile L4-5 zygapophyseal joint and the trochanteric pain can be made only in retrospect.

Treatment

The hypomobility was localized to the L4-5 right zygapophyseal joint, therefore passive stretching could be localized to this joint.

Day 1 (Treatment 1). Posteroanterior oscillatory pressures were applied firmly for 60 seconds to the spinous processes of L4 and L5, and unilaterally over the painful joint. On being questioned, the patient reported no change in his constant trochanteric ache.

Day 2 (Treatment 2). The patient reported that his right trochanteric pain was now intermittent (and continued unrelated to movement or to changes of posture of his trunk). The treatment was repeated giving three applications of posteroanterior pressures lasting 60 seconds each. These were interspersed with gentle large amplitude oscillations to ease the local soreness.

Days 4, 6 and 8 (Treatments 3, 4 and 5). The patient reported continued improvement of his symptoms and the mobilization of L4-5 was progressed in strength and sustained for longer periods to achieve a better stretch on the tight soft tissues (capsule and ligaments). At the last visit, it was necessary to place his lower lumbar spine into full extension and direct the posteroanterior pressures more caudally in order to detect any residual stiffness. By this stage, he experienced only occasional transient aching in his thigh, so treatment was stopped until a review in two weeks.

Day 22 (Treatment 6). When reassessed two weeks later the patient reported that he was symptom free. Passive mobility tests showed no stiffness or thickening of soft tissues on the right of the L4-5 joint.

Zygapophyseal Joint Arthropathy (Intraarticular Problem)

History

A 75-year-old woman complained of a sharp pain to the right of L5 following stepping awkwardly with her right foot into a shallow depression in the pavement one week previously. She had become aware of aching in her back and this worsened with each step until it became constant. As her back was both painful and stiff the following morning, she consulted her doctor. He ordered radiographs to be taken, which revealed narrowing of her lumbosacral disc space and osteoarthritic changes in her lumbosacral zygapophyseal joints. She was given antiinflammatory medication and advised to rest as much as possible. Five days later her pain was no longer constant but certain spinal movements still caused considerable pain and she was referred for manipulative therapy. She had a past history of low backache for many years if she stood for long periods.

Symptoms

Sharp pain just lateral to the spinous process of L5 on the right was provoked by turning in bed from a supine position onto her right side, and when bending to the right when standing.

Physical Signs

All movements of her low lumbar spine were hypomobile. Lumbar extension and lateral flexion to the right reproduced her pain. Pain was experienced at half range, increasing at the limit of these movements.

Palpation of passive accessory movements revealed marked stiffness of L4-5 and L5-S1 segments and posteroanterior pressure and transverse pressure to the left reproduced her back pain. Neuromeningeal tests were negative.

Interpretation

This is an elderly woman with a degenerative, stiff lower lumbar spine. A trivial injury (i.e., a jar up through her right leg) caused the stiff joint to become painful.

This is thought to be an intraarticular problem because pain is experienced with movements that close the right side of the intervertebral joint and because pain is felt early and throughout these movements. Such articular problems respond well to large amplitude passive mobilization, performed carefully to avoid compression of the articular surfaces. Later, when pain is minimal, one may progress to mobilization with the surfaces compressed.

Treatment

Day 1 (Treatment 1). With the patient lying comfortably on her right side in slight flexion, gentle large amplitude left lateral flexion oscillations were produced by moving the pelvis (Fig. 8-5). Care was taken not to cause any discomfort. Following this, extension and right lateral flexion were reassessed. A favorable response was noted in that pain started later in the range of both of these movements. The technique was repeated but no further improvement was noted.

Day 3 (Treatment 2). The patient reported no change in her symptoms but the improvement in the signs gained with the first treatment had been maintained. The Day 1 treatment was repeated twice, following which the pain

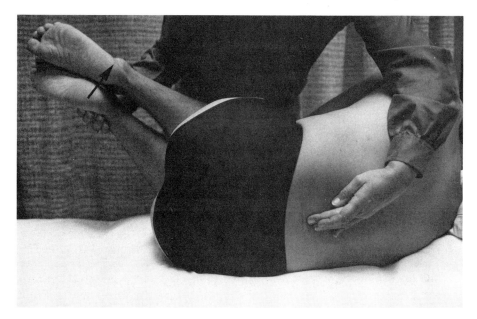

Fig 8-5. Passive left lateral flexion mobilization of the lower lumbar spine is shown, produced by moving the lower limbs and pelvis.

response to right lateral flexion improved, but extension was unchanged. The technique was changed to accessory posteroanterior central pressures to L4 and L5 again employing large amplitude movements. This achieved an immediate improvement in the range of extension and a reduction in the pain response.

Day 5 (Treatment 3). The patient was delighted with her progress in that she had no pain turning in bed and her daily movements were painless. Mild pain was experienced at the limit of both extension and right lateral flexion. By adding extension to right lateral flexion sharp pain was produced.

For treatment, her lumbar spine was placed in the position of slight right lateral flexion combined with extension. In this position, posteroanterior pressures were performed for 30 seconds as a large amplitude movement, causing slight pain at first. During performance of the technique, the pain disappeared, so the spine was placed further into extension and right lateral flexion. Slight pain was again experienced and again this disappeared with another application of the mobilization. On reassessment, combined right lateral flexion with extension was pain free. Slight pain was experienced only on over pressure.

Day 7 (Treatment 4). The patient was still symptom free and right lateral flexion with extension was no longer painful when performed with over pressure. However, when right lateral flexion was added to extension, slight pain was experienced.

The spine was placed in this combined position in the same order (full extension and then full right lateral flexion) and posteroanterior central pressures performed as a strong stretching technique. This caused marked pain and required gentle large amplitude posteroanterior pressures to ease the soreness. Following this the patient complained of aching across her lower lumbar area. Pulsed short wave diathermy for 15 minutes (on a low frequency and low dosage) eased her ache.

Days 10 and 24 (Treatments 5 and 6). The patient remained symptom free but extension plus right lateral flexion still reproduced slight pain to the right of L5. By combining these movements on the left side, a similar pain was produced. This was considered likely to be her normal response and no further treatment was given. This was verified by finding the same signs two weeks later during which time she had remained symptom free.

Postural Pain

History

A 28-year-old mother of three children presented with a six-month history of gradual onset of low back pain. She could not recall an incident that had caused her symptoms. During her third pregnancy two years ago, she had experienced the same pain but this had settled after the birth. There was no history of trauma and her radiographs were reported to be normal.

Symptoms

She was asymptomatic in the morning but by midafternoon her low back began to ache. This ache worsened as the day progressed especially during activities requiring her lumbar spine to be held in sustained flexion (bathing children, making beds, sweeping, vacuuming) and when lifting the children. Sitting and lying eased the pain.

Physical Signs

She stood with an increased lumbar lordosis; she had a full range of painfree movements. Over pressure into full extension was painful and by combining this with lateral flexion to either side the pain was made worse on each side. Testing of intervertebral movements revealed excellent mobility with the exception of posteroanterior gliding of L5 on the sacrum, which was slightly stiff. Tests for the neuromeningeal tissues were normal. Her lower abdominal and her gluteal muscles were slack and weak.

Interpretation

This is a young, mobile spine that became painful when the tissues restraining flexion were stressed (posterior ligamentous structures and zygapophyseal joints). There was poor support by the abdominal muscles, which co-

contract with the erector spinae and gluteals to stabilize the spine during flexion. Pain was relieved by rest (when stress was taken off the painful tissues).

Treatment

Day 1 (Treatment 1). Explanation of the cause of the symptoms, and stress on the need to strengthen the lower abdominals, the gluteals, and erector spinae. Large amplitude accessory posteroanterior mobilization of her L5-S1 joint to restore her normal mobility at this segment will help this joint to become pain free, but the primary objective is to strengthen abdominal, gluteal, and erector spinae muscle groups. This was complemented by postural correction (pelvic tilting) and by giving advice on correct lifting techniques and how to restore the lumbar lordosis after periods of sustained flexion (discussed in more detail in other chapters).

Day 5 (Treatment 2). The patient was seen again to check that she was performing her exercises correctly and regularly. As her strength improved the exercises were progressively increased in difficulty. Her lumbosacral joint was again mobilized. She reported no change in her symptoms. She was urged to continue her exercises regularly.

Day 21 (Treatment 3). The patient reported that she was virtually symptom free, experiencing slight aching if she were excessively busy and tired. On examination, lumbar extension combined with lateral flexion to each side was full and painless, as was posteroanterior accessory gliding of L5. The patient was discharged with the advice to maintain good muscle support of her spine by regular exercise.

Conclusion

Most lumbar dysfunctions have a mechanical component that responds well to carefully applied manipulative therapy. Manipulative therapy is safe, effective, and an important part in the overall management of patients with these conditions. However, the decision to apply manipulative therapy must be based on a thorough examination, sound judgement on which techniques to select, and repeated reassessment of the effects of these techniques if the optimal effect is to be achieved.

REFERENCES

1. Bogduk N, Tynan W, Wilson AS: The nerve supply to the human lumbar intervertebral discs. J Anat 132:39, 1981
2. Bogduk N: The innervation of the lumbar spine. Spine 8:286, 1983
3. Cyriax J: Dural pain. Lancet 1:919, 1978

4. Wyke B: Neurological aspects of low back pain. p. 189. In Jayson MIV (ed): The Lumbar Spine and Back Pain. Sector, New York, 1976

5. Kimmel D: Innervation of the spinal dural mater and dura mater of the posterior cranial fossa. Neurology 10:800, 1961

6. El Mahdi MA, Latif FYA, Janko M: The spinal nerve root innervation and a new concept of the clinicopathological interrelations in back pain and sciatica. Neurochirurgia 24:137, 1981

7. Pedersen HE, Blunck CFJ, Gardner E: The anatomy of lumbo-sacral posterior rami and meningeal branches of spinal nerves (sinu-vertebral nerves). J Bone Joint Surg 38A:377, 1956

8. Simmons FH, Segil CM: An evaluation of discography in the localization of symptomatic levels in discogenic disease of the spine. Clin Orthop 108:57, 1975

9. Grieve GP: Common Vertebral Joint Problems. p. 144. Churchill Livingstone, London, 1981

10. Maitland GD: Vertebral Manipulation. 5th Ed. Butterworth, London, 1986

11. Mooney V, Robertson J: The facet syndrome. Clin Orth 115:149, 1976

12. McCall IW, Park WM, O'Brien JP: Induced pain referral from posterior lumbar elements in normal subjects. Spine 4:441, 1979

13. Edgar MA, Nundy S: Innervation of the spinal dura mater. J Neurol Neurosurg Psychiatry 29:530, 1966

14. Edgar MA, Park WM: Induced pain patterns on passive straight-leg-raising in lower lumbar disc protrusion, J Bone Joint Surg 56B:658, 1974

15. Cyriax J: Textbook of Orthopaedic Medicine. 7th Ed. Vol 1. Ballière Tindall, London, 1978

16. McKenzie RA: The Lumbar Spine. Mechanical Diagnosis and Therapy. Spinal Publications, Waikanae, New Zealand, 1981

17. Kos J, Wolf J: Les menisques intervertebraux et leur rôle possible dans les blocages vertebraux. Ann Med Phys 15:203, 1972

18. Bogduk N, Jull G: The theoretical pathology of acute locked back: a basis for manipulative therapy. Man Med 1:78, 1985

19. Twomey LT, Taylor JR: The lumbar facet joints: a study of age changes and degeneration. p. 116. In Proceedings of Fourth Biennial Conference Manipulative Therapists Association of Australia, Brisbane, 1985

9 | An Interpretation of the McKenzie Approach to Low Back Pain

Mark J. Oliver
James W. Lynn
Jennifer M. Lynn

In this chapter, we will present an outline of the clinical approach to low back pain developed by Robin McKenzie. Several aspects are unique and will be described in some detail. The main features of the McKenzie approach are:

1. A method using repeated movements to classify subgroups in the non-specific spectrum of low back pain
2. The use of the phenomenon of pain centralization
3. Patient self treatment
4. A comprehensive management of low back pain

Special questions relating to contraindications or caution, neurologic examination, and special tests for specific structures are not discussed. These are a vital part of patient examination, but they are not within the scope of this chapter. It is not our intention to give a detailed clinical guideline for patient treatment, this is available from other sources.[1,2] Principles of treatment are discussed, but techniques are not described.

Despite uncertainty about mechanisms responsible for production of recurrent low back pain, a pathologic concept is useful to enable the clinician to visualize the behavior of signs and symptoms when treating patients. Problems only arise when unproven theoretical concepts come to be regarded as factual dogma. McKenzie has hypothesized that the intervertebral disc is responsible for the majority of low back pain symptoms and signs. Whether McKenzie is subsequently proved right or wrong, his principles for syndrome classification and treatment remain valid. The protocol is not dependent on a pathologic concept.

> Only time and much research will reveal the true nature of the mechanism responsible for the production of recurrent low back pain, but the influence of these procedures on that mechanism will be just as effective in fifty years time as they are today.[2]

PATIENT SELECTION

Nachemson[4] describes the common pain syndromes in the low back:

> Acute, sub-acute or chronic low back pain, which is characterised by either a slowly or suddenly occurring rather sharp pain with or without radiation over the buttocks or slightly down the leg, and concomitant restriction of motion. When subsiding to the chronic type, the pain will be a little less severe and continue for more than two months.

These constitute the nonspecific low back pain group and are suitable for treatment by the McKenzie protocol.

McKenzie[2] also includes patients who have intermittent sciatica without neurologic deficit. In other words, there must be times in the day when the patient feels neither sciatic pain nor paresthesia. If there is no position or movement that reduces or centralizes pain, it is unlikely that the patient will respond to mechanical therapy. Patients with true constant severe sciatica and neurologic deficit are unsuited to any mechanical procedure other than perhaps traction according to McKenzie. These patients should be reassessed at a later stage because if symptoms change, mechanical therapy may become appropriate.

MECHANISMS OF PAIN PRODUCTION

In order to clearly describe McKenzie's classification of mechanical pain, some very simple aspects of pain production are outlined.

Wyke[3] states that there are only two possible causes of pain:

1. Normally, the nociceptive receptor system is relatively inactive, but its afferent activity is markedly increased when constituent unmyelinated fibers are depolarized. Pain may be caused by the exposure of unmyelinated fibers to sufficient concentrations of irritating chemical substances in the surrounding tissue fluid. This will occur during infective or inflammatory processes and following trauma.

2. Pain may also be caused by application of mechanical forces suffi to stress, deform, or damage the containing tissue. These include pres: distraction, distension, abrasion, contusion, or laceration. Pain may be voked without damage to tissue and McKenzie uses a bent finger as a sin example of mechanical articular pain.[2] The finger is passively hyperextended until pain is produced, indicating enhanced nociceptive activity. If the force is increased, pain will intensify and eventually become more diffuse and difficult to define, demonstrating how pain alters in response to increased and prolonged mechanical deformation. When the force is removed all pain ceases. All normal joints behave in this way, and those in the lumbar spine are no exception.

THE McKENZIE APPROACH

The McKenzie approach uses pain behavior and its relationship to movements and positions to determine appropriate physical treatment. Interpretation of subjective and objective findings permits classification of the nonspecific spectrum of low back pain into syndromes. Each syndrome is deliberately broad in terms of pathology, but is specific in terms of clinical behavior. Because it is rarely possible to determine which tissue is responsible for the presenting signs and symptoms, no attempt is made to be tissue specific. It is possible, however, to be specific about types of clinical behavior.

McKenzie has classified mechanical pain into three syndromes: posture syndrome, dysfunction syndrome, and derangement syndrome. They are different from each other in terms of presentation and pain behavior, but frequently coexist. These syndromes are defined later in this chapter. Treatment for each syndrome is specific and the techniques utilized for one may be inappropriate or inadequate for the other two. Wherever possible, patients are encouraged to accept responsibility for their own treatment. Emphasis is placed on patient self-mobilization and prophylaxis.

Considerable effort has been made to keep the basis for the concepts and the terminology of this approach within the framework of orthopedic medicine. The reasons for this are:

1. To make aspects of this approach freely open to scientific evaluation
2. To avoid the formation of yet another body of dogma
3. To ensure that the approach is easily comprehended by all groups involved in the treatment of spinal pain

It has been necessary to redefine or modify some existing terminology because phenomena observed could not be adequately described with existing terms. Because it is well recognized that ambiguities in the use of terminology often lead to misunderstandings, we will clearly define the following terms as they are used in this approach.

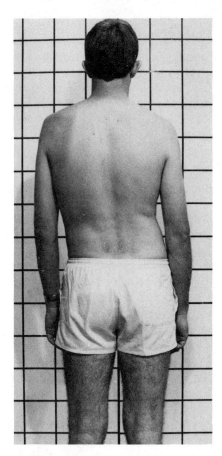

Fig. 9-1. A lumbar lateral shift to the left.

Definitions

Lateral Shift

A lateral shift refers to a lateral displacement of the trunk in relation to the pelvis. It is also called a lumbar scoliosis, or in the presence of symptoms attributed to involvement of the sciatic nerve, a sciatic scoliosis. A left lateral shift denotes displacement of the trunk to the left in relation to the pelvis (Fig. 9-1).

Side Glide

Side gliding is a movement of the lumbar spine combining lateral flexion and rotation in the coronal plane. The patient is instructed to keep the shoulders parallel to the floor when the movement is performed. It is used as an examination and treatment procedure. Figure 9-4 illustrates testing of left side gliding in standing.

Centralization and Peripheralization

In 1961, on retrospective examination of case histories, McKenzie found that patients who responded rapidly to treatment experienced a centralization of pain as improvement took place (personal communication). He called this the centralization phenomenon, and has defined it as, "the situation in which pain arising from the spine and felt laterally from the midline or distally, is reduced and transferred to a more central or near midline position when certain movements are performed. It is permissible for pain to *increase centrally* provided there is a *reduction* in the *lateral or distal* pain."[2]

Centralization of symptoms only occurs in the derangement syndrome. This phenomenon is very reliable for determining which movements reduce mechanical deformation and consequently reduce derangements.[5] Other movements, usually the opposite to those centralizing the pain, will cause peripheralization of symptoms and indicate that mechanical deformation and the derangement are being increased.

Clinically this phenomenon is reliable and repeatable, but to date scientific studies have not investigated its mechanism. From his clinical observations, McKenzie believes that changes in the intervertebral disc are responsible for centralization and peripheralization of symptoms.

Reduce

The definition of reduce according to Dorland's Medical Dictionary is, "to restore to the normal place or relation of parts, as, to *reduce* a fracture."[6] In the context of this approach the term refers to the restoration of normal joint mechanics and function in the derangement syndrome.

Deviation

This term refers to movement of the spine away from the normal movement pathways.

Deformity

Blakiston's Gould Medical Dictionary defines deformity as, "marked deviation from the normal in size or shape of the body or of a part."[7] This term is used by McKenzie in the same way as it used by Charnley[8] who described an acute flattening as a primary deformity of the lumbar spine, probably resulting directly from altered disc mechanics.

Adherent Nerve

Occasionally, referred leg pain or sciatica, presenting with nerve tension signs, may occur as part of the dysfunction syndrome. In this situation, it is possible to be reasonably certain that neural tissue is involved. The symptoms and signs suggest the presence of an adherent nerve root such as those observed on dissection or during surgery.[9–15] It is also referred to as nerve root adhesions[14] or tethering of the nerve root.[15] A postmortem study of several patients with a known history of sciatic pain before death showed dense adhesions between lumbosacral nerves and periosteum at points considerably removed from the spinal canal[13] and these would also present as an adherent nerve. An adherent nerve can be differentiated from the referred pain of the derangement syndrome by the history and by the examination of repeated movements.

Nerve adherence may be a sequela of low back surgery,[15,16] derangement, or trauma. MacNab[15] states that repeated surgical exploration, ". . . inevitably increases scarring with resultant tethering of the nerve root."

SYNDROME CLASSIFICATION OF NONSPECIFIC LOW BACK PAIN

McKenzie has classified nonspecific low back pain into three clinically identifiable syndromes, facilitating the appropriate selection of physical treatment. If a patient's clinical presentation can be classified into one of the syndromes it can be effectively treated by the McKenzie protocol (Fig. 9-2).

Conclusions are drawn from the subjective and objective examination findings. Where pain is found to behave mechanically, the therapist can determine:

1. The classification or syndrome
2. The principle of treatment or direction of movement
3. The need for initial therapist assistance
4. Appropriate prophylactic procedures

These clinical conclusions are subject to change with continued reassessment of the patient's presentation.

Successful application of the protocol is totally dependent on the correct classification of patients. Each of the syndromes has some essential characteristics, which are described in this chapter as *criteria*, and has some nonessential but frequently encountered characteristics, which are described as *associated factors*. A brief definition and outline of the suspected mechanism of mechanical pain production is given at the beginning of each syndrome description.

Posture Syndrome

Postural pain may arise from any pain-sensitive tissue in the lumbar spine. Described simply, postural pain appears eventually by overstretching of normal tissues. The bent finger example described by McKenzie demonstrates the characteristics of this syndrome.

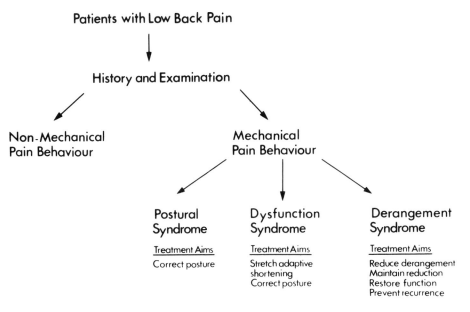

Fig. 9-2.   The classification of patients with low back pain.

Criteria

Pain Distribution and Quality.   It is local, midline, symmetrical, and never referred. Pain is felt as a dull ache.

Onset: Gradual.

Constant/intermittent: Intermittent, never constant.

When worse: Pain is worse with prolonged poor sitting, standing, bending, or lying postures. it is never produced by or felt during movement.

When better: Pain is never felt during, and is abolished by, movement.

Observation: There is no acute lumbar deformity (i.e., kyphosis, lateral shift, or accentuated lordosis), and there is nothing to observe except that the patient adopts a sustained end range position.

Assessment of movement: There is no loss of range, and single or repeated movements do not produce symptoms.

Sustained position: The onset of symptoms is time dependent and only sustained end-range positions produce pain. The patient is instructed to maintain the precipitating posture until the pain is reproduced. This may take more than 15 minutes.

Associated Factors

Patients are usually aged 30 years and under, often having sedentary occupations requiring maintenance of sustained end-range positions. Cervical and thoracic symptoms may occur concurrently. Patients with this sydnrome are sometimes described as hypermobile.

Summary

The only finding is the production of pain if the patient sustains an end range position or posture for a relatively long period of time. There are no signs and no related pathology is implied. The pain is strictly intermittent and time related.

Dysfunction Syndrome

McKenzie uses the term *dysfunction* to describe loss of movement caused by adaptive shortening of soft tissues. Mennell used the same term to describe the loss of movement commonly known as accessory movement or joint play.[17] Dorland's Medical Dictionary defines dysfunction as, "disturbance, impairment, or abnormality of the functioning of an organ."[6]

The mechanism is thought to be similar to that of posture syndrome except that pain results immediately from stretching of adaptively shortened or abnormal tissues. Although tissues may shorten with age asymptomatically, the pain of dysfunction is probably due to a specific shortening or scarring of tissue rather than a general age-related loss of movement.

Criteria

Pain Distribution and Quality. This is local and adjacent to the midline of the spine. The pain from dysfunction is not referred except in the case of an adherent nerve root when the pain may be felt in the buttock, thigh, or calf.

The pain is often described as a stretching discomfort and the intensity is proportional to the vigor of the end range stretch.

Onset: The original symptoms may be due to trauma or derangement. As the injury resolves and adaptive shortening occurs, dysfunction may develop. Postural syndrome may eventually progress to dysfunction syndrome. There is often no history of a specific incident.

Constant/intermittent: Intermittent, never constant.

When worse: Patients with dysfunction syndrome are worse with activities and positions at the end of available movement. There is no pain through range, it is a painful end-range limitation.

When better: The patient is better in positions or during activities that avoid the painful end range. These include walking or running, but if the dysfunction is major, these may eventually produce pain.

Observation: There is usually nothing to see, but the patient may have poor postural habits. If there has been a history of trauma or derangement a chronic nonstructural lumbar deformity may be evident. With extension dysfunction, a common observation is a flattened lumbar spine.

Assessment of movement: There is always a loss of movement or function. This is one of the main factors distinguishing it from the postural syndrome.

Loss of movement may be symmetric when dysfunction coexists with poor postural habit or spondylosis. Following resolution of trauma or derangement, the movement loss may be asymmetric, being full in one direction and partially or completely lost in another. The pain is always felt at the end of the range, never during movement, comes on immediately, and disappears when stress is released. Repetition of test movements does not alter the symptoms. Rapid changes of pain presentation and movement loss do not occur in dysfunction. A deviation may be seen on movement, most commonly during flexion and will not alter with repeated movement.

Sustained position: Sustained positions at the limit of the affected range will produce pain. This occurs immediately and will increase if the position is maintained.

Associated Factors

The patient is usually over 30 years of age, unless there has been a history of trauma or derangement. Poor posture is commonly associated with dysfunction.

Summary

The pain of dysfunction is only produced at the end of available range of movement. It is elicited immediately when the end range movement is stretched and subsides immediately if tension is released. There is loss of mobility preventing full normal end-range movement.

Derangement Syndrome

The pain of derangement is thought to be produced by displacement or altered position of joint structures, resulting in mechanical deformation of pain-sensitive tissues. The change within the joint may prevent the joint surfaces from moving normally, resulting in altered movement patterns.

McKenzie has postulated that in the lumbar spine the derangement syndrome is caused most commonly by a mechanical disturbance of the intervertebral disc. He has divided these into posterior disc and anterior disc derangements because the clinical presentation suggests that one or the other part of the disc is involved. The mechanism of posterior derangement may be similar to that demonstrated by Adams and Hutton.[18]

Criteria

Pain Distribution and Quality. In the low back, pain may be central, unilateral, symmetric, or asymmetric. It may be referred to the buttock, thigh, leg, or foot, and may rapidly vary in area of distribution and in intensity. It is commonly a deep dull ache or an intermittent sharp pain. Paresthesia or numbness associated with nerve root involvement may be present.

Onset: Usually the onset is sudden and may or may not be related to a specific incident. The pain can rapidly worsen within a short period of time.

Constant/intermittent: Pain is often constant but varying in intensity.

When worse: Pain attributed to a posterior derangement is usually worse when the patient is bending, sitting, and/or sustaining positions. Patients commonly experience a sharp pain when rising from a sitting position. If a lateral shift is present, walking will usually aggravate the symptoms. Pain attributed to an anterior derangement is usually made worse by walking and standing. The patient may experience a sharp pain on resuming the lordotic position after sitting in flexion. Patients with derangement syndrome often have difficulty finding a comfortable sleeping position and pain may be worse in the morning.

When better: Patients with a posterior derangement are usually better walking and lying, while those with an anterior derangement are usually better sitting and in other flexed positions. If a lateral shift is due to the derangement, it is unlikely that any position or movement will ease the symptoms for any length of time.

Observation: The patient with derangement syndrome often has an acute deformity. Common deformities are a flattened or kyphotic lumbar spine, a lateral shift, or in the case of an anterior derangement, an accentuated lordosis.

Assessment of movement: There is always a loss of movement and function. Certain movements produce, increase, or peripheralize the pain of derangement. Repetition of these movements will worsen symptoms. Other movements will decrease, abolish, or centralize the pain and repeating them will improve the symptoms. Very severe derangements may be unchanged or made worse by test procedures. One of the most significant features of derangement, particularly in the presence of acute deformity, is difficulty or inability to reverse the lumbar curve (the so-called locked back). In derangement, movement loss is nearly always asymmetric. In flexion, deviation of the lumbar spine may occur to the right or left of the mid-saggital plane. This occurs less frequently in extension.

Sustained position: Sustaining certain positions exacerbates symptoms, but alternatively, sustaining other positions may decrease or abolish them. The effect of sustaining a position is time dependent; the longer a posture is maintained, the more marked will be its effect on symptoms. There is a high correlation between the inability to regain the movement of lumbar extension and surgical findings of posterior intervertebral disc damage in patients with acute low back pain.[19]

Associated Factors

Derangement occurs most frequently in the 20 to 55 year age range, but may occur in the teens or old age. It is seen more commonly in men than women.

The Derangements

The following derangement patterns are commonly seen in the lumbar spine. Many variations of these derangements are possible and not all patients will fit precisely into this listing. The classification is simplified in order to give a clear explanation of principles.

Derangements One to Six have been termed posterior derangements, and are probably progressions of the same syndrome. Behavior of pain during reduction would certainly indicate this.

Derangement One
Central or symmetric pain about L4-5
Rarely with buttock or thigh pain
No deformity.

Derangement Two
Central or symmetric pain about L4-5
With or without buttock and/or thigh pain
With deformity of flat or kyphotic lumbar spine.

Derangement Three
Unilateral or asymmetric pain about L4-5
With or without buttock and/or thigh pain
No deformity.

Derangement Four
Unilateral or asymmetric pain about L4-5
With or without buttock and/or thigh pain
With deformity of lumbar scoliosis.

Derangement Five
Unilateral or asymmetric pain about L4-5
With or without buttock and/or thigh pain
With leg pain extending below the knee
No deformity.

Derangement Six
Unilateral or asymmetric pain about L4-5
With or without buttock and/or thigh pain
With leg pain extending below the knee
With deformity of sciatic scoliosis.

Derangement Seven   (Anterior derangement)
Symmetric or asymmetric pain about L4-5
With or without buttock and/or thigh pain
With deformity of fixed accentuated lumbar lordosis.

Summary

The pain of derangement syndrome can be constant or intermittent. An acute deformity is often present and there is always a loss of movement and function. Pain increases with movement in certain directions and may decrease with movement in other directions. Repeated movements can rapidly alter pain. Sustained positions may increase or decrease pain.

THE HISTORY

In taking a patient's history certain questions must be asked and they form the basis of the subjective examination (Fig. 9-3). The questions are simple so that the patient can easily understand them and so that they provide reliable information. Nelson et al[20] in a study of clinical information reproducibility for low back pain stated that the history, ". . . we conduct on our patients with back and leg pain should be limited and carefully refined in order to minimise the introduction of items which are in fact associated with high observer error."

They concluded that the clinician is left with, ". . . a simple choice. If he wishes to obtain a lot of detailed information then he must appreciate that much of it will be unreliable. On the other hand, if he is prepared to keep the information to simple basic questions . . . then he will increase the reliability of the information obtained."

The initial question in each section is open ended and asked in such a way that a spontaneous reply can be given. This allows the patient to give the information he considers most important. Subsequent questions are more specific and designed to elicit information relevant to the mechanical symptoms.

The first questions relate to working positions and activities, which may be causative factors. Subsequent questions are directly related to the presenting pain.

Q: Where is your pain now?

Detail of the location of pain on a body chart will give an indication of the level and extent of the lesion and the severity of the condition. Location of associated symptoms, such as anesthesia and paresthesia, are noted if present. Then specific areas are cleared with closed ended questions (e.g., Do you have pain in the buttock?) Referred pain suggests derangement syndrome.

Q: How would you describe your pain?

The quality and severity of the pain as described by the patient is noted.

LUMBAR SPINE ASSESSMENT

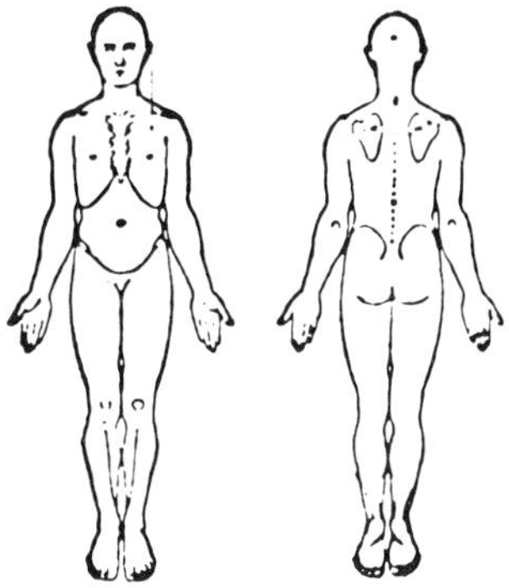

Date ....

Name ....

Address ....

Date of birth ....

Occupation ....

HISTORY

Symptoms now ....

at onset ....

Present for ....

Commenced as a result of ....

No apparent reason. ☐

Constant/Intermittent.

When worse –   bending,   sitting or rising from,   standing,   walking,   lying.

Other ....

When better –   bending,   sitting or rising from,   standing,   walking,   lying.

Other ....

Disturbed sleep – Yes   No   Cough/sneeze +ve −ve

Previous history ....

and treatment ....

X-Rays ....

General health ....   Meds/Steroids ....

Recent surgery ....   Accident ....

Gait ....   Bladder ....

EXAMINATION

Posture sitting ....   Lordosis reduced/accentuated ....

Posture standing ....   Leg length ....

Lateral shift (R) or (L) or nil

....

MOVEMENT LOSS

Flexion: Major.   Moderate.   Minimal.   Deviation (R) or (L) ....

Extension: Major.   Moderate.   Minimal.   Deviation (R) or (L) ....

Side Gliding: (R) or (L) ....

TEST MOVEMENTS

FIS ....   SGIS (R) ....

REP. FIS ....   SGIS (L) ....

EIS ....   REP. SGIS (R) ....

REP. EIS ....   REP. SGIS (L) ....

FIL ....

REP. FIL ....

EIL ....

REP. EIL ....

Neurological ....

Hip joints ....   S.I.

Conclusion: Posture   Dysfunction   Derangement

PRINCIPLE OF TREATMENT

Fig. 9-3. Lumbar spine assessment.

Q: Where did you feel the pain initially?

The location and severity of the pain can change rapidly from the time of onset.

Q: When did the pain start?

This question relates to the present episode only. Duration will give an indication of whether the condition is acute, subacute, or chronic, and may be a guide to the amount of vigor that can be used in the examination. The patient is then asked whether his condition is now improving, worsening, or remaining the same.

Q: How did the pain start?

The patient may be able to relate a specific incident, but many do not know how their pain started. The onset of pain may be gradual or sudden.

Q: Is the pain constant or intermittent?

If pain is constant there is no time of day or night when it is not present. Constant pain may be produced by chemical irritation or mechanical deformation. Pain of chemical origin is always constant and no mechanical procedure can significantly reduce it. Chemical pain following trauma reduces steadily as healing takes place. Mechanical pain may be constant or intermittent. If mechanical pain is constant, it will vary with movement and position, but will never completely disappear. If pain is intermittent, there will be a movement or position that will totally abolish it. The derangement syndrome can be associated with constant pain, whereas the postural syndrome and dysfunction syndrome are characterized by intermittent pain.[2] If constant pain commences for no apparent reason, and is gradually and insidiously becoming more severe, particularly if the patient looks or feels unwell, then serious pathology should be suspected. The patient should be referred for appropriate investigation.

Q: What makes the pain worse? and; What makes the pain better?

Following these initial questions the patient is specifically asked about: bending, sitting, rising from sitting, standing, walking, and lying.

Bending: Patients complaining of pain worsened by bending will be worsened by all flexion movements.

Sitting and rising from sitting: McKenzie contends that poor sitting posture alone may eventually produce back pain[20,21] and, "will frequently enhance and always perpetuate the problems in patients suffering from low back pain."[2] The great majority of patients complain of an increase in pain while sitting or on rising from sitting. Unless a lumbar support is used, relaxed sitting allows the lumbar spine to adopt a fully flexed end range position. A sharp pain on rising from sitting and difficulty reversing the lumbar curve strongly suggests derangement syndrome. If symptoms decrease as a result of sitting it is likely that flexion reduces mechanical deformation.

Standing: Relaxed prolonged standing can place the lower lumbar spine in full end-range extension. If pain is produced or made worse by this position, it suggests that sustained end-range extension may be causing mechanical deformation. If pain is decreased, the position may be reducing mechanical deformation.

Walking: Walking accentuates extension. If walking is painful it is likely that extension will produce or worsen the symptoms. Walking will also worsen pain in the presence of a lateral shift. If pain is decreased, extension may be reducing the mechanical deformation.

Lying: The position of the lumbar spine is influenced by the surface of the bed. The effect of position is summarized by McKenzie:[2] lying supine on a firm surface, the lumbar spine falls into extension, whereas on a soft surface the degree of extension is decreased, and in some cases flexion may be produced. Lying prone on a firm or a soft surface the lumbar spine is always near or at full end range of extension. In side lying, side gliding of the lumbar spine occurs towards the bed, more so when the surface is soft.

Q: Have there been previous episodes of low back pain?

This question gives an indication of the frequency and duration of episodes and the effects of previous treatment. Episodic history suggests derangement, which may be associated with subsequent dysfunction.

THE EXAMINATION

The purpose of the objective examination is to evaluate static postures, movements and the effect of repeated movements on pain (Table 9-1).

Examination of Static Postures

Posture Sitting

The patient is asked to sit unsupported on the edge of the examination table. After a few minutes most people will assume a posture that fully flexes the lumbar spine. A forward leaning posture has been shown to be a significant

Table 9-1. Description of the Effects of Repeated Movements on Symptoms

Increases	Symptoms already present are increased in intensity.
Decreases	Symptoms already present are decreased in intensity.
Produces	There are no symptoms at rest. Movement creates symptoms.
Abolishes	Symptoms are present. Movement eliminates symptoms.
Worsened	Symptoms present or produced are increased with each movement, and remain worse as a result.
Not worsened	Symptoms present or produced are increased with each movement but do not remain worse as a result.
Pain during movement	Pain appears or increases as movement occurs. Pain disappears or reduces when movement stops.
Pain at end range	Pain does not appear until end range is reached. Pain disappears when end range is released.
In status quo	Movement has no effect on symptoms.

(Modified from Hoyt K, Kelley D: A comparative study of the effect on symptoms of single versus repeated performance of flexion and extension movements in patients with low back pain. p. 57. Unpublished research project, Kaiser Permanente Medical Center, Hayward, California, 1980)

risk factor for low back pain.[23] Bendix et al,[24] in a study simulating posture of assembly workers with poor leg space found that while sitting, the lumbar spine moved towards kyphosis, even without backward pelvic rotation. If low back pain is present, a forward-leaning posture is by far the greatest aggravating factor.[25]

Posture Standing

In standing, the patient is examined for postural faults and spinal deformity. A person may stand with a reduced or an exaggerated lordosis either of which may be significant in the production of symptoms. The eye balling of posture is unreliable,[26] but the observation may have some significance when other factors are considered.

Spinal deformities that may be seen include a lumbar lateral shift, a lumbar kyphosis, or an accentuated lordosis. A lateral shift is present if the lumbar spine is seen to deviate laterally from the midline in relation to the pelvis. This may be due to derangement of lumbar joints, or to bone asymmetry such as a leg-length discrepancy,[27] congenital anomaly, tropism of lumbar zygapophyseal joints, or idiopathic scoliosis. Small lateral shifts are sometimes difficult to detect but, if caused by a lumbar derangement, must not be overlooked. Extension procedures performed in the presence of a lateral shift are ineffective and may worsen the condition. A nonstructural lumbar kyphosis or exaggerated lordosis may be due to a mechanical derangement or major dysfunction.

Examination of Movement

The range of movement is assessed and any deviation from the normal movement pathway is noted. At this stage the effect of movement on pain is not assessed. Only one movement is repeated in each direction because movement repetition or sustaining a particular position may significantly alter symptoms and signs.

Flexion

Loss of flexion may manifest itself by either end-range limitation or deviation from the normal pathway of movement. If movement loss is major, a lumbar lordosis may still be present even after the patient has bent forward at the hips as far as possible. Deviation from the midline in flexion may occur:

1. In an arc-type movement, with the spine continuing to divert from the midline as flexion progresses; or
2. The spine may initially deviate from the midline then return to the midsagittal path as flexion progresses.

A deviation from the normal movement pathway may occur in derangement syndrome, dysfunction syndrome, or result from a structural abnormality.

Extension

Extension is very difficult to assess because of its relatively small range. A painful loss of extension may occur in either dysfunction syndrome or derangement syndrome. A major derangement may cause deviation in extension, usually away from the side of pain.

Side Gliding

If side gliding is restricted, the movement loss is usually unilateral. In the presence of a lateral shift, side gliding is restricted or completely blocked in the direction opposite to the shift.

Examination of Movement Related to Pain

At this stage of the examination movements are performed to determine their effect on pain. The behavior of the pain is different in each syndrome and indicates the appropriate classification. Pain that behaves mechanically must be affected by movement or position. Certain movements or positions produce, increase or peripheralize symptoms, while others abolish, decrease, or centralize them. Test movements are performed in both standing and lying because (1) gravitational forces on the lumbar spine are greater in standing than lying, and this may alter the behavior of symptoms; and (2) movements in standing are essentially active, while those performed in lying are passive. Frank et al[28] define passive joint motion as, ". . . any movement of an articulation that is 'produced by some external force.' The source is any force other than the neuromuscular units that would normally be powering the joint under voluntary control (active joint motion)."

Passive motion of lumbar segments in lying is produced by distal body levers (Fig. 9-5). To produce a passive force, local active muscle contraction in the lumbar spine must be avoided because active movements may cause different mechanical effects and alter pain behavior.

A single movement will not demonstrate the behavior of pain. This can only be achieved by repeating the movement. If the derangement syndrome is present, repetition of movement in certain directions will result in progressive increase in symptoms and/or peripheralization of symptoms, indicating that the derangement is being made worse. Repeated movements, usually in opposite directions, may progressively decrease or centralize pain, indicating that the derangement will be reduced by these movements.

If the dysfunction syndrome is present, performance of repeated movements in directions that stretch adaptively shortened tissues will produce pain at the end of range, but repetition will not make symptoms worse. The pain rapidly disappears when the neutral position is resumed. In the postural syndrome, pain will not be experienced on the initial or subsequent repetitions of any test movements. A position must be sustained in order to reproduce symptoms.

A set of repeated movements in each direction is performed in the sequence listed below. After each repetition, the patient returns to the neutral starting position. During and after the initial movement, the effects on pain are recorded. The movement is then repeated up to ten times, and the effects of repetition are recorded. Maximum stretch should be achieved in the last few repetitions. If the patient is in severe pain, the examination is limited accordingly. The test movements are performed in the following sequence:

	FIS	(flexion in standing)
Rep	FIS	(repeated flexion in standing)
	EIS	(extension in standing)
Rep	EIS	(repeated extension in standing)
	SGIS	(right and left side glide in standing)
Rep	SGIS	(repeated right and left side gliding in standing)
	FIL	(flexion in lying)
Rep	FIL	(repeated flexion in lying)
	EIL	(extension in lying)
Rep	EIL	(repeated extension in lying)

Flexion in Standing

The patient is asked to run his hands down the front of both legs as far as pain will allow, then return to the neutral position.

Extension in Standing

The patient stands with the hands in the small of the back to act as a fulcrum and bends backwards as far as possible.

Side Gliding in Standing

When performing the test, both shoulders should remain parallel to the floor. Left-side gliding is said to occur when the shoulders move to the left and the pelvis moves to the right (Fig. 9-4). If a lateral shift is present, this movement will determine its relevance to the patient's symptoms. The importance of this test movement cannot be overstated, particularly in the presence of a derangement.

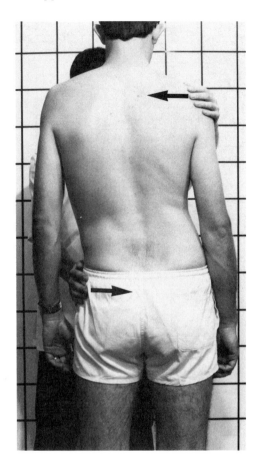

Fig. 9-4. Testing of left-side gliding in standing.

When side gliding is painful and restricted, a lateral shift is probably present, and therapist assistance may be required to reduce it. If side gliding is painful but unrestricted, there is probably no lateral shift.

If a shift is present it may be considered relevant (i.e., results from the same mechanical disturbance that produces the patient's pain) when the side gliding movement alters the site or intensity of the pain. If left- or right-side gliding does not alter the pain, the lateral shift or scoliosis is probably not relevant.

Flexion in Lying

The patient, in supine lying with knees flexed and feet flat on the treatment table, is asked to bend the knees onto the chest. Maximum lower-lumbar flexion is applied by the patient clasping the knees with the hands, then the starting position is resumed.

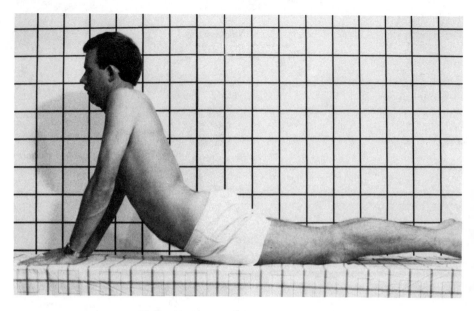

Fig. 9-5.   Passive extension in lying.

Extension in Lying

The patient, in prone position lying with the hands on a flat surface directly beneath the shoulders, raises the top half of the body by straightening the arms while allowing the thighs and legs to remain on the table. If the pelvis lifts, the low back must be allowed to sag as much as possible (Fig. 9-5). The patient then returns to the starting position. It is important that the lumbar erector spinae muscles remain inactive to ensure that the procedure is passive.

Examination Conclusions

By correlating the information gained from history, examination, and test movements, it should be possible to determine which syndrome is present, and to establish the principles of treatment. These mechanical diagnostic procedures, plus careful assessment of the response to treatment, can distinguish patients with back pain of nonmechanical origin, and expose unsuitable conditions and serious pathologies. The procedures can, therefore, play an important part in assessment of some complex orthopedic problems. This has been demonstrated in a recent study by Kopp et al.[19]

Palpation

Palpation of movement restriction at a spinal level must reproduce the patient's symptoms. Palpation may be useful for localizing levels of involvement,[29] but does not constitute an essential part of this examination approach.

It has been hypothesized that provocation and reproduction of pain is the key factor in reliable identification of the injured level, not tissue compliance features.[30] A recent review of reliability in clinical arthrometrics by Matyas and Bach,[30] "cast some doubts as to the appropriateness of the passive accessory intervertebral movement tests as reliable inter-test or inter-therapist indicators."[31]

Other examination procedures are used, but it is not within the scope of this chapter to describe them. These include a neurologic examination and special tests for specific structures.

TREATMENT

General Principles of Treatment

Self-Treatment and Prophylaxis

The concept of patient self-treatment originated in response to early attempts at treating lumbar derangement syndromes. McKenzie found that acute kyphotic, lordotic, and/or scoliotic deformities could be substantially reduced in the clinic, but in many cases regressed soon afterwards. Only when patients were instructed to perform appropriate reductive procedures regularly throughout the day, was correction maintained. It also became evident that if the patient performed the wrong movements or adopted the wrong positions, relapse often followed. The stressing of self-treatment during the acute phase, results in self-reliance rather than dependence upon therapy, and provides the patient with a program of prophylactic self-mobilizing procedures, which can be used to prevent recurrence and treat future episodes.

Low back pain tends to be self-limiting. Dixon[32] cites Fry who found that of patients consulting their family practitioner with low back pain, 44 percent were better within one week, 86 percent within one month, and 92 percent within two months. Hirsch et al[33] and Horal[34] in studies of acute low-back pain found that 90 percent of symptoms resolved within two months. They also found that 90 percent of patients had recurrence of symptoms. Horal found that subsequent attacks typically lasted longer, were more painful, and led to more lost work hours. One of the major risks for recurrence of low back pain appears to be a history of low back pain. McKenzie contends that reduction in recurrence rate is the most meaningful indicator of successful treatment. A survey of patients with low back pain demonstrated that a reduction in recurrence was achieved by application of the prophylactic advice based on the McKenzie protocol.[22]

Because patients have a prophylactic routine that can control their pain, most are able to continue normal working and recreational activities. The blanket instruction do not bend is not necessary in most cases. If patients have a history of low back pain aggravated by flexed activities, they are taught to fully extend regularly at intervals while working, before the onset of pain. If lumbar discomfort is present, the self-mobilizing procedures will usually lessen pain quickly.

Technique

One of the main features of the McKenzie approach is that it is possible and desirable for patients to treat and control their low back pain. McKenzie[2] states:

> In order to achieve this it is necessary to depart from the traditional methods of mechanical treatment, whereby the therapist does something to the patient to bring about change. In that case the patient attributes his recovery rightly or wrongly to what was done to him and for all future episodes of low back pain he commits himself to the care of the therapist. By avoiding the use of therapist technique in the initial stages of treatment and substituting patient-technique, the patient will recognise that his recovery is clearly the result of his own efforts. Only a few patients fail to assume responsibility for active participation in their treatment.

Although McKenzie's maneuvers are referred to as exercises, most of the procedures are passive, and when performed at a certain frequency and in such a way that a rhythmic passive stretch is produced, become a form of mobilization. The exercises are more accurately described as self-mobilization procedures.

The therapist and patient techniques described by McKenzie are totally unsophisticated and nonspecific, certainly affecting many spinal segments. Most techniques are performed to the maximum possible end range, and followed by a brief pause of total relaxation. The actual therapist technique used is considered unimportant as long as the behavior of the patient's symptoms and signs are appropriate. Mobilization and manipulation are regarded as progressions of self-mobilizing procedures. Techniques used to treat the derangement syndrome must decrease, eliminate, or centralize the patient's pain while those used to treat the dysfunction syndrome must reproduce it. The arguments for or against movement in certain directions based on theoretical concepts of pathology and biomechanics become obsolete if these principles are applied.

Reassessment

Treatment is guided by continual reassessment of symptoms and signs. Patient response to the initial treatment over a 24 hour period will confirm a diagnosis. Treatment can be continually progressed or modified in response to alteration of symptoms and signs and improvement can be assessed by changes in the intensity, frequency or site of pain. All patients must be warned that if self-mobilization increases peripheral pain, the procedure should be discontinued until reassessed by the therapist. This is important because even if the prescribed procedures are inappropriate, the patient will not worsen the condition. If adequate instruction and careful explanation of treatment aims are given, the self-treatment concept is safe and effective.

Treatment of the Postural Syndrome

If the patient's pain is caused solely by poor postural habits, a clear explanation and demonstration of the postural problem is the most important aspect of treatment. In order to demonstrate the relationship between posture and the pain, it is necessary to adopt the position that will produce the symptoms. The patient is then shown how to correct or modify the posture, which will immediately relieve the pain. This demonstration must be repeated on several occasions to reinforce the lesson. Postural pain may be produced by sustained end-range lying, standing, or sitting postures, but the latter, involving full lumbar flexion, is encountered most often. Many people find active modification of sitting posture very difficult, and without passive support, will adopt end range flexion very quickly. A simple study has shown that use of a lumbar support pillow changes sitting posture by increasing lumbar lordosis.[35] Use of lumbar pillows to control sitting posture is vital in any situation where prolonged sitting produces pain. Poor postural habits may predispose the patient to development of the dysfunction or derangement syndromes. Instruction on prophylactic exercise in addition to posture correction may help prevent this.

Treatment of the Dysfunction Syndrome

It is postulated that the pain of the dysfunction syndrome is caused by the stretching of adaptively-shortened pain-sensitive soft tissues. It has been found in practice that to be effective, treatment must involve some reproduction of the pain or discomfort felt at end range in the painful direction. The principles of treatment for this syndrome are based on the mechanisms of tissue healing, and the response of soft tissue to application of controlled forces.[28,36–38,40,41] Pain will remain until there has been sufficient stretching of the involved tissues. This cannot occur quickly and may require weeks or months of diligent self mobilization. End-range stretches must be performed regularly to achieve worthwhile long-term improvement.

Correction procedures used for the posture syndrome are also taught to those patients with the dysfunction syndrome. Correction of posture may markedly decrease pain because the patient will learn not to adopt uncontrolled end-range positions. The behavior of the pain in response to treatment determines:

1. The amount of force used in a stretch.
2. The number of repetitions per routine.
3. The number of times the routine is performed daily.

Ideally, as the mobilization is performed the patient should experience a stretch pain similar to the bent finger example. When the stretch is released the pain should stop almost immediately. After completion of an exercise routine, the localized pain should completely cease within 10 to 20 minutes. If it does not cease, the stretches may be too vigorous, or the frequency of the routine and/ or the number of repetitions too high. The combination of new postures and stretching will inevitably lead to transient aches in other areas, and the patient must be warned that this will occur.

It is essential that patients with dysfunction continue to perform appropriate self-mobilization, even when symptoms have resolved. If adaptive shortening has occurred, the normal activities of daily living and general back exercises will often be insufficient to maintain an adequate range of movement and prevent recurrence of symptoms.

Differentiation between Sciatica Caused by Adherent Nerve and Derangement Syndrome

Nerve adherence has the same insidious onset and pain behavior as dysfunction in other tissues.

If flexion in standing produces or increases referred sciatic leg pain, it may be due to derangement syndrome or to dysfunction syndrome in the form of nerve root adherence. During this movement, if an adherent root is present, it will often cause deviation of the spine from the median sagittal plane, by pulling the patient's torso towards the painful side. Deviation may also be due to derangement, or dysfunction of nonneural tissues. Repeated flexion in standing may increase peripheral pain and change the deviation caused by derangement, but will not alter the pain and deviation caused by root adherence. Flexion in standing fully lengthens and stretches the nerve roots, producing effects similar to the Straight Leg Raise test and Slump test described by Maitland.[41] However, flexion in lying simultaneously flexes the hip and knee, and the nerve root will not be fully stretched. Leg pain produced or increased by flexion in lying can be caused by derangement, but not by nerve adherence. Discrepancies between the pain produced by flexion in lying and flexion in standing facilitates differentiation of adherence and posterior derangement.

The principles of treatment for dysfunction syndrome are used for adherent nerve and peripheral symptoms should be produced during stretching.

Treatment of the Derangement Syndrome

The derangement syndrome is treated by using movements and positions that decrease, abolish, or centralize pain, and by avoiding those that worsen or peripheralize it. Constant repetition of the corrective procedures is necessary, and time must be allowed for reduction to occur. Because certain positions will worsen symptoms, it is essential that appropriate postural correction be instituted without delay. This will form part of the patient's prophylactic program.

If the patient is unable to reduce the derangement with self-mobilization procedures, therapist technique is required in the initial stages of treatment.

Treatment of lumbar derangements can be based on either extension principle or flexion principle, after correction of a related lateral shift. The use of extension or flexion principle simply means that the techniques employed are those that emphasize the direction of movement that decreases pain. An acute lateral shift or lumbar scoliosis must be corrected before sagittal movement procedures are used. In the presence of a lateral shift, extension will not be effective. McKenzie[2] states that, ". . . to a large extent, the disrepute surrounding the application of extension exercises has developed because of failure to detect minor lumbar scolioses and determine their relevance to symptoms."

Once the derangement has resolved, symptoms of dysfunction syndrome may become apparent and are treated appropriately.

The ability to achieve extension in the presence of a posterior derangement appears to be a good sign for predicting response to conservative treatment.[19,43]

SUMMARY

Many theories have been proposed for the mechanisms of spinal pain, but these remain unsubstantiated. Until the true nature of mechanical low back pain is understood, treatment can only be based on the behavior of symptoms and signs. The McKenzie approach is not dependent on a pathologic concept. It uses the behavior of pain and its relationship to movement and position to determine appropriate treatment. Patients are encouraged to be responsible for prevention of back pain, for their own treatment, and to become independent of the therapist. Preliminary investigations indicate that future clinical studies of the McKenzie approach are warranted.[19,43–46]

REFERENCES

1. McKenzie RA: Treat Your Own Back. Spinal Publications, Waikanae, New Zealand, 1980
2. McKenzie RA: The Lumbar Spine: Mechanical Diagnosis and Therapy. Spinal Publications, Waikanae, New Zealand, 1981
3. Wyke B: The neurology of low back pain. p. 265. Jayson M (ed): The Lumbar Spine and Back Pain. 2nd Ed. Pitman Medical, Kent, 1980
4. Nachemson A: A critical look at conservative treatment for low back pain: p. 453. Jayson M (ed): The Lumbar Spine and Back Pain. 2nd Ed. Pitman Medical, Kent, 1980
5. Donelson R, Murphy K, Silva G: Centralisation phenomenon: Its usefulness in evaluating and treating sciatica. Proceedings of International Society for the Study of the Lumbar Spine, Dallas, 1986

6. Dorland's Illustrated Medical Dictionary. 25th Ed. WB Saunders, Philadelphia, 1974

7. Blakiston's Gould Medical Dictionary. 4th Ed. McGraw-Hill, New York, 1979

8. Charnley J: Orthopaedic signs in the diagnosis of disc protrusion. Lancet 260:186, 1951

9. Dandy WE: Concealed ruptured intervertebral discs. JAMA 117:821, 1941

10. Frykholm R: Lower cervical vertebrae and intervertebral discs. Surgery, anatomy and pathology. Acta Chir Scand 101:345, 1951

11. Russell WR: Discussion on cervical spondylosis. Proc R Soc Med 49:197, 1956

12. Rexed B, Wennstrom KG: Arachnoidal proliferation and cystic formation in the spinal nerve-root pouches of man. J Neurosurg 16:73, 1959

13. Goddard MD, Reid JD: Movements induced by straight leg raising in the lumbo-sacral roots, nerves and plexus, and in the intrapelvic section of the sciatic nerve. J Neurol Neurosurg Psychiatry 28:12, 1965

14. Fahrni WH: Observations on straight leg-raising with special reference to nerve root adhesions. Can J Surg 9:44, 1966

15. MacNab I: Negative disc exploration. JBJS 53A:891, 1974

16. Burton CV, Kirkaldy-Willis WH, Yong-Hing K et al: Causes of failure of surgery on the lumbar spine. Clin Orthop 157:191, 1981

17. Mennell J McM: Joint Pain. Diagnosis and treatment using manipulative techniques. Little Brown, Boston, 1964

18. Adams MA, Hutton WC: Gradual disc prolapse. Spine 10:524, 1985

19. Kopp JR, Alexander AH, Turocy RH et al: The use of lumbar extension in the evaluation and treatment of patients with acute herniated nucleus pulposis. A preliminary report. Clin Orthop 202:211, 1986

20. Nelson MA, Allen P, Clamp S, et al: Reliability and reproducibility of clinical findings in low back pain. Spine 4:97, 1979

21. Magora A: Investigation of the relation between and occupation. Ind Med Surg 41:5, 1972

22. McKenzie RA: Prophylaxis in recurrent low back pain. NZ Med J 89:22, 1979

23. Nachemson A: The lumbar spine. An orthopaedic challenge. Spine 1:59, 1976

24. Bendix T, Krohn L, Jessen F et al: Trunk posture and trapezius muscle load while working in standing, supported standing and sitting positions. Spine 10:433, 1985

25. Biering-Sorensen F: A one year prospective study of low back trouble in a general population. Dan Med Bull 31:362, 1984

26. Waddell G, McCulloch J, Kummel E et al: Nonorganic physical signs in low back pain. Spine 5:117, 1980

27. Giles LGF, Taylor JR: Low-back pain associated with leg length inequality. Spine 6:510, 1981

28. Frank C, Akeson WH, Woo S et al: Physiology and therapeutic value of passive joint motion. Clin Orthop 185:113, 1984

29. Jull GA, Bogduk N: Manual examination: An objective test of cervical joint dysfunction. Proceedings of the Manipulative Therapists Association of Australia, Brisbane, 159, 1985

30. Matyas TA, Bach TM: The reliability of selected techniques in clinical arthmetrics. Aust J Physiother 31:175, 1985

31. Twomey LT: Editorial. Aust J Physiother 31:174, 1985

32. Dixon A StJ: Diagnosis of low back pain: p. 135. Jayson M (ed): The Lumbar Spine and Back Pain. 2nd Ed. Pitman Medical, Kent, 1980

33. Hirsch C, Jonsson B, Lewit, T: Low back symptoms in a Swedish female population. Clin Orthop 63:171, 1969

34. Horal J: The clinical appearance of low back disorders in the city of Gothenburg, Sweden. Acta Orthop Scand suppl 118, 1969

35. Majeske C, Buchanan C: Quantative description of two sitting postures with and without a lumbar support pillow. Phys Ther 64:1531, 1985

36. Akeson WH, Amiel D, LaViolette D et al: The connective tissue response to immobility: an accelerated aging response. Exp Gerontol 3:289, 1968

37. Akeson WH, Amiel D, Woo S: Immobility effects of synovial joints: the pathomechanics of joint contracture. Biorheology 17:95, 1980

38. Peacock E, Van Winkle W: Wound Repair. WB Saunders, Philadelphia, 1976

39. Donatelli R, Owens-Burkhart H: Effects of immobilisation on the extensibility of periarticular connective tissue. J Orthop Sports Phys Ther 3:67, 1981

40. Evans P: The healing process at a cellular level. Physiother 66:256, 1980

41. Woo S, Matthews JV, Akeson WH et al: Connective tissue response to immobility: correlative study of biomechanical and biochemical measurements of normal and immobilised rabbit knees. Arthritis Rheum 18:257, 1975

42. Maitland GD: The slump test: Examination and treatment. Aust J Physiother 31:215, 1985

43. Kopp JR, Turocy RH, Levrini MG et al: Predictive values of the physical examination for patients with acute discogenic low back pain. Surgical Forum 33:532, 1982

44. Ponte DJ, Jensen GJ, Kent BE: A preliminary report on the use of the McKenzie protocol in the treatment of low back pain. J Orthop Sports Phys Ther 6:130, 1984

45. Nwuga G, Nwuga V: Relative therapeutic efficacy of the Williams and McKenzie protocols in back pain management. Physiother Pract 1:99, 1985

46. Fredrickson B, Murphy K, Donelson H et al: McKenzie treatment of low back pain. A correlation of significant factors in determining prognosis. Proceedings of International Society for the Study of the Lumbar Spine, Dallas, 1986

10 | Muscles and Motor Control in Low Back Pain: Assessment and Management

Gwendolen A. Jull
Vladimir Janda

Low back pain is a multifactorial problem and currently there is no regimen of treatment that has singularly and successfully met the challenge of its prevention and management. The number of treatment methods available for the back pain sufferer reflects the problems that still exist in the assessment and understanding of all etiologic and pathologic processes.

There can be no dispute about the fundamental role played by the trunk and pelvic musculature in the normal functioning of the vertebral column. Muscles produce and control motion. They are the dynamic stabilizers of the spine and are an integral component of protective mechanisms that relieve the spine of the large loads that can be inherent in normal functioning. Taking the normal pattern of joint and muscle innervation into account, it is not unreasonable to expect that muscle function will be compromised in the presence of injury or pain in a motion segment, or that impaired muscle function may produce or perpetuate pain and strain in the lumbar motion segments. Good muscle function is a primary defence against pain and recurrent low back disorders. Not surprisingly, authors writing on the management of patients with low back pain stress the importance of exercise in the rehabilitation program.[1-5] However, the effectiveness and rationales for many standard regimens of back exercises have been difficult to substantiate.[6,7]

This situation may reflect the problems encountered in (or indeed question the validity of) testing the efficacy of one treatment mode in the multifactorial problem of back pain. Conversely, exercise regimens that stress one aspect of treatment for all patients (for example, flexion, extension, or strengthening), incorrectly imply that pathologies, muscle composition, body types, and functional demands are identical among all back pain sufferers. They may also fail to acknowledge the interdependence of the central nervous and musculoskeletal systems in normal and abnormal function.

Knowledge of how muscles react and consequently of how to exercise them efficiently is incomplete. In recent years, emphasis has been placed increasingly on the importance of achieving coordinated activity between all muscles within a balanced muscular system for the prevention and management of chronic pain syndromes.[8,9] Within this text, factors based on clinical observation, which have influenced this change in emphasis in exercise therapy, will be pursued. Methods of clinical assessment that may reveal deficits in muscle function, as well as the need for an integrated and individualized approach to treatment, will be discussed.

MUSCULAR RESPONSES IN LOW BACK PAIN

To view a patient's back disability as primarily affecting one structure or one motion segment ignores the basic interdependence of all the structures and systems involved in the production and control of motion in both normal and pathologic states. Movement of noncontractile elements, such as osseous, articular, and neural tissues, is produced and controlled by muscle activity. Ultimately, however, it is the central nervous system in response to various stimuli that controls the activity of muscles and thus the pattern of motion in an individual's musculoskeletal system. It is important to correctly conceptualize this integrated and interdependent neuromusculoarticular system when assessing the cause and effect of disability in low back pain patients. Dysfunction in any component of this system can affect the activity of muscles and thus the control of motor response.

The nature, source, and duration of adverse stimuli on the muscular system can evoke several and variable (but frequently interdependent) responses (Fig. 10-1). For this reason, there are several dimensions for the involvement of muscles in the production and perpetuation of low back pain.

Muscles as a Source of Pain

Muscles can be the source of both local and referred pain. While primary and traumatic muscle lesions have a doubtful place in the etiology of acute lumbar dysfunction,[10] painful trigger points, referred tenderness in muscle, and

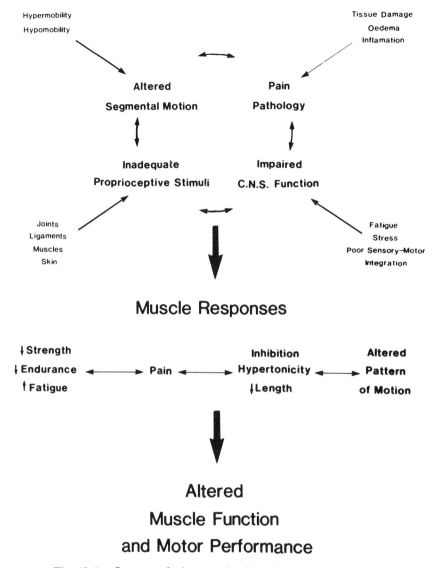

Hypermobility
Hypomobility

Tissue Damage
Oedema
Inflamation

Altered
Segmental Motion

Pain
Pathology

Inadequate
Proprioceptive Stimuli

Impaired
C.N.S. Function

Joints
Ligaments
Muscles
Skin

Fatigue
Stress
Poor Sensory–Motor
Integration

Muscle Responses

↓Strength
↓Endurance
↑Fatigue

Pain

Inhibition
Hypertonicity
↓Length

Altered
Pattern
of Motion

Altered
Muscle Function
and Motor Performance

Fig. 10-1. Sources of adverse stimuli and muscular responses.

musculotendinous lesions are not uncommonly seen in low back pain patients.[11–13] Muscle spasm as a defence reaction against pain and pathology may of itself be asymptomatic or be a source of muscle pain.[14] Paradoxically, its presence may cause excessive compressive or tensile strains on the tissues of motion segments thereby producing new pain syndromes. Muscle spasm can also be the primary mechanism involved in referred pain as encountered, for example, in the piriformis syndrome.[13,15,16]

Impairment of Muscle Function

Trunk muscle activity can be inhibited to prevent motion into a painful posture or direction and to avoid stresses on motion segment pathology.[17] Conversely, the trunk muscles may go into spasm to fulfil a similar protective role. Such reactions are commonly seen clinically in low back pain patients. However, there is less certain information about muscle reactions in the long term and therefore the role of muscles in chronic and recurrent low back pain.

The strength of trunk musculature has received quite considerable attention. Absolute trunk strengths have been measured under isometric, isotonic, and isokinetic conditions and comparisons made between acute and chronic back pain sufferers and matched controls. Results are diverse. Some studies have reported no difference in the strength of trunk flexion and extension between back pain and normal control subjects.[18,19] However, the majority have found the reverse to be true (i.e., reduced trunk muscle strength in back pain subjects compared to controls.[17,20-24] The duration of symptoms appears to be an important factor for it was in the chronic back pain subjects that reduced strength compared to controls was more consistently found.

There is a natural imbalance in or inequality between the strength of muscle groups controlling the trunk; extensor strength exceeding flexor strength.[24-26] Some studies report that this strength ratio does not change in back pain patients.[20,26] However, Addison and Schultz[22] and McNeill et al[17] found that on testing patients with sciatic pain, muscle strength in attempted extension was less than that in flexion. They considered that this was probably a result of protective inhibition to avoid either large tensions in the posterior soft tissues or large compressions on the lumbar motion segments rather than an absolute strength deficit. Other studies have reported a selective loss of trunk flexion strength in low back pain patients.[21,27,28]

The variety of opinion about strength of trunk musculature may be attributable to differences in testing methods, equipment, and the types of subjects tested.[24,27] Indeed, it is always difficult to draw positive conclusions about the strength of the abdominal and erector spinae muscles from experiments that measure trunk flexion and extension strength. This is because it is difficult to isolate the tests to these specific muscles, without involving pelvic musculature.

Parameters other than strength of trunk muscles have also been investigated. Endurance of trunk musculature is an important functional consideration. In studying a normal population, Hasue et al[29] showed that trunk muscles were fatigued more easily by a sustained contraction than by repeated contractions. The abdominals fatigued more easily than the back extensors, and in back patients they fatigued more readily than in control subjects under isokinetic endurance conditions.[26] The extensor muscles did not behave differently comparing back pain and control groups. Nevertheless, in electromyographic studies of activity in the trunk extensors in their more postural and static role, De Vries[30] found that there was a difference in the fatigue curves between back-pain and non-back-pain subjects. The increased muscle activity with time was associated with the experience of back pain in those subjects. Kravitz et al[31] also found that there was increased muscle activity in trunk extensors in back pain subjects compared to controls when both groups were required to contract other muscles.

In addition to considering the contractile properties of muscles, one must give attention to the effects of insufficient muscle length. There is a close biomechanical relationship between the muscles of the lumbar spine and pelvis. Tightness of muscles can influence both static postures and dynamic function of the lumbopelvic complex. Reduced trunk mobility and lack of extensibility of such muscles as the hamstrings and iliopsoas are frequently reported from studies of low-back pain patients.[32-34]

However, it needs to be questioned whether the observed reactions in muscle, such as strength deficits, susceptibility to fatigue, increased motor unit activity, and apparent or real muscle shortening, occur randomly and independently or are part of a general muscle reaction. It is currently believed that when they occur, these changes are part of a general muscle reaction, which presents in typical patterns, and which is intimately involved with the motor regulatory influences of the central nervous system.

The Concept of Muscle Imbalance

Muscle reactions to pain and pathology are frequently encountered at peripheral joints. For example, degenerative hip pathology is regularly associated with tightness in the iliopsoas and hip adductors, while atrophy and weakness are found in the glutei. These muscle reactions are not random but are consistent and it is considered that such typical responses of muscle tightness and weakness occur throughout the whole muscular system.[35,36]

The way in which muscles tend to react (either by overactivation and tightness or by inhibition and weakness) appears to be fairly consistent for the particular muscle concerned. The tightness or weakness may vary in degree between subjects but rarely in distribution. Motion is secured by muscles from both groups but muscles which have a tendency to become tight are usually those that span more than one joint (Table 10-1). Explanations for these differing reactions cannot be found in differences between the physiologic characteristics of these muscles and whether there are differences in innervation between one and two joint muscles is unknown at this present time. In general, muscles prone to tightness are approximately one-third stronger than those prone to inhibition. This ratio could be considered as a natural, physiologically balanced imbalance between these two systems. However, electromyographic studies demonstrate that muscles prone to tightness are readily activated during various movements,[8,37] and in subjects with altered or poor movement patterns, their degree of activation even increases.[8] Therefore, the possibility has to be considered that a difference may exist in the central nervous system's motor control of those muscles that are readily activated and prone to tightness and of those prone to inhibition and weakness. This concept is further reinforced by the observation that the typical muscle responses seen with articular path-

Table 10-1. Functional Division of Muscle Groups

Muscles Prone to Tightness	Muscles Prone to Weakness
Gastrocsoleus	Peronei
Tibialis posterior	Tibialis anterior
Short hip adductors	Vastus medialis and lateralis
Hamstrings	Gluteus maximus, medius, and minimus
Rectus femoris	Rectus abdominis
Iliopsoas	Serratus anterior
Tensor fasciae latae	Rhomboids
Piriformis	Lower portion trapezius
Erector spinae (especially lumbar,	Short cervical flexors
thoracolumbar, and cervical portions)	Extensors of upper limb
Quadratus lumborum	
Pectoralis major	
Upper portion of trapezius	
Levator scapulae	
Sternocleidomastoid	
Scalenes	
Flexors of the upper limb	

ologies are identical or very similar to those that are seen in some structural lesions of the central nervous system.[38] For example, in spasticity of capsular origin, as in cerebral vascular accidents or cerebral palsy, muscles that develop spasticity or even spastic contractures are those that commonly respond by tightness in musculoskeletal conditions. Therefore, the typical hemiplegic posture may be an extreme expression of the imbalance between the muscular chains that exists to some extent under normal physiologic conditions.

It is considered that muscle imbalances may develop via two avenues and may be a prominent factor in the onset or perpetuation of low back pain syndromes. Any acute pain and pathology in the lumbar motion segment can initiate muscle responses which, if they persist, can alter the patient's pattern of motion and in turn perpetuate adverse strains in the lumbar spine. Furthermore, these altered motor patterns may facilitate a chain reaction in the whole motor system and cause strain and pain in other areas of the spine. Interestingly, Horal[39] found that over 50 percent of 212 subjects with low back pain developed cervical symptoms on average six years after their first episode of low back pain. These findings may reflect the existence of such chain reactions in the muscular system.

The second mechanism leading to muscle imbalance is considered to be an impairment in motor control from the central nervous system. This may even provoke the onset of low back pain either by the overactivity of the muscle itself[30,40] or from the adverse mechanism induced in the lumbopelvic and thoracolumbar regions through poor patterns of movement.[41] If the concept of impairment of central nervous regulation of posture and motion is to be accepted, then it is reasonable to question the mechanism for its onset. Definitive data is not available, however, there are several reasoned theories. Increased muscle tone is an important factor influencing the evolution of painful musculoskeletal conditions.[40] The highest level of the nervous system regulating muscle tone is the limbic system.[42] This in turn can be influenced by such psychic reactions as stress, fatigue, pain, and emotional states. It has been observed that in such states, there are demonstrable changes in muscle tone that can be accompanied by poor quality and control of motion and the symptom of pain.[8,40]

In exploring the hypothesis that chronic back pain may be associated with poor patterns of movement and thus some impairment in the central nervous system's motor regulating mechanisms, Janda[8,43] studied a group of 500 chronic low back pain subjects. The subjects included in the study were those who had developed back pain early in adulthood, who had suffered from pain for many years, and who were unexpectedly resistant to treatment. It was determined that approximately 80 percent of this patient group showed slight but distinct signs considered to be characteristic of the disorder recognized in childhood as minimal cerebral dysfunction.

The importance of adequate sensory input, proprioceptive control and proper function of sensorimotor integration has probably been underestimated in the pathogenesis of low back pain. Inadequate proprioceptive stimulation from joints, muscles, skin, and other structures means that no level of the sensorimotor system is facilitated to work properly. In this way, joint and muscle dysfunction can directly impair the central nervous system's motor regulation. In addition, more highly mechanized and sedentary life-styles lead to a reduction in the variety of movement. This in itself may decrease the proprioceptive stimulation essential for the performance of good motor patterns. For this reason, proprioceptive facilitation techniques should be included in the therapeutic programs for those suffering from low back pain syndromes and postural defects.[44]

The Significance of Muscle Imbalance and Altered Movement Patterns

The classic muscle strength test involves the resisted attempt of a movement in the direction considered to be characteristic for the specific muscle or muscle group tested. Yet more often than not it is a series of muscles acting as prime movers, synergists, or stabilizers that combine to produce the movement. It is considered that the quality of performance of the movement may be of greater importance than the test for strength. For example, the hamstrings, glutei, and erector spinae (lumbar and thoracolumbar portions) are active in the performance of hip extension.[45] The strength of hip extension may appear to be normal, but if it is being provided by the hamstrings and erector spinae with little activity being contributed by the glutei, then the quality of performance or movement pattern is poor. Poor movement patterns can have adverse effects on joint and muscle mechanics. This will be discussed in the following section.

The importance of the presence of muscle imbalance is thought to lie in its influence on the motor patterning process. A tight muscle can influence a movement performance in several ways. The irritability threshold of tight muscles is lowered and this can lead to the situation where the tight muscle is activated much more than is expected during a movement. As a result, the movement cannot be performed properly and muscles that should be used during the movement are not activated to the required degree. At the present stage of our knowledge it is difficult to determine whether the tight overactive muscle directly inhibits its antagonist (in accordance with Sherrington's law of reciprocal innervation) or whether a general reprogramming of the motion occurs, in which the subject performs a trick movement to gain the desired result (e.g., in a curl-up exercise using iliopsoas predominantly, rather than the abdominals). Regardless of the mechanism, an important reaction has been shown to occur.[8] When the inhibited and weakened muscle is resisted (with the aim of strengthening the muscle) its activity tends to decrease rather than increase. If the tight muscle is stretched and its normal length is achieved, a spontaneous disinhibition of the previously inhibited muscle occurs. Additionally, there is a return to the normal responses when resistance is increased.[8] For these reasons, emphasis in therapeutic programs should be placed initially on regaining normal length of the tight muscles so that exercises directed towards facilitating and strengthening weakened muscles and achieving good motor patterns can be successful.

SYNDROMES INVOLVING THE MUSCLES

Common Syndromes

As discussed earlier, it is believed that a certain muscle will respond in a typical way to a given situation whether this be pain, impaired afferent input from the joint, or impairment in central motor regulation. It is held that the tendency of muscles to respond by either overactivity and tightness or by inhibition and weakness is not random, and typical patterns of muscle reactions can be identified. However, two important features should be recognized. Muscle reactions may not remain confined to the local symptomatic region. They may facilitate a chain reaction, which can eventually involve the whole motor system, thus causing symptoms in other areas. Conversely, the low back pain may be the symptom of muscle imbalance elsewhere and thus be a local expression of general muscle and motor dysfunction.

Pelvic Crossed Syndrome

There are two regions where muscle imbalance is more evident or in which it starts to develop. One is the pelvic-hip complex and the other the shoulder-neck complex.

The pelvic crossed syndrome is characterized by the imbalance between shortened and tight hip flexors and lumbar erector spinae and weakened gluteal and abdominal muscles (Fig. 10-2). Such an imbalance can adversely affect

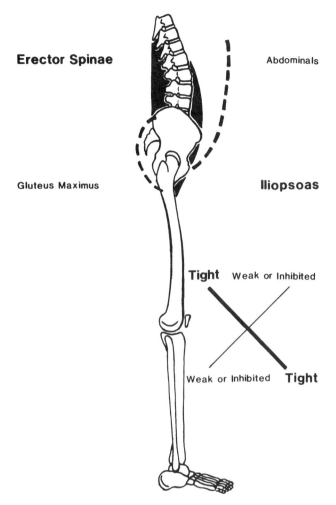

Erector Spinae

Abdominals

Gluteus Maximus

Iliopsoas

Tight Weak or Inhibited

Weak or Inhibited **Tight**

Fig. 10-2.   Depiction of the pelvic crossed syndrome.

both the static posture and dynamic function of this region, notably during walking. This imbalance promotes a forward pelvic tilt, increased lumbar lordosis, and a slightly flexed position of the hip. If the lordosis is deep and short, the imbalance is principally located in the pelvic musculature. If it is more shallow but longer, extending into the thoracic area, the imbalance is more marked in the trunk musculature. The hamstrings are frequently found to be tight in this syndrome. This may be a compensatory mechanism to lessen pelvic tilt[9] or the overactivity and tightness could be a functional compensation for the inhibited glutei. The latter factor emphasizes an important point. Not only should the pattern of muscle imbalance be viewed in its ventrodorsal crossed antagonist pattern, but also the relationship between adjacent muscles must be considered. Overactivity and tightness of the erector spinae in the presence of

Muscle Hypotrophy   Muscle Hypertrophy

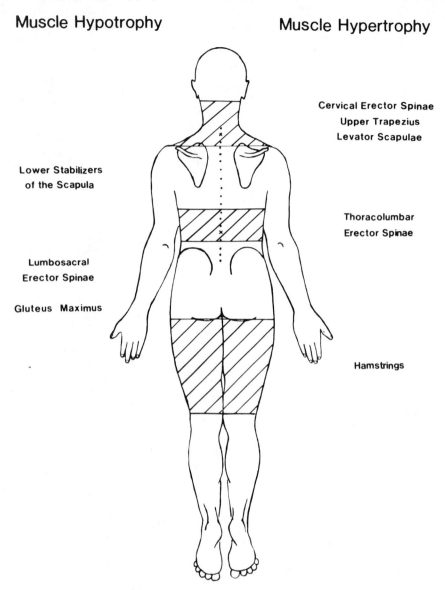

Cervical Erector Spinae
Upper Trapezius
Levator Scapulae

Lower Stabilizers
of the Scapula

Thoracolumbar
Erector Spinae

Lumbosacral
Erector Spinae

Gluteus Maximus

Hamstrings

Fig. 10-3. Depiction of the layer syndrome.

an inhibited or weakened gluteal muscles will alter the pattern of hip extension—a fundamental gait pattern. A tight or overactive iliopsoas in the presence
of inhibited or weakened abdominals will alter the movement pattern of the
curl up from the supine to the sitting position.

An imbalance can also exist in the lateral lumbopelvic musculature. If
weakness occurs in the gluteus medius it can be compensated for by overac-

tivity and tightness in the ipsilateral quadratus lumborum and tensor fasciae latae.

The postures resulting from the imbalances in this syndrome can change the distribution of forces in both the lumbar motion segments and the hip joint. This can occur not only in standing but also in locomotion. If the hip loses its ability to extend to the range of motion required in the last stages of the stance phase, there will be a compensatory increase in forward pelvic tilt and in extension of the lumbar spine. Similarly imbalances in lateral pelvic musculature can overstress the lumbar spine. It is notable that Magora[32] reported that at least slight limitation of hip movement was not an uncommon examination finding in his study of 429 back pain patients. Significantly, the symptomatic complaint of these patients was back pain not hip pain.

In the erect posture, an increase in forward pelvic tilt and lumbar lordosis causes changes in posture in other areas to maintain a postural equilibrium. An increased thoracic kyphosis and a further compensatory increase in cervical lordosis develop in efforts to balance the body against gravity and to keep the head and eyes in the upright position. Such compensatory posture changes in the thoracic and particularly the cervical spine may underly the future development of symptoms in these areas.

The Layer Syndrome

It is considered that this syndrome of muscle imbalance is symptomatic of quite marked impairment of the central nervous system's motor regulation and is accompanied by poor movement patterns. This syndrome is characterized by alternating "layers" of hypertrophic and hypotrophic muscles, and may be most clearly observed from the dorsal aspect of the subject.[41] The layers are depicted in Figure 10-3. In this syndrome, there is also weakness of the abdominals, particularly of the rectus abdominis and the transversus abdominis. The oblique abdominals appear in contrast to be overactive. Inherent in this pattern of muscle imbalance is poor muscular stability in the lumbosacral region, a situation that can predispose to development or perpetuation of low back pain.

ASSESSMENT OF MUSCULAR DYSFUNCTION

There is no place for the routine prescription of standard lists of exercises in the management of patients with low back pain. Before starting any rational exercise program, the patient must be thoroughly examined, and the presence, nature, and stage of any problems and the factors contributing to them duly noted. At the least, inappropriate exercises can be ineffectual but more importantly can be harmful to the patient's condition.

Low back pain is a problem in an integrated and interdependent neuro-musculoarticular system. Problems in these systems occur concurrently, and residual problems in any system can inhibit the return to normal function of another component thus increasing the risk for recurrent episodes of pain. It is essential that the therapist adopts a methodical and disciplined differential diagnostic approach to the examination of the low back pain patient in order to reveal all components of the problem. Emphasis here will be placed on the assessment of muscle dysfunction, as approaches to the examination of articular problems have been discussed elsewhere in this volume.

The assessment of muscle dysfunction is undertaken in three stages; evaluation of standing; examination for muscle tightness; and examination of movement patterns. Timing of the assessment is important. In patients with nonacute or chronic back pain, assessment of muscle function can be incorporated in the overall examination from the outset. However, for patients in acute pain with or without a deformity, pain or pathologic factors may distort posture and muscle function to such a degree that tests yield invalid information. In such patients, the assessment should be conducted when the acute episode has subsided and stabilized, and the patient has regained habitual posture and movement status.

Evaluation of Standing

The evaluation of the standing posture and the appearance of the muscles can give the therapist an overall view of the patient's muscle function. As time in a busy clinic is always at a premium, the evaluation of standing can also give the indications for the tests that need to be performed in detail and for those that can be safely omitted. A full examination of the standing posture will also encourage the therapist to think comprehensively about the patient's whole motor system and not limit attention to the local level of the lesion only.

Abnormalities of posture commonly occur in the low back pain patient. When observing, the therapist must attempt to differentiate between possible provocative causes as many factors including structural variations, age, altered joint mechanics, muscle imbalance and residual effects of pathology can underly a postural deviation. Certain signs may be observed that reveal whether or not muscle impairment is causing or contributing to the patient's postural attitude and these signs should be present if muscles are involved. Such signs include changes in the size and/or shape of the superficial muscles known to react either by overactivity and tightness or by weakness and inhibition. Muscles will often be involved in such patterns as occur in the pelvic crossed or layer syndromes. The role of deeper muscles in postural deviations may need to be confirmed or negated in later muscle length tests.

Initially the therapist should look at the patient as a whole to gain an overall impression of posture. Attention should then be directed towards the position of the pelvis, as abnormalities in other structures, such as the lumbar spine, sacroiliac joints, and lower limbs, are frequently reflected in pelvic position. Common changes include an increase or decrease in sagittal tilt, a lateral shift, forward or backward pelvic rotation, and iliac torsions. In seeking muscular origins for these deviations, the pelvic crossed syndrome may be responsible for the increased anterior tilt of the pelvis, which is usually accompanied by an increase in lumbar lordosis. A lateral shift may occur with acute or chronic lumbar motion segment pathology.[3,46] A shift frequently masks an oblique tilt of the pelvis resulting from a true leg-length difference. However, imbalance in the lateral pelvic musculature may also produce an apparent leg length difference, which is compensated by a lateral pelvic shift. When rotation of the pelvis is present, there may be shortness in the piriformis, while iliac torsions are often associated with tightness in the piriformis and iliopsoas.

The actual shape and quality of the muscles must be observed also for this can reveal possible compensations in function and motor control. Observation should begin from the posterior view and proceed in an orderly manner.

Ideally the glutei should be symmetrical and well rounded. If they are weak or inhibited, the muscle tends to "hang" loosely. Such a situation may confirm their part in the pelvic crossed syndrome, and may indicate that the pattern of walking is not ideal. Asymmetry of the gluteals may indicate a partial pelvic crossed syndrome, a sacroiliac joint problem, hip pathology, or leg-length inequality.

The hamstrings are usually well developed but it is important to look at their bulk relative to that of the glutei, for when the latter are inhibited the hamstrings often become predominant. This is readily evident when there is unilateral inhibition of the gluteus maximus. Tightness of short hip adductors can be visualized as a distinct bulk of muscle in the upper third of the thigh, while tightness of the gastrocnemius-soleus is characterized by the prominence of the soleus, particularly on the medial side of the tendocalcaneum.

Careful attention should be paid to the back muscles. The bulk of the erector spinae should be compared from side to side, as well as from the lumbar to the thoracolumbar regions. There should be no difference in bulk between sides and regions. Prevalence of the thoracolumbar portions of erector spinae is a poor sign. It may indicate that there is poor muscle stabilization in the lumbosacral region and it may constitute a component of the layer syndrome.

The therapist should progress to view the posture of the thoracic and cervical spine to seek compensatory changes for altered lumbar posture and loss of bulk of muscles in the interscapular region. The latter in association with tightness in the trapezius and levator scapulae are features common in neck pain patients.

In viewing the patient from the front, the quality of the abdominals should be examined first. Ideally, the abdominal wall should be flat. A sagging and protruding abdomen may reflect generalized weakness of the abdominals. When the obliques are dominant, a distinct groove will be seen on the lateral side of the recti. This indicates that there may be a decrease in the stabilizing function of the recti in the anteroposterior direction, an important factor for stabilization of the spine.

The two anterior thigh muscles, which can influence the lumbopelvic posture, are the tensor fasciae latae and the rectus femoris. Normally the bulk of the tensor should not be distinct. This sign coupled with the appearance of a groove on the lateral side of the thigh usually indicates that this muscle is overused, and both it and the iliotibial band may be tight. When the rectus femoris is tight, the position of the patella moves slightly upwards and also laterally if there is concurrent tightness of the iliotibial band.

From this initial observation of standing, the therapist should have gained an overall impression of the patient's muscle status. Important syndromes such as the pelvic crossed or layer syndrome may have been identified and the assessment can lead the therapist to specific tests of both muscle length and movement patterns.

Examination of Muscle Length

Once the therapist has become experienced in the observation of muscle dysfunction in standing, muscle length tests can be confined to those where tightness is suspected. However, in the initial stages, it may be prudent to test all muscles that have a tendency to tightness (Table 10-1). This can be valuable not only for the therapist to gain experience in the patterns of muscle involvement, but for the patient. Signs of imbalance in other regions may be a precursoral sign for pain in these regions. With such information, the therapist is well equipped to institute a comprehensive preventative program.

When considering muscle tightness, the muscles of most importance in the inferior half of the body are the lumbar erector spinae, hip flexors, hamstrings, quadratus lumborum, piriformis, short hip adductors, and the gastrocnemius-soleus group. Full descriptions of all length tests have been published elsewhere[45] and discussion here will be confined to those tests that may not be routinely familiar.

Hip Flexors

An appreciation of the length of iliopsoas, rectus femoris, tensor fasciae latae, and the short hip adductors can be gained from the one test. The starting position is shown in Figure 10-4. The therapist should initially observe the position of the leg.

Normal Findings. The thigh is horizontal and the leg hangs vertically. The patella has a very slight lateral orientation, and the outer side of the thigh is flat or slightly grooved.

Signs of Tightness. A flexed position of the hip joint indicates tightness of the iliopsoas, while a diagonal position of the lower leg shows shortness in the rectus femoris.

There may be simultaneous tightness in both muscles. A laterally deviated patella in association with a definitely grooved appearance of the lateral side of the thigh points to a tight tensor fasciae latae and iliotibial band.

Confirmation of Tightness. The therapist is able to confirm observations of tightness when excessive soft-tissue resistance and a decreased range of

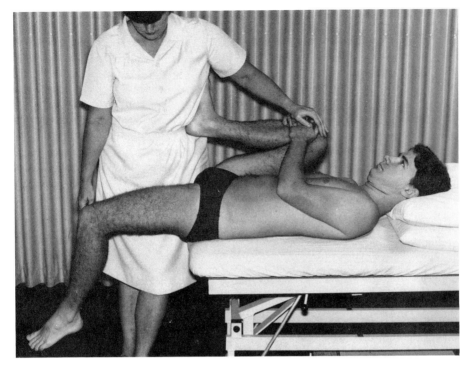

Fig. 10-4. Length test for the hip flexors. The leg to be tested must hang free of the couch. The opposite hip and knee are maintained in a flexed position to tilt the pelvis backward and to eliminate the lumbar lordosis.

movement are encountered on application of pressure in the following directions:

Hip Extension. Less than 10 to 15 degrees—iliopsoas. A simultaneous extension of the knee joint points to shortening of the rectus femoris.

Knee Flexion. Less than 100 to 105 degrees—rectus femoris. The tendency for compensatory hip flexion should be controlled during the test.

Hip Adduction. Less than 15 to 20 degrees—tensor fasciae latae and iliotibial band. There will be an associated increased deepening of the groove on the outside of the thigh.

Hip Abduction. Less than 15 to 20 degrees—short hip adductors. The tendency for compensatory hip flexion should be controlled during the test.

Quadratus Lumborum

The therapist may first suspect tightness of the quadratus lumborum when examining lumbar lateral flexion to the contralateral side in standing. Normally, a smooth lateral curvature of the spine is seen. However, when the lumbar

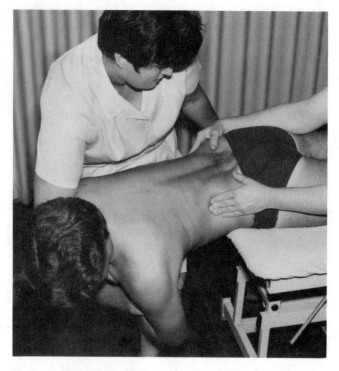

Fig. 10-5. Length test for quadratus lumborum. One examiner stabilizes the pelvis and legs and simultaneously palpates the tension in quadratus lumborum during movement. The second examiner supports the upper trunk and produces the movement of lateral flexion.

spine appears straight, with motion occurring only from the thoracolumbar region upwards, tightness of the quadratus lumborum may be suspected. This involvement of the whole lumbar region is in contrast to blockage at one or two levels, which may result from motion segment dysfunction.

The standing test lacks some validity because quadratus lumborum contracts eccentrically during this motion. The ideal testing position for this muscle is shown in Figure 10-5.

Normal Findings. There should be a smooth and symmetric lateral curve of the spine with side bending to each direction.

Signs of Tightness. When the quadratus lumborum is tight, the lumbar spine remains straight and a compensatory increase in movement occurs in the thoracolumbar region. Simultaneously, abnormal tension can be felt on deep palpation of the muscle.

When two examiners are not available for this testing procedure, an insight into quadratus lumborum tightness can be gained by positioning the patient in a half side-lying position (Fig. 10-6). Changes in the shape of the lateral curve of the spine are again sought.

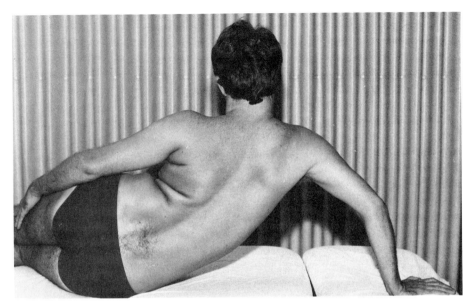

Fig. 10-6. Alternative test position for quadratus lumborum. The patient pushes up sideways to the point where the pelvis begins to move. (There should be no flexion or rotation of the trunk.)

Piriformis

Tightness of the piriformis can be revealed by a restriction in adduction and lateral rotation when the hip is flexed. However, palpation of the muscle is usually a more reliable indication than the stretch test. A deep palpation is performed in the region of the greater sciatic foramen across the muscle fibers (Fig. 10-7).

Normal Findings.   The buttock tissue is soft and the piriformis is not palpable.

Signs of Tightness.   When the piriformis is tight, the tense muscle belly can be palpated as the examiner's fingers move over the region. The patient often complains of acute tenderness.

Examination of Movement Patterns

Poor quality and control of movement can be of major importance in either the production or perpetuation of adverse stresses in the lumbar spine. Attention should not be limited to testing the strength of individual trunk and pelvic muscles but assessment must include observation of the coordination and sequencing of muscle activity during movement.

Movement patterns are very individualized and a person can be charac-

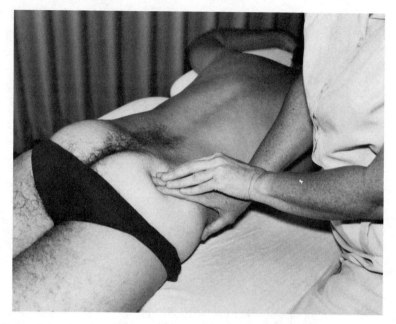

Fig. 10-7. Palpation for tightness of the piriformis. Any piriformis can be made to spasm through poor technique. Excessive tenderness and false-positive results can be avoided if downward pressure is applied through the examiner's relaxed lower fingers.

terized, for example, by the way they walk. There is, therefore, a range of "normal" for a suitable, nonstressed motor performance but in the presence of muscle imbalance or poor central nervous system motor regulation, some typical abnormal patterns of muscle activation have been observed.[43]

Six basic movements can give the therapist a good overall indication of the quality of an individual patient's motor control patterning. Those of most importance for the lumbar spine are the patterns of hip extension, hip abduction, and the trunk curl up. Poor patterns of hip extension and abduction can cause over stress to the lumbar spine during gait, while a poor relationship between iliopsoas and the abdominals during a curl up can indicate poor muscular stability of the lumbar segments.

Examination of Hip Extension

The pattern of hip extension is examined with the patient in the prone lying position. Three muscle groups are principally activated to lift the straight leg from the couch. These are the hamstrings and gluteus maximus acting as prime movers, and the erector spinae, which stabilize the lumbar spine and pelvis. The first sign of altered patterning is when the hamstrings and erector spinae are observed to be readily activated during the movement, while contraction of the gluteus maximus is very delayed. The poorest pattern occurs when the erector spinae initiate the movement and activity in the gluteus maximus is delayed and weak. In this situation, the whole motor performance is changed. There is little if any extension in the hip joint. The leg lift is achieved through forward pelvic tilt and hyperextension of the lumbar spine, which undoubtedly must over stress this region.

Examination of Hip Abduction

When abducting the leg from the side lying position, the gluteus medius and minimus and the tensor fasciae latae act as prime movers, while the quadratus lumborum stabilizes the pelvis. The first sign of weakness in this lateral pelvic musculature can be observed when the patient's leg laterally rotates during the upward movement. This indicates that tensor fasciae latae has initiated and even dominated the movement performance. A patient may further compensate for weakness in the glutei by allowing the leg to fully externally rotate during the lateral leg lift. This indicates that the patient has substituted hip flexion and iliopsoas activity for a true abduction movement.

Perhaps the poorest pattern of hip abduction occurs when the quadratus lumborum acts not only to stabilize the pelvis but also to initiate the movement through lateral pelvic tilt. This pattern again can cause excessive stress to the lumbar and lumbosacral segments during walking.

Examination of the Trunk Curl Up

Examination of the patient's ability to sit up from the supine position allows the therapist to examine the relationship between the abdominal and iliopsoas. The test is conducted from the crook lying position. Initially the therapist should observe the patient's spontaneous pattern of sitting up. If the iliopsoas is strong and dominant, there will be little flexion of the trunk and the movement performed is essentially hip flexion. The therapist can also palpate the iliopsoas to determine how early in the attempted sit up it becomes the dominant prime mover.

A further indication of the actual strength of the abdominals (or conversely an indication of the reliance of the patient on iliopsoas activity to perform a sit up) can be obtained by inhibiting or minimizing the early activity of iliopsoas. This can be achieved by making the patient keep his feet on the couch while actively plantar flexing his ankles.[45] The therapist should then instruct the patient to curl up through progressive flexion of his cervical, thoracic, and lumbar spines. The moment the patient begins to use iliopsoas, his feet will lift from the couch. The weaker or more inhibited the abdominals, the earlier in the curl up this will occur. Normally, the patient should be able to curl up so that the flexed thoracic and lumbar spines are clear of the couch before the feet lift. Excellent strength is demonstrated by the patient who can perform a full curl up to the sitting position while maintaining foot control.

Through the observation of standing and the examination of muscle length, strength, and these basic patterns of motion, the therapist can gain a good appreciation of the quality of a patient's motor function. Furthermore, the results of such an examination give the therapist definitive aims for a patient's individualized exercise therapy program.

TREATMENT APPROACH

The philosophy of this exercise approach is to maintain good balance between muscle groups in terms of length and strength, coupled with coordinated, controlled motion, and good posture. These aims are fundamental to the prevention of adverse mechanical stresses and pain in articular and muscular structures.

Remedial measures that may be required to achieve good quality and control of motion and posture are presented in Figure 10-8. The therapist must assess the patient carefully to determine whether or not such motor deficits are present and, if so, analyze the nature and extent of the motor impairment. An exercise program appropriate for the particular patient should be established, and it will require continual modification as the patient progresses.

The exercise program can be broadly divided into three stages:

Restoration of normal length of muscles, which are overactive or are tight.
Strengthening of muscles that have been inhibited and are weak.
Establishing optimal motor patterns to secure the best possible protection of the spine.

The program requires individual adaptation and more emphasis may be placed on one or more of these stages depending on the patient's problem.

Some basic principles should be followed when introducing exercise into the overall treatment program. Many exercises can induce high loads on the lumbar spine.[47] Therefore, a patient's condition should be stable before exercise can be safely commenced. Furthermore, if the patient is in pain or an exercise is painful, muscle activity can be inhibited.[17,21] Importantly, if the exercise is painful, the patient may compensate and perform a trick movement to achieve the desired goal. Thus the therapist may be inadvertently creating or perpetuating a patient's poor movement pattern. Pain and stiffness in a lumbar motion segment can also impair the important proprioceptive input required for good motor control. Therefore, every endeavor must be made to achieve normal and pain free movement in the lumbar motion segments to achieve successful motor rehabilitation.

In accordance with the earlier discussion on the adverse effects of tight muscles on motor performance, attention in the exercise program is initially directed towards normalizing the length of muscles. Having assessed that a

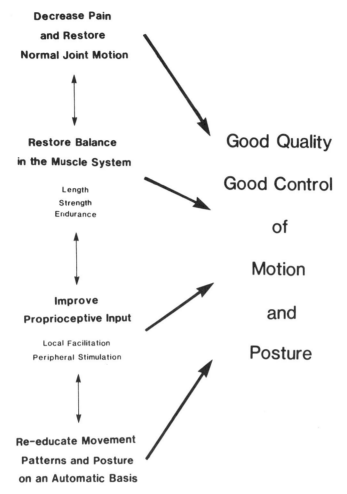

Fig. 10-8. Remedial measures used to achieve good motor control. (One or several of these treatment measures may be required to gain full rehabilitation.)

muscle is tight, the therapist must further differentiate whether the muscle is in spasm or whether structural changes, including shortening of connective tissue, have occurred. The latter is particularly common in chronic low-back pain patients. Such an assessment will direct the therapist to the treatment technique that should be used to achieve normal muscle length.

In principle the treatment of tight muscles can be divided into two parts. The muscle activity must be inhibited, and in the inhibitory period the muscle should be stretched. For muscles that have been assessed to be predominantly hypertonic, minimal facilitation and minimal stretch, such as is employed in the muscle energy technique[48] or a slightly greater activation followed by a moderate stretch, can be successful. However, when true muscle shortness is present, it is usually necessary to use strong resistance to activate the maximum number of motor units followed by a rather vigorous stretch if the desired increase in muscle length is to be achieved. Stretching by the therapist in the clinic should be complemented by the patient at home.[9,41]

Once the inhibitory influence of muscle tightness has been removed, there will often be a spontaneous improvement in muscles that were previously assessed to be inhibited and weak. Concomitantly, there is frequently an automatic improvement in the patient's motor pattern. In this situation, the patient's future preventative program is centered on a stretching routine.

Strengthening and particularly endurance training of muscles that have true weakness is quite a delicate procedure. Vigorous strengthening should initially be avoided. If a muscle is weak and the patient is forced to perform a strongly resisted exercise, he will often achieve the exercise through a compensatory "trick" movement. In doing so, muscles that are strong will be activated and those that are weak will not be used. A clear example is evident in the patient who can perform a sit up exercise, but principally uses his iliopsoas rather than his abdominal muscles to move from the supine to the upright trunk position. Such "uncontrolled" exercise will reinforce a poor pattern of movement, which is not only contrary to the aim of treatment, but may ultimately harm the patient's spine. Similarly, an exercise that is too vigorous does not allow the patient to control the movement properly and exercising into fatigue may also support a switch to a compensatory rather than a pure movement. Therefore, the therapist must carefully design the exercise so that the correct muscle is activated. Furthermore, the patient should have a perfect understanding and awareness of both the feeling of muscle activity and the exercise. The emphasis must be on quality of performance and not on speed, number of repetitions, or maximum resistance at this stage. Eventually, the exercise can be progressed as the quality of performance improves.

It is not only important to regain muscle length, endurance, and strength, but to ensure that the patient has good coordination and control of muscle activity.

There are a number of patients within the group who suffer from chronic and recurring pain, in whom good muscle activity is neither spontaneously nor easily achieved, and signs of poor motor control are evident. Their rehabilitation is not easy and reeducation of good movement patterns and postural control takes time and a cooperative and conscientious effort on the part of the patient. There is no "recipe" approach to this rehabilitation program. The motor performance of different patients varies and methods to achieve well coordinated muscle activity and postural awareness will vary between individuals. However, guidelines to the approach can be offered.

The reeducation program can be broadly divided into two stages. The patient must learn conscious control of muscle activity and movement; muscle function and posture will require reeducation on a subcortical or automatic basis.

Initially, the therapist must devise exercises that produce the desired joint movement and appropriate activity of the particular muscle or muscle group assessed to have impaired function. Emphasis commonly needs to be placed on gaining good and accurate control of lumbopelvic movement as this is fundamental to good posture. Specific and direct reeducation of the basic patterns of hip extension and abduction and the trunk curl up are also frequently necessary. Reeducation of motor control is often commenced in the stable lying position. The therapist should employ appropriate facilitatory techniques, such as vibration, stretch, traction, or compression to stimulate the correct muscle activity and pattern of movement. The patient must gain the feeling of the muscle contraction and sense the correct movement. Care should be taken not to exercise to fatigue, but to incorporate frequent short rests. Practice and repetition of the exercises are essential to the learning process,[49,50] and ultimately to the spontaneous use of the muscle during normal function.

When the patient can consciously perform and control good patterns of movement in lying, exercise and activity are progressed to the standing position. The next stage is to develop automatic control of the correct muscle activity, movement and posture. Therapeutic methods that will facilitate central nervous system motor regulation at subcortical levels are introduced. Such methods might include stimulating the patient's basic righting reactions and while doing so ensuring that correct muscle activity is achieved. The program may begin using the method of rhythmic stabilization, facilitating first through the pelvic region and later through the upper trunk and shoulder region. The speed with which the patient must make automatic postural adjustments may be improved by introducing short, sharp pushes to the pelvis and shoulders in the anteroposterior, lateral, rotational, and diagonal directions.

As discussed earlier, inadequate abnormal peripheral afferent stimulation is considered to be an important factor underlying the deterioration of movement patterns in some chronic low-back pain patients. Freeman[51,52] investigated the use of balance boards to provide afferent stimulation to improve muscle cocontraction and coordination following ankle ligament trauma. Similar proprioceptive training programs can be given to the low back pain patient once good control of normal movement patterns has occurred. Unstable surfaces, such as balance boards and mini trampolines, can be successfully used to facilitate good muscle activity in the lumbopelvic and hip-pelvic complexes, and to improve automatic postural reactions.[44] Importantly, such activities are facilitating muscle responses on an automatic or reflex basis.

Only some of the methods that therapists have at their disposal to reeducate movement have been mentioned but it is hoped they serve to illustrate the aim of this exercise approach. In summary, attention should initially be directed towards normalizing the length of any muscles which are overactive or are tight so that their detrimental influence on the motor patterning process is removed. Rather than concentrate only on strengthening exercises, emphasis in the rehabilitation program is placed on reeducation and achievement of good quality and control of muscle contraction using economical and nonstressful patterns of motion. It is considered that good motor control is an essential natural defence against low back pain.

CONCLUSION

Multiple factors are inherent in the symptom of low back pain. Whatever the underlying cause, pain in the lumbar spine will invariably produce either an acute or chronic impairment of muscle function. Individual muscles appear to react in a fairly predictable way and the imbalance in the level of activity between certain muscle groups is considered to underly the development of poor patterns of movement that often involve the whole muscle system.

The assessment of impairment of muscle function must be conducted on an individual basis. As poor quality of motor control is considered to be of primary importance in either the production or perpetuation of low back pain syndromes, the ultimate aim of any exercise program should be directed towards the achievement of well coordinated muscle activity and movement. Clinical experience has shown that attention should first be directed towards gaining the normal length of muscles that are overactive or tight. Once their inhibitory influence has been removed, the activity of muscles that were previously inhibited or weak should be actively facilitated.

Finally and most importantly, attention must be directed towards gaining voluntary and then automatic control of good coordinated muscle activity and movement.

REFERENCES

1. Cailliet R: Low Back Pain Syndrome. 3rd Ed. FA Davis, Philadelphia, 1981
2. Grieve GP: Common Vertebral Joint Problems. Churchill Livingstone, Edinburgh, 1981
3. McKenzie RA: The Lumbar Spine. Mechanical Diagnosis and Therapy. Spinal Publications, Waikanae, New Zealand, 1981
4. Nachemson A: Work for all. For those with low back pain as well. Clin Orthop 179:77, 1982
5. Woolbright JL: Exercise protocol for patients with low back pain. JAOA 82:919, 1983
6. Davies JE, Gibson T, Tester L: The value of exercises in the treatment of low back pain. Rheumatol Rehabil 18:243, 1979
7. Jackson CP, Brown MD: Is there a role for exercise in the treatment of patients with low back pain? Clin Orthop 179:39, 1983
8. Janda V: Muscles, motor regulation and back problems, p. 27. In Korr IM (ed): The Neurologic Mechanisms in Manipulative Therapy. Plenum, New York, 1978
9. Lewit K: Manipulative Therapy in Rehabilitation of the Motor System. Butterworth, London, 1985
10. Frymoyer JW, Pope M: The role of trauma in low back pain: A Review. J Trauma 18:628, 1978
11. Fairbank JCT, O'Brien JP: The iliac crest syndrome: A treatable cause of low back pain. Spine 8:220, 1983
12. Travell JG, Simons DG: Myofascial Pain and Dysfunction. The Trigger Point Manual. Williams & Wilkins, Baltimore, 1983

13. Dvorak J, Dvorak V: Manual Medicine: Diagnostics. Georg Thieme Verlag, Thieme-Stratton Stuttgart, 1984
14. de Vries HA: Quantitative electromyographic investigation of the spasm theory of muscle pain. Am J Phys Med 45:119, 1966
15. Janda V: Pseudoradikuläre Syndrome Bei Muskelfunktionsstörungen in Becken-bereich. Zschr Physiother 28:113, 1976
16. Kirkaldy-Willis WH, Hill RJ: A more precise diagnosis for low back pain. Spine 4:102, 1979
17. McNeill T, Warwick D, Andersson G, Schultz A: Trunk strengths in attempted flexion, extension and lateral bending in healthy subjects and patients with low-back disorders. Spine 5:529, 1980
18. Pedersen OF, Petersen R, Staffeldt ES: Back pain and isometric back muscle strength of workers in a Danish factory. Scand J Rehabil Med 7:125, 1975
19. Berkson M, Schultz A, Nachemson A, Andersson G: Voluntary strengths of male adults with acute low back syndromes. Clin Orthop 129:84, 1977
20. Alston W, Carlson MD, Feldman DJ et al: A quantitative study of muscle factors in the chronic low back syndrome. J Am Geriatr Soc 14:1041, 1966
21. Nachemson A, Lindh M: Measurement of abdominal and back muscle strength with and without low back pain. Scand J Rehabil Med 1:60, 1969
22. Addison R, Schultz A: Trunk strengths in patients seeking hospitalization for chronic low-back disorders. Spine 5:539, 1980
23. Smidt G, Herring T, Amundsen L et al: Assessment of abdominal and back extensor function. Spine 8:211, 1983
24. Langrana NA, Lee CK, Alexander H, Mayott CW: Quantitative assessment of back strength using isokinetic testing. Spine 9:287, 1984
25. Davies GJ, Gould JA: Trunk testing using a protype Cybex II dynamometer sta-bilization system. JOSPT 3:164, 1982
26. Suzuki N, Endo S: A quantitative study of trunk muscle strength and fatigability in the low back pain syndrome. Spine 8:69, 1983
27. Thortensson A, Arvidsson A: Trunk muscle strength and low back pain. Scand J Rehabil Med 14:69, 1982
28. Hemborg B, Moritz U: Intra-abdominal pressure and trunk muscle activity during lifting. II chronic low-back patients. Scand J Rehabil Med 17:5, 1985
29. Hasue M, Fujiwara M, Kikuchi S: A new method of quantitative measurement of abdominal and back muscle strength. Spine 5:143, 1980
30. de Vries HA: EMG fatigue curves in postural muscles. A possible etiology for idiopathic low back pain. Am J Phys Med 47:175, 1968
31. Kravitz E, Moore M, Glaros A: Paralumbar muscle activity in chronic low back pain. Arch Phys Med Rehabil, 62:172, 1981
32. Magora A: Investigation of the relation between low back pain and occupation. Scand J Rehabil Med 7:146, 1975
33. Biering-Sorensen F: Physical measurements as risk indicators for low back trouble over a one year period. Spine 9:106, 1984
34. Mayer TG, Tencer AF, Kristoferson S, Mooney V: Use of noninvasive techniques for quantification of spinal range-of-motion in normal subjects and chronic low-back dysfunction patients. Spine 9:588, 1984
35. Janda V: Postural and phasic muscles in the pathogenesis of low back pain. Proc XI Congress ISRD, Dublin 553, 1969
36. Rhode J: Das Muskelmuster. In Proceedings VI International Congress, FIMM, Baden-Baden, 1979

37. Richardson C: The role of knee musculature in high speed oscillatory movements of the knee. Proc IV Biennial Conf Manip Ther Assoc Aust Brisbane:59, 1985
38. Janda V: Comparison of spastic syndromes of cerebral origin with the distribution of muscular tightness in postural defects. Rehabilitacia Supp 14–15:87, 1977
39. Horal J: The clinical appearance of low back disorders in the city of Gothenburg, Sweden. Acta Orthop Scand suppl 118:15, 1969
40. Kraus H: Clinical Treatment of Back and Neck Pain. McGraw-Hill, New York, 1970
41. Janda V, Schmid H: Muscles as a pathogenic factor in back pain. Proc I'.' Conf IFOMT, Christchurch, New Zealand 1, 1980
42. Bannister R: Brains Clinical Neurology. 64th Ed. Oxford University Press, London, 1985
43. Janda V: Störungen Des Motorischen Lernens und Rückenschmerzen. Man Med 27:74, 1984
44. Janda V: Motor learning, proprioceptive training and back pain. Physio Can 1985 (in press)
45. Janda V: Muscle Function Testing. Butterworths, London, 1983
46. Farfan H, Kirkaldy-Willis WH: The present status of spinal fusion in the treatment of lumbar intervertebral joint disorders. Clin Orthop 158:198, 1981
47. Nachemson A: Lumbar intradiscal pressure. p. 341. In Jayson MIV (ed): The Lumbar Spine and Back Pain. 2nd Ed. Pitman Medical, Tunbridge Wells, Kent, 1980
48. Mitchell FL: Concepts of Muscle Energy. Proc Vth International Conference IFOMT, Vancouver, 1, 1984
49. Marteniuk RG: Motor skill performance and learning. Considerations for rehabilitation. Physiol Can 31:187, 1979
50. Kottke F: From reflex to skill: The training of co-ordination. Arch Phys Med Rehabil 61:551, 1980
51. Freeman MAR: Co-ordination exercises in the treatment of functional instability of the foot. Physiother 393, 1964
52. Freeman MAR: Instability of the foot after injuries to the lateral ligament of the ankle. J Bone Joint Surg 47B:660, 1965

11 | Back Schools and Ergonomics

Colleen B. Liston

BACK SCHOOLS

History

In 1825 Delpech[1] established an orthopedic institute for the treatment of spinal deformities. Patients who were managed in this "back school" lived in and performed "amazing feats" on rope ladders, floating stairs, bars, and rolling chairs. The apparatus was placed both inside a gymnasium and outside along maze pathways. In addition, a pool was used as part of the treatment regimen. Delpech believed in a holistic approach emphasizing fresh air and a series of balancing and climbing exercises "performed with propriety." Although patients remained in the program for one or two years, there are no records of program outcomes.

While McClurg Anderson's[2] ideas on functional analysis form the basis of current programs used in back schools, the first formal back school was set up in Sweden by Zachrisson-Forsell.[3] This followed the "educational approach" to treatment for back pain instigated by Fahrni and Orth,[4] who advocated the use of pelvic tilting in all postures. Zachrisson-Forsell's school was established in Danderyd Hospital, Stockholm, to teach body mechanics, and this has progressively developed into the "Swedish Back School." In a prospective controlled study with patients referred from industry, Berquist-Ullman and Larsson[5] were able to establish that the Swedish Back School program substantially reduced the number of days lost from work when compared with traditional physical therapy treatment (heat and exercise). The success of this ergonomic instructional approach prompted the establishment of over 300 more such programs throughout Scandinavia.

The three goals of the Swedish Back School as identified by Fisk et al[6] are:

1. To create self-confidence so that patients may most effectively adjust to and manage their own back conditions.

2. To avoid potentially harmful treatment and, particularly, unnecessary surgery through better patient judgment.

3. To reduce the continually increasing cost of medical care for low back problems.

While the Scandinavian approach is basically aimed at an ergonomic change to life-style, the Canadian Back Education Units established in Toronto by Hall in 1974 promote attitudinal change in life-style. The responsibility for health or ill health is to be assumed by the patient. By providing accurate information about the physical and psychological factors involved, the patient's attitude to their low back pain can be altered. In small groups, instruction about basic anatomy of the spine, body mechanics, specific exercises, pain and stress management, and relaxation techniques is given.

Hall[7] reports on the rates of symptom reduction and patient satisfaction and in 1983[47] in his review of 6,418 participants in Canadian Back School programs, he found that there was a significant subjective improvement in 69 percent of the participants. When only those patients who had experienced back pain for six months or less were considered, subjective improvement increased to 80 percent. Of greater interest was the establishment of a statistically valid positive correlation between this subjective improvement and the retention of information.

A behavioral approach reinforcing health behavior at the expense of ill health behavior was pioneered by Mooney at Rancho Los Amigos Hospital, California.[8] Elements of reward, competition, group work with peer pressure, and feedback led to 75 percent of patients reporting an increase in their activity levels and decrease in their back pain. Mooney reports in his paper that 62 percent of patients returned to work.

The first true back school in the United States was established in California by White in 1976. The aims of the program are described as being to elicit patient compliance in self care and management skills.[5] The program makes use of an obstacle course as its evaluation tool for measuring physical performance. In reviewing the first 300 patients retrospectively, Mattmiller[9] found that although 64 percent reported no significant change in lifestyle, 95 percent resumed normal activity and 89 percent did not seek further medical treatment.

In 1978, a back school was established at the Derbyshire Royal Infirmary, England.[10] A retrospective survey of patients' random comments considered the ratio of positive to negative responses. Results were not detailed but in the sample answers provided the ratio of subjective positive responses to negative responses was 6:1. A return rate of patients for treatment of low back pain of only 10 percent is reported.

More than 40 schools have since been established in Britain, all providing education, ergonomic advice, postural correction, gymnasium exercises, relaxation therapy, and hydrotherapy, with some also providing sexual counseling. These activities follow a thorough clinical examination, functional and subjective assessment by physical therapists and treatment for acute pain. Patients do not attend back schools in the acute phase.

Beryl Kennedy[11] pioneered back schools in Australia. She proposed the term *dynamic abdominal bracing* (DAB). This technique makes use of intra-abdominal pressure to give stability and protection to the lumbar spine, both in weight-bearing postures and in movement. In 1982, the Australian Physiotherapy Association ran a back schools' workshop in New South Wales bringing together those involved in developing back schools in that State.[12] No objective data are available, nor have outcomes been reported to date from any Australian back schools.

Rationale of Back Schools

Since low back pain statistics on incidence, epidemiology, social implications, and economic costs indicate a problem of staggering magnitude,[13] the development of back schools as conservative management for these patients must address all of these concerns. Incidence of back pain is reported to be as high as 80 percent of all adults of both sexes at some time between the ages of 30 and 55.[14-21]

Psychological factors, including personality, have been investigated and addressed many times.[22-30] Pain perception affected by thoughts and emotions varies with personality type. By learning to initiate, control, and work with pain fear subsides. Thus information concerning pain and the use of group work to provide cognitive instruction is advocated.[30,31]

Social factors are less often identified and discussed, and have been found to revolve around dissatisfaction with work, marriage status (divorced and widowed persons have a reportedly higher incidence), lower educational level, and increased age.[15,16,32] Psychological and social factors overlap in their influence on low back pain.

Rehabilitation of the long-term low-back pain patient may be regarded as the successful combination of improved attitudes and behavior with social, vocational, and physical activity.[33]

Benefits of Back Schools

Those who may benefit from attendance at a back school fall into several categories.

The Workforce

Men and women between the ages of approximately 20 to 60 years, with a multiplicity of different needs dependent upon their injury, their employment, and their social and psychological status.

Pregnant Women and New Mothers

Women between the ages of approximately 18 to 30 years, with a reported incidence of significant backache of 48 percent.[34] In this situation, there is an opportunity to provide a preventive back program early in pregnancy as suggested by Glover[35] and Mantle et al.[36]

The Elderly

Men and women from the age of 65 years and onward with varying degrees of age-related structural changes; with various mental and physical fitness levels, and disabilities. In addition, the usual influence of social and psychological factors merits consideration.

The Disabled

Individuals with secondary or tertiary low back pain. Males and females in a wide age range (whole of life) with a large variety of possible causes of their back pain. The chances of creating an overall program are limited in part by the particular needs of each patient. The above-mentioned factors for each of the other categories also apply.

The Compensable

The accident victims of both sexes and all ages, those who have much to gain by continuing to "have pain," and those who have genuine pain, but who often carry a stigma associated with compensation.

Preoperative and Postoperative Patients

Those with primary, secondary, or tertiary low back pain who require education, support, and a change of life-style in order to return to work after successful surgery and/or rehabilitation. This is essential if they are not to become another low back pain patient statistic.[37-39]

Others

Other groups who may derive benefit from a different style of back school are those involved in caring for patients and other specific occupational groups interested in the prevention of low back pain. These include:

Workplace Personnel. This group should involve architects and designers of the work places, ergonomists, planners, and board members, as well as unionists. The most important are those in management who should ensure that specific information is provided for each category of worker, and that the workplace is properly designed to provide a safe environment.

School Children. In view of the wide prevalence of back pain in our society, back education should begin in school and back education programs are currently being included in school curricula in Australia.[40] The Back School concept can be and is being readily adapted to provide a program for children.

Health Professions. Nursing staff, therapists, orderlies, and those involved with lifting patients, instructing patients with low back pain, and handling the disabled should be given adequate back school information. Occupational Health nurses and therapists involved in teaching and treating those in the work place require special skills to enable them to convey messages and assist in preventive work place programs.

Recreational Skills Personnel. Sportsmen and women, fitness groups, aerobics instructors and participants, coaches, umpires, and health studio staff constitute another category of those who require specific back school information. In this situation, the aim is to enhance particular awareness of the low back and the prevention of unnecessary stresses and injury.

Referral to a back school or requests for back schools may come from doctors, individual clients, industry (safety officers or management), teachers, health studio management, sporting clubs, insurance companies, workers' compensation boards, and other government agencies. Reasons for referral to a back school vary from its use as "the last resort," through awareness, self help, confidence, prevention of back injury, and increased fitness; to cost savings in worker's compensation insurance payments.

For whatever reasons, the use of the back school should achieve all of these stated ends giving clients an active role in the management or prevention of low back pain.

Aims of Back Schools

As previously mentioned, historically the aims of the various back schools have differed slightly. It is important to assess outcomes regularly to ensure that specific program aims are being met and to bring to light any new aims that may have been overlooked. Depending upon the clients of each school, the aims will necessarily vary. A check list of possible aims should include the following, which have been categorized under various headings:

Provision of Information

1. *Anatomy*—basic–of the back
2. *Biomechanics*—as related to the back
3. *Pain*—the control mechanisms, its effect or function, methods of relief
4. *Drugs*—uses and abuses
5. *Sex*—and low back pain
6. *Stress*—management–relaxation techniques
7. *Physical fitness*—including general health and diet
8. *Holistic health*—pulling together all of the above
9. *Availability of other resources*—professionals and agencies

Rehabilitation/Prevention

1. *Posture*—to teach postural awareness, correction (in all positions), postures that minimize strain and stress in the lower back.
2. *Awareness*—to be alert to the shape of the body, patterns of breathing, tension versus relaxation, fatigue, attitude.
3. *Movement*—to teach awareness of movement patterns that minimize strain and stress in the lower back.
4. *The Interrelatedness of body and mind*—to teach organization of movement in order to achieve greater efficiency and flexibility.[41]
5. *Self-help*—to teach the importance of and skills in self-reliance, motivation to be responsible for one's own back care, avoiding fatigue, self-control, confidence, symptomatic relief, happiness and independence.
6. *Physical intervention techniques*—to teach the relevant exercises (coordination, stretching, relaxation, strengthening, aerobic), trigger point massage, use of heat and cold to assist in achievement of the preceding aims.

Teaching Ergonomic Principles

1. *Human characteristics*—to teach the importance of recognizing that physical abilities, working postures, and mental alertness influence the ability to learn the best way to accomplish a given task.
2. *Environmental conditions*—to teach the analysis of the environment to assess problem areas and be able to recommend methods to rectify the problems (e.g., lighting, noise, vibration, heat, ventilation, pollutants in the air).
3. *Work dynamics*—to teach the importance of recognizing the influence of workload, layout of the work place and work station, stress and fatigue on errors, accidents, safety, endurance, and efficiency.
4. *Human–machine relationships*—to teach the relevance of the position and status of the worker to the work performed (e.g., controls, automated panels, display units, keyboards, loads to be moved, bench, and seat heights).

General Multidisciplinary Aims

Thus the overall aims for back schools should broadly encompass education, postural awareness, stress management and relaxation, attitudinal change, and exercise.

More specifically, the physical therapist's role in this multidisciplinary approach to the management of low back pain should include:

1. Development of a positive attitude, responsibility, and self help
2. Prevention of back injury
3. Life-style change for greater productivity, efficiency, and self satisfaction
4. Community and interprofessional education concerning the scope of the physical therapist's contribution in this area
5. Support for relevant social, work place, and environmental changes that would improve management of low back pain

Methods Used in Back Schools

While some schools concentrate on biomechanics (e.g., the Swedish Back School) some emphasize operant conditioning and greater psychological input (e.g., pain clinics/schools). Others utilize the correct ergonomic performance approach (e.g., the California, San Antonio, and Mississippi Back Schools).[42] In Australia Kennedy advocates the greater role of exercise; strength and fitness are seen as being the main aim by some,[43] while the Canadian Back Education units seek to alter patient attitude. In all schools, there is some overlap in approach and methodology. The efficacy of different programs has been investigated.[3,7,9,10,11,21,44,45,46,47] Most advocate the inclusion of all methods and aims in the optimum combination for the particular clients in attendance at each school.

Variables that determine the selection of a method include:

1. Presence or absence of pain
2. Type of pain (i.e., acute versus chronic)
3. Duration of pain (e.g., eight days versus five years)
4. Intensity of pain (e.g., transient to unbearable)
5. Age, gender, lifestyle, and occupation of participants
6. Personality, psychological, and social status of participants
7. Educational standard and language skills of participants
8. Class size (e.g., one-on-one versus up to 25)
9. Intensity and frequency of treatment sessions
10. Personnel, facilities, and location available

It is difficult to compare methods used and results obtained from the various back schools unless the above-mentioned variables are consistent within each program. Information should be collected via questionnaires and tests given at individual schools, and the selection criteria for participants, as well as demographic data on participants, should be faithfully recorded. Assessment pre- and post-back schools should include clinical and functional examination using standardized assessments. These should include a pain rating scale[24,48] and psychological tests. Analyses of such data using correlation and/or analysis of variance statistics would permit back school organisers to ensure that each back school was conducted on a cost-effective, therapeutically effective, and efficient basis, and was subjectively acceptable to clients.

The method chosen varies, as suggested above, but generally consists of classes at variable intervals usually one week apart, over a four to ten week period, with each class lasting from 45 to 90 minutes, and including a follow-up review lecture some six to eight weeks after the conclusion of the program. Information is collected prior to commencement, at the conclusion of the series, and retrospectively over a number of years. The retrospective data enables the presenters to assess retention of material and skills learned by participants.

The classes are held one week apart to ensure that adequate time is given for participants to absorb and assimilate information, thus prompting ongoing interest and the desire for more information. The format of each class requires some active involvement of the participants, particularly if the class is lengthy (e.g., 90 minutes). Information given may be demonstrated using audiovisual aids, or by the physical therapist, and clients may then practice techniques (e.g., lifting, relaxation, exercises, etc.).

The number of participants should be limited so that interaction is possible, and the expression of fears, problems, differences, and similarities can be enhanced within a manageably sized group.

Some back schools provide an intensive inpatient program (like that devised in Bath, England, for those with ankylosing spondylitis), while others give a one hour session each weekday for two weeks. These programs provide formal lecture sessions of instruction and participation three days a week. Relaxation, exercise, and hydrotherapy occupy the alternate two days.

Whether the back school is intensive or intermittent over a longer period of time, the overall aims remain the same.

The quality of the instructors and their instruction, the setting out of clear goals and objectives, which must be understood by the instructors and participants, and the statement of realistic expected outcomes are all important considerations. Instructors should be well versed in small group teaching skills and act as facilitators for the participants.[49–51]

The use of audiovisual aids should enhance teaching but the aids must be relevant, clear, uncluttered, interesting, and of good quality. They must also be presented at a suitable level, in understandable language, and in a format that is consistent with the rest of the presentation. Ideally films, videotapes, or slide-tape shows should be short, punchy, and depict information in an active reinforcing manner. Some back schools do not use audiovisual aids as they fear lack of identification of the participants with their instructors. Charts, models, diagrams, and skeletons are then used more widely as an adjunct to teaching.

Lectures, discussions, and practical sessions should be complementary and build on those that preceded them. It is best to establish key personnel, but a multidisciplinary team where all members fulfill the desirable criteria and work well together reinforces the holistic nature of health. The educational component concerning anatomy, physiology, and pathophysiology may be best given by an anatomist or orthopedist; the biomechanics, self-help relief methods, and postural information by the physical therapist. A psychologist or psychiatrist could best discuss the pain mechanisms, emotional influence on the body musculature, depression, anxiety, stress management, relaxation techniques, and uses and abuses of drugs. A dietitian is best qualified to present the importance of diet in a healthy life-style, an occupational therapist can suggest ways in which to modify activities of daily living to minimize stresses on the low back, a sexologist can advise on the best management of sexual life-style, and an ergonomist could make recommendations for changes to the work place.

Since it is unlikely that such a comprehensive team would be readily available on a regular basis, it may fall to the lot of a physical therapist to fulfil all of these roles. Liaison with appropriate health professionals will ensure that accurate and up-to-date information is given. The basic training received by most physical therapists, supplemented by ongoing reading and appraisal of the literature on back schools, would render the physical therapist capable of conducting a back school in its entirety.

Demonstration, instruction, and supervision of the practical skills that form part of the program include postural correction, relaxation exercises, handling skills (e.g., lifting), and specific exercises. Techniques of aerobic exercise and life-style adaptations can be explained.

Postural correction should form an important part of the program and be stressed as being not just "standing up straight." Postural awareness with the mind alert to the position of the body at all times will ensure that there is no undue stress is imposed on joints, bones, muscles, and ligaments. With body-mind awareness, good posture becomes a way of life; circulation, joint proprioception, function of organs, and muscle tone are enhanced, and the risk of back pain is minimized. Positions of rest should also be explained, e.g., the use of a footrest to prevent "sway back" during ironing, sewing, etc., resting the calves on the seat of a chair while lying on the back.

Optimum standing, lying, sitting, driving, and benchworking postures can be explained, demonstrated, and practiced.

Relaxation exercises may be given with the use of tapes using autogenic phrases, which encourage active involvement of participants in the relaxation process. These exercises may be practiced at home. Physical fitness and its contribution to the ability to relax should be emphasized. Regular aerobic activity using the large muscle groups of the body for 20 minutes without prolonged rest so as to increase heart and lung efficiency can be suggested. The most appropriate may be swimming, but walking, or static or active cycling are often acceptable alternatives. Warning must be provided and fitness levels tested before suggesting vigorous, sustained aerobic exercise.

Lifestyle adaptations for activities of daily living, work, play, rest, and recreation should be explained. For gardening, it may be appropriate to recommend the use of long-handled tools, altering the weeding or planting position at least every 20 minutes, raking leaves into one pile, and reducing twisting, flexion, and other stresses on the low back. This entails bending the knees to pick up leaves and other debris while facing the heap and then placing it to the front of the wheelbarrow. The wheelbarrow load is then closer to the fulcrum thereby giving greater efficiency to the lever. By standing in a position between a hole being dug and the pile of soil being created, minimum twisting is required.

For the handyman, a midtrunk height bench and footstool (4 to 5 in high) to rest one leg when standing for lengthy periods will minimize back strain. A forward-backward sawing motion using a wide-based stance will provide a more effective force. When painting, the task should be within easy reach to avoid over-stretching and consequent stress on the back. A sturdy chair or a trestle will assist in painting ceilings.

Housework should be performed in an environment designed to minimize back strain. Awareness of correct posture, fitness, and rest periods are useful preventive measures. When making beds, a person should bend the knees and keep the back as straight as possible. Do away with sheets and blankets in favor of continental quilts wherever possible (theoretically no bedmaking required). Castors on the bed will assist the making of a bed positioned against a wall. A trolley for moving the clothes basket to and from the line will avoid stretching to and from a basket on the ground, and obviate lifting and carrying the basket. Long-handled, light vacuum cleaners, polishers, brooms, and mops are important. An ironing board of adjustable height used with a footstool for one foot for those who like to stand, or at the correct height for those who prefer to sit when ironing, will decrease the strain on the back and allow the person to work with the lumbar spine in a more normal lordotic posture for that position. Workbenches, ovens, and freezers should be at waist height wherever possible to avoid unnecessary bending and reaching. Cleaning the bath should be done in a half kneeling position with a long-handled brush. It would be easier to clean the bath (or the shower) from within after use!

The pregnant woman must be particularly aware of the vulnerability of her back. Attention to posture will assist in avoiding the stress on the low back produced from the added load of the unborn child. The avoidance of high-heel shoes and prolonged standing should be emphasized. Strong abdominal and pelvic floor muscles are essential as well as instruction in relaxation positions (e.g., sitting, standing, and lying to optimize posterior tilting of the pelvis).

In purchasing equipment at this time, the height of the change table, trolley for the carry basket, bassinet or crib, carriage or buggy handle, and baby bath should be such that bending is not required. Slings are commercially available and these are a safe way to carry the baby, initially in front and later on the back. If the baby is carried close enough and as high as possible, strain on the low back and upper limbs is reduced. Lifting skills should be taught in pregnancy and continually reinforced especially during the first six postnatal months.

Lifting is a topic that has to be addressed by all back schools. Reinforcement of previously learned concepts concerning the importance of adequate rest and diet, physical fitness, and general good health should be provided. Back education participants must understand how important alertness and fitness are for safe lifting. It is also important to avoid unnecessary risks when lifting loads. It does not save time to lift a heavy load unaided.[52-54] Risk taking includes lifting too quickly, in an unprepared environment, without obtaining help where it is required, and lack of care in judging or assessing the size and weight of the load to be lifted. For large awkwardly shaped objects, assistance from lifting devices or another person should be sought. Pulleys, levers, hoists, and inclined planes may all be of help.

There is evidence[55-58] to suggest that stress on the spine is at its greatest when lifting from ground level or above waist height and least when lifting from hip height or between the knees. If the load is in front of the knees, however, the stress is increased. Likewise, if the load is to the side of the knees, twisting will be necessary and stress on the lumbar spine is increased.

Because a mechanical disadvantage is created in assuming a forward stooped position, the forces transmitted to the lumbosacral spine are great. Compression of the vertebrae and discs is reduced if the lift is performed without delay, smoothly, and at a steady rate.[56] Intrathoracic and abdominal pressure can also help reduce stress as can slight flexion of the lower back. Side flexion and rotation should never be allowed during the lifting of large weights, since this increases the total stress considerably.[55]

Most injuries during lifting occur when:

1. Judgment of the force required is incorrect
2. The load is lifted too quickly or too slowly, or where the surface is uneven or slippery
3. The lift is performed incorrectly (e.g., with the knees straight, the back bent, and the load too far from the body)
4. Uncoordinated lifting where more than one person is involved, one person should give clear instructions; incorrect use of assisting machines
5. Clothing obstructs the lift (e.g., flapping skirts, tight trousers, slippery gloves)
6. Unaccustomed repetitive lifting

Good habits for lifting should be learned early. For example, young children lifting kindergarten chairs and boxes of toys should be encouraged to lift and carry correctly. Older children should be taught in school the principles of correct lifting. The manual handling hazards arising from a lack of understanding of the principles and from bad lifting habits and the subsequent risk of low back injury in the work place should be reduced.

The Basic Rules of Lifting

Stance

The lifter should be well balanced over a stable base, with feet apart, and placed one further forward than the other facing in the direction of the lift. This position enables the lifter to maintain balance during the lift.

Posture

The shoulders and pelvis should remain in alignment to eliminate axial rotation and side flexion of the spine. If a turn is necessary, the lifter should pivot on the feet or step around. The back must be kept as straight as possible, with the abdomen braced and the pelvis tilted slightly backward. Keep the shoulders as far as possible directly above the pelvis and avoid stooping.

Grip

If there are handles, it is safer to curl the fingers around the handle. Otherwise the use of the palm and flat fingers in an intrinsic grip is best, but this is tiring. The grip should be firm, and use as much of the fingers as possible.

Picking Up

If the load is on the floor, the lifter should bend the knees and move to a squatting position. The load should be straddled between the knees and gripped firmly. Should the load be high, then the lifter must either be positioned as close as possible to it or must pull the load as close to the body as possible. Pulling is less stressful than pushing, as the horizontal force applied can be maintained close to the long axis of the spine.

Lifting the Load

At all times the load should be held as close to the body as possible. The lift must be powered with the large leg muscles when the load is on the ground. The back must remain straight, erect, and evenly loaded. Dividing a load may be possible (e.g., one bucket or case in each hand).

Moving the Load

By keeping the load close to the body, the lifter can more readily make use of the kinetic energy in the movement of the load, and by leaning back to balance the load use body weight to reduce effort to assist in moving the load to its required position.

Replacing the Load

If the load is to be placed on the floor, then the reverse action of bending the knees and straddling the load between the knees must be used. At all times the load should remain close to the body and jerky, rapid movements should be avoided. When placing a load on a platform or bench it should be at hip height to avoid the necessity of lifting upward. The lifter must allow the surface to take some of the weight and slide the load on to the bench. By using arms, trunk, legs, and thoracoabdominal bracing, the stress is spread, reducing the forces acting on the spine. By keeping the load close to the body, the lifting force required by spinal extensor muscles is reduced. By keeping the spine straight, it is maintained in a posture less vulnerable to injury. The lifting motion should be achieved by straightening the legs and powering the lift through the leg muscles.

Exercise

An exercise program designed for the reasonably fit average person should form the basis for specific programs for patients recovering from low back pain and form an essential part of any preventative program. It should include principles of DAB[11] to assist with lifting skills, flexibility, strength, mobility, and balance around the pelvis and low back.

A selection of three to five exercises repeated up to ten times provides a program of average length (15 minutes). Alternative exercises to achieve the same aims should be given to provide variety in the program and ensure continuing interest and compliance.

Important aspects of exercise programs follow.

Strength

Abdominal Exercises. The following are utilized in an exercise program: pelvic tilting; partial sit up (with knees bent); and curl up. Abdominal exercises assist to "brace" the lumbar spine in lifting and straining. Pelvic tilting, using the abdominal muscles combined with breathing exercises will provide the DAB[11] in slight flexion for lifting activities. Progression of exercises to include bridging, cross-arm knee pushing, knee raising, double knee raising, sit ups, oblique sit ups, and alternate straight leg raising and lowering with the opposite knee bent and the foot resting on the floor should be provided.

Extension Exercises. These strengthening exercises must avoid hyperextension and if contraindicated be performed within a functional range: single leg lifts to back level in prone over an abdominal pillow; single leg lifts from floor to back level with the trunk prone on a table; and raising head, shoulders, and arms to back level if prone over an abdominal pillow. These exercises may be progressed to double leg lifts.

Pelvic Floor Contractions.   This exercise should be performed in conjunction with abdominal exercises to assist with intraabdominal pressure and spinal bracing.[11]

Flexibility

Stretching of Hamstrings. The following exercises are used in exercising this muscle:

1. Long sitting with one hip in flexion, abduction, and external rotation to stabilize the pelvis. Stretch forwards to bring the face to the straight knee;
2. Supine lying, with knees bent, straightening one leg and pulling it up towards the head;
3. Alternate flexion of the knee to chest while the other leg is straight.

Mobility of the Low Back

Flexion.   In acute disc pathology, large ranges of flexion should be avoided as the lumbar roots may be compressed if a posterolateral nuclear prolapse is present (when this occurs, it is most usual for it to be in a posterolateral direction). In subacute and chronic conditions, or in preventive programs, flexion mobility exercises are useful:

1. Supine lying, clasping one bent knee to the chest alternately;
2. Clasping both knees to the chest;
3. Kneeling on all fours, with alternating back arching and flattening.

Exercise progression includes rocking in the knees on chest position, all fours, alternate knee to head with alternate leg extension to level and straight leg overs in shoulder stand position with the low back supported by the hands.

Extension.   Active lumbar extension exercises may be useful when there is increased intradiscal pressure due to loss of the lumbar lordosis. Restoration of the normal lordosis can greatly relieve pain.

Rotation.   Alternating the following exercises may be useful:

1. Supine, knees bent, feet on the floor rolling both knees together to alternate sides keeping the shoulders on the floor;
2. Knees to chest, rolling these together to alternate sides keeping the shoulders flat;
3. Crocodile—supine, one leg straight one bent—rolling the bent leg to opposite side and pressing it to the floor with the opposite arm.

Side Flexion.   Some mobilization of side flexion occurs during rotational work. It may be best achieved in standing by bending sideways ensuring body alignment with the arm on the bending side moving down the leg. In supine lying, with friction eliminated, the same mobilization may be performed with less intradiscal pressure and postural muscle activity superimposed. (NB: It is important to avoid those exercises that require excessive neck flexion in patients with rheumatoid arthritis or anyone with advanced cervical spine pathology.)

It would be appropriate to suggest that a daily exercise routine should include one exercise from each category repeated slowly ten times. By alternating these with others through the week all muscle groups and movement ranges would be exercised. If a particular muscle group is weak or mobility is reduced in a particular direction then the individual should be advised to concentrate more in that area.

Advice and information about progressions of exercises, as well as the checking and rechecking of exercise technique, must be undertaken regularly to ensure efficacy, accuracy, and compliance.

ERGONOMIC PRINCIPLES

Work habits, related laws and customs—the way humans perform work— this defines *ergonomics*.[59] Thus an account of ergonomic principles must look at the workplace and its relationship with humans. The problems attached to work must be addressed not only in industry but in other workplaces. These include the home, the office, the garden, the highways, and the classroom. The recreational workings of the body, such as in sport, travel, hobbies, even watching TV, must also be considered.

A realistic approach to the science of ergonomics requires cooperation between engineers, architects, tool makers, designers, medical and paramedical personnel, management, and sports administrators.

As previously mentioned, physical therapists have an important role to play in addressing ergonomics within their back schools. Physical therapists are also involved in assessment of prospective personnel in the workplace and advising about optimum techniques for working—including rest periods, adjunct exercise breaks, prevention of prolonged repetitive activity, and static postures. The physical therapist treats low back pain and must determine the cause in order to advise the patient on methods of preventing recurrence of the injury. The patient must not be allowed to believe that a job of work done must necessarily give back pain. By analyzing the task, performance of it by the worker, environmental factors, and attitudinal factors, the physical therapist should be able to offer appropriate suggestions for a solution.[60]

In assessing the task and its performance the following points should be considered:

1. Access to the work area
2. Space available for the task to be performed safely
3. Work height—suitability and adjustability

4. Placement of materials and controls—for easy reach and sequencing of the task

5. Comfort and stability—postural changes permitted, availability of foot rests, back supports, etc.

6. Nature of the task—repetitive, static, prolonged, degree of precision required

7. Rest periods—practicability, availability, possibility of changing use of muscle groups

8. Limitations of the work—does the task require too much speed, strength, accuracy, range of movement, repetition?

When assessing personnel, gender, posture, body size, strength, fitness, endurance, mobility, and past history of low back pain should all be considered. If the workplace provides benches, seats, equipment, and tasks for the average person with no adjustability or flexibility, then it will not be possible to select anyone but an average person for the job. Obviously attitudes must be changed so that designers plan adjustable equipment and installations and management ensure the provision of such an environment.

Unnatural, strained postures lead to discomfort, muscular tension, overload, fatigue, and ultimately to pain. Advice given regarding optimum heights for equipment must be considered along with the individual worker's posture.

For example when considering chairs and desks, there are several points to consider.

The Chair

1. Mobility—preferably castors with some friction on five legs
2. Comfort—rounded edges on an upholstered seat and back
3. Adjustability—adjustable height of seat and adjustable height and angle of lumbar support
4. Stability—base diameter larger than seat diameter
5. Arm rests—provide arm support with 90 degree elbow flexion

The Desk

1. Adjustability
2. Space—between the under surface of the desk and knees
3. Depth—adequate enough to allow for legs and feet
4. Top—not larger than the reach
5. Height—to allow elbows and forearms to be at the height of the work or rest on the chair arm rests

It is important to always consider the purpose of the chair and the user as well as teaching its correct use. Suggested dimensions in detail are to be found in the *Australian Journal of Physiotherapy*,[61] in an article by Barbara McPhee addressing ''Work Chairs and Seating.'' ''Ergonomics and Seat Design" has been addressed by Miriam Brunswic[62] in, *Physiotherapy*, January, 1984, and in the same journal, Mandal[63] discusses, "The Correct Height of School Furniture."

Alternative sitting posture via the Balans seat gives stability while enhancing good spinal alignment in sitting, but it gives no back support. It should be used with an angled desk to overcome any forward slump and only if it is suitable for the individual concerned (*not* for those with knee problems, because support is provided by the infrapatellar region).

When advising on the selection of a chair for relaxing, it is more difficult to specify dimensions. The choice must be personal, but consideration of the following points will be useful:

1. The chair design should make allowance for postural changes.
2. Back support in the lumbar region is an important feature.
3. Seat slope should enable the user to stay in the chair with the lumbar spine applied to the lumbar support without conscious effort, but not create difficulty in rising out of the chair (i.e., no more than 15 degrees of backward tilt).
4. Seat height and length should not be too great in relation to the length of the limb segments, as this causes ejection of the user by the chair.
5. The front edge of the seat should be rounded to prevent undue popliteal pressure.
6. The angle formed by the thighs and trunk should not be less than 105 degrees.
7. If the angle formed by the back rest with the vertical is greater than 30 degrees, the chair should support the head.
8. Padded armrests parallel with the seat and wide enough to support the arms are desirable.

Since good posture is the maintenance of the comfortable arrangement of body parts with the minimum of effort and no reduction of normal flexibility and function, then individual posture is highly variable. Seating must always make allowances for such postural variation.

Occupational back pain was reported by Snook[13] to have plagued the ancient Egyptians and in the seventeenth century was the main reason for Bernadino Ramazzini founding occupational medicine.[64]

Prevention of low back injury in industry requires a combined approach using a number of strategies:

1. Problem Identification
   a. the nature of the problem
   b. the cause of the problem
2. Training Program
   a. education that will lead to attitudinal and behavioral change
3. Testing of Personnel
   a. health status

b. functional ability
c. risk factors for injury
4. Ergonomic Improvements
a. engineering changes to equipment design, selection, and specifications
b. changes to systems designs
c. changes to task designs
5. Post-injury Return to Work
a. adequate assessment and treatment of injury
b. return to work gradual, not too soon, and to altered task and/or system

For example, suggestions may be offered regarding manual handling tasks. These pose a problem because lifting, holding, carrying, pushing and pulling are activities giving great stress to the spine. Having identified manual handling as the nature of the problem, the cause of risk to the low back may be inadequate assistive devices and/or no education program.

A specific Back School could be implemented in the workplace and workers tested to ascertain their current health status, abilities, attitudes, and risk factors likely to cause them to suffer a back injury.

An ergonomic assessment of the manual handling of materials may reveal that all four activities (lifting and lowering, holding, carrying, pushing and pulling) must be performed. Changes can be suggested as follows:

Lifting and Lowering

1. Use of assistive devices such as a crane, hoist, forklift, or platform. Where this is impracticable then ensuring that loads are at waist height before and after having to be lifted and lowered again.
2. Reduction in the size and weight of each load.
3. Changing to a less stressful method of moving of the load (e.g., pulling the load or pushing with the back against the load using the leg muscles).
4. If an assistive device is to be used, the weight (and size) of the load may be increased so that the frequency of lifting is decreased.
5. Changing from lifting and lowering to pushing and pulling using trolleys.

Holding

1. Use of mechanical loading and unloading to reduce holding time.
2. Use of jigs and fixtures to eliminate the need to manually hold.
3. Reduction in the size and weight of the load.

Carrying

1. Use of assistive mechanical devices (e.g., conveyor-belt, slide, fork lift, trolley, traymobile, etc.).

2. Elimination, if possible, by redesigning the workplace.
3. Use of two personnel carrying loads of reduced weight and size.
4. Reduction of distance over which loads are carried.

Pushing and Pulling

1. Elimination, and the use a conveyor-belt, fork lift, or other vehicle.
2. Reducing the size and weight of the load.
3. Use of aids (e.g., cable, wheels, pulleys, conveyer, etc.).

By analysis of the task, the physical therapist may discover a combination of factors capable of causing low back problems. Limitations of the workplace layout, equipment design, and the work, as well as individual anthropometric constraints may cause unnatural postures and excessive static or repetition work, leading to fatigue and pain in the low back. Appropriate modifications can be suggested and education of the worker in the correct use of equipment and performance of the task will reduce the number of workers' compensation claims for low back disorders. Coupled with a preventive Back School program, combining attitudinal, educational, ergonomic, and lifestyle changes, as well as exercise components as previously outlined will maximize the changes of preventing back pain. Regular monitoring of workplace ergonomics would, therefore, be a cost-effective exercise to be arranged by management.

The comfort, safety, happiness, and ability of the individual to work will be assured and the well being of the entire community enhanced.

SUMMARY

The evaluation of Back Schools is an ongoing requirement, but empirically they appear to have a valuable role in the nonsurgical and preventive management of low back pain. At this stage, it is appropriate to review their advantages and some related problems of a logistic and practical nature. Advantages may be outlined under these headings: philosophy, efficacy, economic factors, and group work.

Philosophy

Back Schools promote a philosophy of self-help. By increasing the individual's knowledge of a back condition and the importance of adaptations to life-style, each individual can take personal responsibility for the maintenance of low back health or management of a continuing problem.

Efficacy

Increased knowledge provides a greater awareness of body mechanics, including that of anatomy and posture. By conducting back schools, the general public, at a variety of levels, may be made more aware of the importance of back care and prevention of back injuries. Public awareness of the role of the physical therapist and the value of one-on-one treatment of acute problems may also be promoted. It is important for the public to be aware of the complementary roles of the medical practitioner, physical therapist, and other health professionals in the provision of such forms of health care. Back schools, at their most effective, decrease the requirement for surgery and medication as well as teaching self responsibility.

Economic Factors

Back schools are cost effective in a variety of ways. By working with groups there is a saving in time and work load for the health care provider. The saving for the community and especially for the individual (in terms of reduction of incidence of back injury and subsequent pain and disability) is obvious.

Group Work

In a group there is the opportunity for group interaction. Participants are able to contribute, ask questions, and benefit from the experience of others. This is especially so with homogenous groups (e.g., carpenters, a group with low back pain after lifting incorrectly, an antenatal group, a school class). The social contact will assist in providing group motivation and enthusiasm and compliance is more readily obtained. More time can be spent on education in a group and there is a greater possibility of interprofessional interaction (e.g., orthopedic specialists with psychologists, etc.).

The success of the back school depends upon the avoidance of problems with: the group; the leader; or of a practical nature. Examples of such problems are included below:

The Group

Some one within the group may have a specific problem requiring special attention. There is not enough time to spend with the individual, so this problem may not be addressed. Within the group there may be people with personality difficulties and differences; of different ages, cultures, and intellects. The difficulty of generalizing to a mixed audience may require the group to be reduced in size and divided so that there is more homogeneity.

Other complications include management of the dominant, disruptive, or overreactive participant. Occasionally someone is unable to adapt to the group situation or there may be destructive, unreasonable competition between group members.

The Leader

It is important that the leader should recognize potential problems and circumvent them. The leader must also have the necessary skills in conducting small groups, be an effective facilitator, and possess confidence and an adequate level of knowledge.

Practical Considerations

The suitability of a venue is an important consideration. If a hospital base is chosen then this may reinforce an illness concept particularly in a patient resistant to being helped or wishing to remain sick. This type of venue may be unpopular with healthy members of the public. Should a suitable venue be decided upon, it may not be available at a convenient time. If workers are involved then an evening school may be preferred. Back school times should be arranged to ensure that they are available to most clients. It may be necessary to schedule a day school and an evening school. The venue should be accessible, light, bright, comfortable, and large enough to allow room for practical work, but not so large as to discourage group interaction.

There may be problems with red tape, (e.g., obtaining permission, the referral system, methods of advertising allowed). To procure the best premises and personnel the cost of actually running the school may be prohibitive. Some compromises must be made as the costs can be covered in a short time.

Overall, the problems outlined are not insurmountable and the advantages far outweigh them.

REFERENCES

1. Peltier LF: The classic: The "Back School" of Delpech in Montpellier. Clin Orthop 179:4, 1983
2. McClurg Anderson T: Human kinetics and analysing body movements. Heinemann, London, 1951
3. Zachrisson-Forsell M: The Swedish back school. Physiother 66(4):112, 1980
4. Fahrni W, Orth M: Conservative treatment of lumbar disc degeneration: Our primary responsibility. Orthop Clin North Am, 6:1, 1975
5. Berqvist-Ullman M, Larsson U: Acute low back pain in industry. Acta Orthop Scand suppl 170:73, 1977
6. Fisk JR, Dimonte P, Courington SMcK: Back schools: past, present and future. Clin Orthop 179, Oct, 1983
7. Hall H: The Canadian back education units. Physiother 66(4):115, 1980
8. Mooney V: Alternative approaches for the patient beyond the help of surgery. Orthop Clin North Am 6:331, 1975
9. Matmiller AW: The California back school. Physiother 66(4):118, 1980
10. Hayne CR: Back schools and total back care programmes—a review. Physiother 70(1):14, 1984a

11. Kennedy B: An Australian programme for management of back problems. Physiother 66(4):108, 1980
12. Higgs J, Kemp P: What goes into a back school? A workshop report. Aust J Physiother 29(3):107, 1983
13. Snook SH: The design of manual handling tasks. Ergonomics 21(12):963, 1978
14. McBeath A: The problem of low back pain. Wisc Med J 69:208, 1970
15. Magora A: Investigation of the relations between low back pain and occupation: psychological aspects. Scand J Rehabil Med 5:191, 1973
16. Nagi SZ, Riley LE, Newby LG: A social epidemiology of back pain in a general population. J Chronic Dis 26:796, 1973
17. Anderson G: Low back pain in industry: epidemiological aspects. Scand J Rehabil Med 6:104, 1974
18. Wood PHN: Epidemiology of back pain. In Jayson MIV (ed): The Lumbar Spine and Back Pain. Pitman Medical, London, 1976
19. Kelsey JL: An epidemiological study of acute herniated lumbar intervertebral discs. Rheumatol Rehabil 14:144, 1975
20. Cochrane AL: Working group on back pain. Lancet 1:936, 1979
21. Frymoyer JW: Epidemiological studies of low back pain. Spine 5:419, 1980
22. Wiltse L, Rocchio P: Pre-operative psychological tests as predictors of success of chemonucleolysis in treatment of low back syndrome. J Bone Joint Surg 57A:478, 1975
23. Freeman C, Calsyn D, Louks J: The use of the Minnesota multiphasic personality inventory with low back patients. J Clin Psychol 32:294, 1976
24. Ransford AO, Cairnes D, Mooney V: The pain drawing as an aid to the psychologic evaluation of patients with low back pain. Spine 1:127, 1976
25. Caldwell AB, Chase C: Diagnosis and treatment of personality factors in chronic low back pain. Clin Orthop 129:141, 1977
26. Sternbach R: Psychological aspects of chronic pain. Clin Orthop 129:150, 1977
27. Pheasant H, Gilbert D, Goldfarb J et al: The MMPI as a predictor of outcome in low back surgery. Spine 4:78, 1979
28. Dennis MD, Greene RL, Farr SP et al: The Minnesota multiphasic personality inventory: general guide to its use and interest in orthopaedics. Clin Orthop 150:125, 1980
29. Pope MH, Rosen JC, Wilder DG et al: The relation between biomechanical and psychological factors in patients with low back pain. Spine 5:173, 1980
30. Herman E, Baptiste S: Pain control: Mastery through group experience. Pain 10:79, 1981
31. White A: Instructional course lectures, back school. 184. CV Mosby, St. Louis, 1979
32. Westrin JC: Low back pain sick-listing: a sociological and medical insurance investigation. Scand J Soc Med suppl 7:1, 1970
33. Aberg J: Evaluation of an advanced back pain rehabilitation programme. Spine 9(3):317, 1984
34. Mantle MJ, Greenwood RM, Currey HLF: Backache in pregnancy. Rheumatol Rehabil 16:95, 1977
35. Glover JR: Prevention of back pain. In Jayson MIV (ed): The Lumbar Spine and Back Pain. Pitman Medical, London, 1976
36. Mantle MJ, Holmes J, Currey HLF: Backache in pregnancy II: Prophylactic influence of back care classes. Rheumatol Rehabil 20:227, 1981
37. Beals RK, Hickman NE: Industrial injuries of the low back and extremities. J Bone Joint Surg 54A:1593, 1972

38. Kelsey JL, Pastides H, Bisbee G: Musculo-skeletal disorders: their frequency of occurrence and their impact on the population of the United States. New York Prodist 1978
39. Holmes H, Rothman R: The Pennsylvania plan: an algorithm for the management of lumbar degenerative disc disease. Spine 4:156, 1979
40. Liston CB: Back education begins at school. Paper delivered to Australian Physiotherapy Association Paediatric Seminar, Adelaide, South Australia, May, 1982
41. Feldenkrais M: Awareness through movement—health exercises for personal growth. Harper & Row, New York, 1972
42. Attix EA, Tate MA: Low back school: a conservative method for treatment of low back pain. Miss Med Assoc J 20:4,1979
43. Cady LD, Buschoff DP, O'Connell GR et al: Strength and fitness and subsequent back injuries in fire fighters. J Occup Med 21:269, 1979
44. Doran DML, Newall DJ: Manipulation in treatment of low back pain: a multicentre study. Br Med J 2:161, 1975
45. Cairnes D, Thomas L, Mooney V et al: A comprehensive treatment approach to chronic low back pain. Pain 2:301, 1976
46. Mooney V, Cairnes D: Management in the patient with chronic low back pain. Orthop Clin North Am 9:543, 1978
47. Hall H, Iceton JA: Back school: an overview with specific reference to the Canadian back education units. Clin Orthop 179: Oct, 1983
48. Huskisson EC: Measurement of pain. Lancet 11:1127, 1974
49. Boulton-Davies I: Physiotherapists–teachers of the public. Physiother 65(9):280, 1979
50. Hamilton-Duckett P, Kidd L: Counselling skills and the physiotherapist. Physiother 71(4):179, 1985
51. Berry AR: An introduction to interviewing techniques. Physiother 71(5):225, 1985
52. Asfour SS, Ayoub MM: Effects of training on manual lifting. American Industrial Hygiene Association Abstracts, 152, 1980
53. Mital A: Task variables in manual materials handling. J Safety Res 12:163, 1980
54. Niosh Tech. Report. Work practices guide for manual lifting. U.S. Dept of Health and Human Services, Cincinnati, 81, 1981
55. Nachemson A: Towards a better understanding of low back pain: a review of the mechanics of the lumbar disc. Rheumatol Rehabil 14:129, 1975
56. Charlesworth D, Hayne CR, Troup JDG: Lifting instructors' manual. Back Pain Association, Middlesex, England, 1978
57. Troup JDG: Biomechanics of the vertebral column. Physiother 65(8):238, 1979
58. Wood PHN: Understanding back pain. In Jayson MIV (ed): The Lumbar Spine and Back Pain. 2nd Ed. Pitman Medical, London, 1980
59. Bullock MI: Ergonomics: What is its role in health care. Patient Management 5(8):25, 1981
60. Hayne CR: Ergonomics and back pain. Physiother 70(1):9, 1984b
61. McPhee B: Occupational health: workchairs and seating. Aust J Physiol 28(5):30, 1982
62. Brunswic M: Ergonomics of seat design. Physiother 70(2):40, 1984
63. Mandal AC: The correct height of school furniture. Physiother 70(2):48, 1984
64. Teniswood C: Back injury prevention in metalliferous mining operations. Institute for Accident Prevention Seminar Paper Perth, Western Australia (Unpublished), 1982

12 | The Lumbar Spine, Low Back Pain, and Physical Therapy

Lance T. Twomey
James R. Taylor

Few people escape back problems and associated pain during their lives and all vertebral columns show changes with age that make them less able to cope with the variety of physical stresses of daily life. It is claimed that 80 percent of adults in Western societies suffer back pain at some point in their lifetime, and that in terms of work loss and treatment costs back pain is the single most expensive ailment in Western society.[1,2] Backache is as universal as headache but it is frequently impossible to be precise about the exact source of mechanism of the pain, as most demonstrable pathology is also visible in the symptom-free population.[3,4]

In the absence of an adquate knowledge of the pathogenesis of back pain, many of the diagnostic labels attached to patients are uncertain, and treatment remains largely empirical.[5] However, recent biologic studies continue to increase our knowledge of normal structure and function, and of the patterns of age changes and related pathology in the spine. Recent research (Ch. 3) demonstrates the anatomical basis of low back pain in terms of innervation of spinal structures,[6,7] and outlines a variety of possible mechanisms of pain production including poor posture, trauma, wear and tear, and degenerative changes in various parts of the mobile segment. Recent clinical studies have also monitored the response of particular clinical syndromes to a variety of treatment approaches.

A principal purpose of this final chapter is to consider the still developing link between the biologic sciences and physical therapy. Although the previous chapters demonstrate a diversity of treatment approaches, there is much in common among them. Each method utilizes a systematic, ordered approach to patient diagnosis and the progression of treatment based on meticulous consideration of signs, symptoms, and responses to treatment. All treatment methods emphasize movement (passive, active, or both) and advocate life-style changes.

In reviewing the physical therapy procedures described, this chapter considers the important contribution made by each approach to meeting the complex problem of low back pain. This will be done under the general headings of: diagnosis and assessment; prevention; and treatment.

DIAGNOSIS AND ASSESSMENT

Since so many physical therapists are now primary contact practitioners, diagnostic skill and technique have become of the utmost importance to them. The ideal situation remains that the referring physician should have the primary responsibility in diagnosis, with a close interaction maintained between physician and physical therapist. However, reality dictates that this will not always be possible. Whenever possible, and certainly when there is any suspicion that spinal pain or dysfunction may have a nonmechanical origin, the patient must be seen by a physician. Whatever the case, the physical therapist has to assume full responsibility for all physical treatment procedures utilized.

Diagnostic skills are required by physical therapists, not only for primary diagnosis, but also for more "refined" diagnosis of the anatomical origin of back pain or dysfunction in patients referred from physicians. It is usual for such physicians to simply exclude the nonmechanical origins in a painful condition and refer the patient as a case of low back pain. Diagnostic skills and accurate, objective clinical observation (Ch. 5) are also essential to assess the appropriateness of treatment methods by noting and measuring the patient's response to treatment. This provides the basis for judgement of the appropriateness of particular treatments and for the progression and development of a treatment plan with a particular patient. The process of diagnosis/initial treatment/reassessment/treatment modification is one of the major contributions that Geoffrey Maitland (Chs. 5 and 8) has made to the ordered, logical, physical treatment of low back pain and dysfunction.

Behavioral Aspects of Chronic Low-Back Pain

Since this book is primarily concerned with back pain of mechanical origin, full discussion of behavioral aspects is outside its scope. However, one must recognize that in chronic low-back pain, the reaction of the patient to pain is an important consideration. This is influenced by many developmental, family, social, and environmental factors related to the particular individual's circumstances. The suggestion that the refractory nature of a chronic low-back condition may be due to nonphysical factors is often resented by patients who may think that they are being accused of hypochondria, or that the doctor or therapist is looking for excuses for failures in diagnosis or treatment. When the stigma attached by many patients to the idea of behavioral causes for chronicity of pain disappears, they may be better able to come to terms with their condition. However, a positive rather than a negative attitude should always be taken in seeking solutions to a patient's pain problem.

The psychological effects of chronic pain provide a powerful motivation to health professionals to prevent chronicity by initially implementing effective therapy. Nachemson[8] points out that the chances for successful rehabilitation are reduced to 40 percent in patients in whom pain persists for more than six months, as persistence of pain for more than three months alters the psychological make-up of the patient.

The physical therapist should never be so blinded as to have narrow diagnostic horizons, which consider only mechanical or organic causes for back pain. Conversely, response to treatment may sometimes be attributable not only to the treatment used, but also to the optimism and ebullience of the therapist's personality inducing faith in the patient.

PREVENTION, EDUCATION, LIFE-STYLE AND RISK FACTORS

Education

Enough is known to support the view that education regarding a healthy life-style can make a vital contribution to back health. By developing an adequate knowledge of the structure and function of the spine, individuals can learn to maintain correct posture in all activities of daily living and develop muscle fitness. This would involve learning correct lifting techniques, avoidance of unnecessary hazards in work or sport due to unwise techniques or inadequate preparation for particularly stressful demands on the spine. By these and other means, we can reduce wear and tear on the spine and maintain a normal and useful range of pain-free spinal mobility into old age.

In the prevailing epidemic of back pain in our society, everyone should have a reasonable understanding of the structure and function of the back and of the age changes to which it is subject throughout the lifespan. They should understand the vulnerability of the spine to stress (e.g., loading in extreme flexion or in full extension) as in lifting loads or in certain sporting activities (Ch. 2), and the potential pathologic consequences of such activities.[9] Conversely, the hazards of a sedentary life-style in promoting poor fitness, poor posture, and predisposing to osteoporosis in later life should be understood if they are to be prevented. Information should be provided at a suitable level, to school children during their formative years, to adults in general, and also to particular occupational and sporting groups, which may be at particular risk.

All back education programmes (Ch. 11) should stress these features. While structure and function of the segmented rod that is the vertebral column is necessarily complex to meet the requirements of support, flexibility, and protection of neural structures (Chs. 1 and 2), it is relatively easy to convey the essentials of its structure and function to a lay audience.

There are many common misconceptions about the spine that should be laid to rest. The vertebral column is not inherently weak due to poor adaptation to the erect posture, although the lumbosacral angle involves stresses predisposing it to spondylolysis. Intervertebral discs do not slip, but the anulus may bulge in a degenerated disc, or the nucleus may prolapse through a ruptured anulus. There is no evidence that intervertebral joints "go out" or sublux repeatedly, requiring regular replacement, though muscle spasm normally accompanies acute back pain and is frequently relieved by spinal mobilization. A more informed and intelligent understanding of the normal spine and its reaction to trauma and degenerative change is essential, not only to prevent injury but also both to understand the need for different forms of treatment and to learn to live with an aging or damaged spine.

Nutrition and Body Weight

Excessive body weight unnecessarily overloads the spine, accelerates wear and tear, and increases the risk of trauma to spinal components.[10,11] It increases the rate and amount of "creep" in the mobile segment, with potentially painful results when poor posture is maintained for relatively long periods. A sensible informed approach to nutrition and regular exercise are appropriate, both in prevention of obesity and in treatment of obesity. Counseling by a psychologist, or membership in a group addressing itself to controlled weight loss may help. Many sufferers from chronic low-back pain would benefit by weight reduction, but seem unable to achieve this on their own.

Posture

The importance of good lumbar posture is repeatedly emphasized in this book, highlighting the general view that poor posture is a prelude to back pain. It is vital to maintain good posture in standing, sitting, and in bed. The normal lordotic posture of the lumbar spine assists in the efficient transmission of axial loads and provides the most efficient position from which to move the spine.[10,11] Flattening of the lumbar lordosis has been associated with aging and particularly with low back pain.[5,13,14] An essential feature of the McKenzie approach to treatment is the maintenance of a normal lumbar lordosis (Chs. 6 and 9). In standing it is important to stress the close relationship between pelvic and lumbar posture.[5] Physical therapists involved in both preventive programs and in treatment of back pain should stress this, help patients to develop an awareness of lumbar spinal posture (Ch. 2), demonstrate how changes in pelvic posture change lumbar posture, and how abdominal and gluteal muscles can effect these changes. Thus, they should ensure that patients understand how they can easily maintain a normal lumbar lordosis. In prolonged sitting, maintenance of good lumbar posture should be assisted by ergonomically designed seating or by the use of a lumbar roll. In Western societies, many of us spend a considerable amount of time driving a car. It is well known that professional drivers frequently suffer from chronic low-back pain and that long-distance drivers are prone to back injuries when lifting after long periods of driving. These particular problems probably relate to lengthy maintenance of bad posture, usually in a forward slumped position, with resultant "creep" of the soft tissues of the lumbar spinal joints into abnormal positions with abnormal states of fluid distribution in the tissues. In addition, tensions associated with driving on congested highways may provoke muscle tensions and some vibration may accentuate the effect of axial loading. The stresses placed on the spine by the abnormal posture itself, by continual use of the limbs, in steering, gear-changing and other maneuvers or by lifting procedures all contribute to pain or trauma to the spine rendered more vulnerable by these postural and "creep" changes. Better seat design and proper ergonomic positioning of the seat in relation to the controls would improve the position of the lumbar spine and its ability to cope with the stresses of driving (Ch. 11). In addition, regular changes of position (e.g., by stopping, getting out of the car, and doing stretching exercises at regular intervals during a long drive) would help to prevent or reverse "creep" changes. At the same time, a realization of the vulnerability of the spine after a long drive would alert individuals to the associated dangers of lifting stresses before recovery.

Mobility and Musculoskeletal Strength

Mobility

Prolonged inactivity or reduced activity lead both to muscle atrophy with loss of strength and to reduced range of movement with adaptive soft-tissue shortening.[15] A reduction in the range of lumbar spinal movement reduces the potential of the spine to respond to sudden demands of loading and movement and consequently increases its vulnerability to injury. Loading of the spine in a position well within the normal range for a normal individual, but close to end range for an individual with reduced range, puts contracted soft tissues under stress. Since the situation is compounded by reduced muscle strength, the joints may be forced beyond end range with consequent injury. Reduced muscle strength associated with altered spinal posture leads to similar problems with loading of the spine in unfavorable spinal postures.

Recent experiments on joint healing after injury provide a rationale for much current physical therapy. For instance, they show that immobilization hinders cartilage repair, while repetitive passive movements accelerate repair.[14–18] Synovial fluid circulation in the articular cartilage is essential for its nutrition and this circulation is favored by the stirring and alternate pressure and relaxation of passive movements. Other studies confirm that a considerable range of passive movement is necessary for proper repair of damaged cartilage.[19,20] The corollary would be that nonstressful active movement through the full range helps to keep a joint healthy.

Physical therapeutic procedures using active and passive movements of the lumbar spine aid nutrition of both the intervertebral discs and the zygapophyseal joint cartilages, while helping to preserve the full range of movement and the normal strength and flexibility of periarticular soft tissues, ligaments, and tendons. In other words, they prevent adaptive shortening of these tissues and stiffness of the joint.[17] A healthy life-style should include regular activities involving a full range of movements with exercise of the muscles moving and controlling the posture of the lumbar spine. This is equally applicable to prevention and treatment of low back disorders.

Muscle Strength

Muscles grow in mass and strength as the individual grows. Full strength is maintained in early adult life, but tends to decline slowly in middle life and more rapidly in old age. However, muscle endurance increases with increase in age in adults and quite high levels of muscle strength can be maintained into old age by regular exercise.[21-23]

Of the muscles controlling the lumbar spine, the extensors are usually the strongest and the abdominal flexors are often comparatively weak.[24] In an obese person, a protruding abdominal wall may reduce the mechanical efficiency of the abdominal muscles and thus diminsh their protective effect on the loaded lumbar spine (Ch. 2). Raised intraabdominal pressure, particularly as produced by the transverse and oblique abdominal muscles, is a potent force reducing the effect of heavy loads on the lumbar spine. This is achieved both by the "balloon effect" exercising a distractive force anterior to the vertebral column, and also by tension effects on the lateral margins of the extensor aponeurosis, which would reduce the extensor force required from the erector spinae to maintain the lumbar spine in an extended lordotic posture.[25,27] Thus, abdominal muscle strengthening exercises are mandatory in treatment of most low back pain and highly desirable as a preventive measure. Patients with low back pain should understand the importance of abdominal muscle "bracing" for many of the activities of daily living, particularly lifting.

Bone Strength

It is probably by the intermediary of muscle activity that bone strength is maintained.[25,26] Loss of transverse trabeculae from lumbar vertebral bodies is the first sign of osteopenia with aging.[29] In postmenopausal women, bone-mineral loss can be prevented by exercise programs.[28,31,32] Lifetime habits of regular exercise, maintained into old age as appropriate, would help to diminish the osteoporosis, which for too long has been regarded as an inevitable accompaniment of old age. Regular exercise needs to be accompanied by an adequate intake of dietary calcium. In some individuals, hormonal replacement therapy may also be required for some time after the menopause.[33,34] The incidence of back pain, vertebral body fractures, and increasing kyphosis could be substantially reduced by widespread application of these measures.[26]

Loading at End Range (i.e., Working at the Limit of the Normal Range of Motion)

Flexion

As discussed in Chapters 1 and 2, our posterior release studies, "creep" studies, studies of age changes in lumbar zygapophyseal joints, and Nachemson's intradiscal pressure studies[46] all point to the dangers of loading the spine in full flexion. Prolonged loading in flexion causes soft-tissue "creep," with redistribution of tissue fluid and change of shape in the mobile segment, so that the collagenous elements in the disc and facet joint cartilages are abnormally stressed in conditions of sustained high intradiscal pressures. In full flexion the spine is also hanging on its facet joints and the effects of this loading are reflected in the selective age changes in the coronal components of these joints.[30] Particular occupational groups, such as bricklayers' and stonemasons' work for extended periods in a fully flexed posture, susceptible to injury when the spine has to bear any further sudden increase in loading at the limit of flexion. It is not surprising that they have a much higher incidence of low back pain than other occupational groups.

Back education is essential for such workers, and should include warning of the dangers of prolonged loading in flexion, advice to maintain a straight spine, and to work at waist height whenever possible. They should be instructed of the need for back mobility exercises, particularly extension stretching exercises at regular intervals during the working day,[13] and coached in abdominal muscle strengthening exercises to be done on a regular basis. Expert attention to the ergonomics of the tasks involved may also help to minimize the problem (Ch. 11), but there will always be some risk attached to those occupations where some loading in flexion is inevitable.

Extension

Relatively few occupations require working for long periods in full extension, but a number of sporting pursuits may either require, or may involve through wrong technique, short- or long-term loading of the lumbar spine in extension. These would include serving at tennis, fast bowling in cricket, gymnastic exercises, and wind surfing. In tennis or fast bowling, movement into full extension is accompanied by explosive loading of the lumbar spine. Then rapid active flexion of the lumbar spine follows. Sometimes this combination of movement and peak loading results in stress fracture or spondylolysis of the pars interarticularis of a lower lumbar vertebra. Such conditions of loading should be avoided wherever possible. Otherwise regular rigorous abdominal muscle strengthening exercises may prove protective of the spine at risk.

TREATMENT

Self-Treatment

Since we are all liable to suffer from back pain occasionally, we should all learn how mild, recurrent episodes can be prevented or managed. McKenzie argues that repeated visits to a manipulative physical therapist are unnecessary if patients can be taught and given responsibility for the management of their own back problems. He emphasizes the need for the maintenance of the "normal" lordotic lumbar curvature through all daily activities, and for preserving a full range of lumbar extension. To this effect, clients are shown how to assume positions of full extension, how to maintain them (e.g., by use of a lumbar roll when sitting) and when this is appropriate. There is an increasing body of evidence that supports this premise, and that demonstrates the efficacy of this approach (Chs. 6 and 9).

On the other hand, we would suggest that backache that develops after standing for prolonged periods is probably due to the effects of axial and extension creep due to gradual adoption of a sway-back posture (Ch. 2). This would be best managed initially by the patient going gently into full lumbar flexion. Tyrell et al[36] showed in a recent study that rehydration of discs and soft tissues after prolonged standing occurred most rapidly in a flexed position, allowing the height of lumbar intervertebral discs to return to their usual values. The rationale for the management of back pain following either flexion or extension creep after prolonged loading in either of these postures is that it requires the opposite movement to reverse the "creep" effect. McKenzie's experience suggests that "creep" in flexion is more common and possibly more troublesome than "creep" in extension. Individuals whose work involves them in prolonged periods of time in full lumbar flexion should regularly interrupt their work for "pause exercises," with a particular emphasis on extension movements.

Even some of the basic principles and techniques of spinal mobilization can be taught to patients for self management. A full range of all lumbar spinal movements is desirable, and low back pain often responds rapidly to gentle, mobilizing exercise (both passive and active) performed in the outer range of lumbar movements. Such self-mobilization, which may be accompanied by joint clicks is easily taught to patients and is often particularly useful.

Lumbar traction can also be self-administered in a number of ways. Clients can be taught to apply traction while sitting in an armchair by taking their body on their extended arms with the trunk and lower limbs relaxed; they can be shown how to hang from their arms; or they can use sophisticated autotraction devices[37] or "gravity" traction.[38] The rationale for the worth of traction again depends on improving soft-tissue hydration and allowing the intervertebral discs to "re-inflate."[36]

Intervention—Physical Treatment

It is beyond the scope of this book to consider the many physical agents and modalities that may be used in the treatment of low back pain. There are strong advocates within physical therapy who emphasize a role for heat, cold, electrophysical agents, acupuncture and acupressure, various massage modalities, and a variety of peripheral techniques for this complex problem. However, this section will discuss only those physical therapy techniques described in Chapters 5–11, which emphasize treatment intervention by active or passive movement.

Active Movement

The rationale for the use of either flexion or extension exercises, or generalized full-range active exercises has been discussed earlier in this chapter. The same principles apply as in self-treatment. Since so many daily activities result in lumbar flexion creep, extension exercises are most often of importance. In addition, there is recent evidence to suggest that treatment by active and passive extension movements is beneficial for cases of proven disc degeneration.[14]

In the absence of specific pathology, lumbar rotation, lateral flexion, and combined mobility exercises will usually accompany exercise regimes, which are predominantly flexion or extension directed. They emphasize a fuller range of motion, provide compression and relaxation of articular cartilage and intervertebral discs, and assist in the stirring of synovial fluid in the zygapophyseal joints, all of which are necessary for cartilage nutrition. The effect that joint movement has on articular cartilage, ligaments, and tendons has been described previously and is well reviewed in a recent paper by Frank et al.[19]

Passive Movement

Much of the acute physical treatment of low back pain is by the passive movement of spinal segments (Chs. 5, 7, and 8). The techniques involved range from very gentle movements or mobilization through to forced passive movement at the end of range (i.e., manipulation). The efficacy of this form of treatment has been the subject of much recent critical review.[35,40,41] The reasons provided for the effectiveness of manipulative therapy range from the restoration of range of motion,[40,41] to complex neurologic explanations.[35,42] Our recent studies of age changes in the lumbar zygapophyseal joints indicate that in some individuals articular cartilage may be partially stripped away from the underlying subchondral bone in the posterolateral region of the joints (Ch. 1). It is postulated that such a piece of hard articular cartilage may be caught between opposing joint surfaces (like a torn meniscus in the knee), causing joint locking and acute back pain. This may account for the group of patients with acute back pain who respond so dramatically to a single manipulation. A manipulative procedure is best used when techniques of self-help (before) and gentle passive movement do not bring about the expected increase in range of movement or decrease in joint pain.[35,40] It is still impossible to logically differentiate between the use of self-help and active movement on the one hand, and operator-assisted mobilization and manipulation on the other, since devotees of both methods advocate their use for similar joint pain problems (Chs. 5–10).

Manipulative therapy is an empirical form of treatment favored by very many clinicians from a variety of medical and nonmedical backgrounds, and patronized by a vast public. The results of clinical trials of manipulation have largely been disappointing, although in recent years, a number of trials have shown a useful application in the early stages of acute low back pain.[43–45] There is no doubt that more carefully controlled, blind clinical trials of manipulative therapy need to be carried out on large populations if the efficacy of this most popular form of physical treatment is to be properly understood.

Traction

The rationale for the use of traction as physical treatment in low back pain has been briefly considered under the section Self-treatment. Traction may be continuous or intermittent, mechanical or manual. Intermittent mechanical traction is also said to increase local circulation, and by axial movement to improve joint function.[41] Continuous traction has been claimed to assist in the reduction of some forms of herniated nucleus pulposus.[37] Traction usually forms part of a physical treatment program, which may also include active or passive movement or both.

LOOKING AHEAD

Attempts are made in this book to correlate basic scientific research with successful treatment methods, to see the place of different treatment approaches in overall patient care and to emphasize the vital importance of proper diagnostic methods and assessment of responses to treatment with disciplined record keeping.

Given adequate attention to self-education by health professionals, on advances in knowledge of spinal function and pain pathogenesis, continuing vigilance in development of diagnostic skills and objective evaluation of treatment, there is much room for optimism that the perennial problems of back pain will not remain intractable. Modern diagnostic methods like magnetic resonance imaging (MRI) and selective nerve block procedures are already providing more accurate anatomical diagnoses. It is gratifying that the hands of expert physical therapists can be just as accurate in localizing the source of pain (Ch. 3).

It is already obvious that there is no universal recipe for the treatment of low back pain, and that treatment methods alone will not be the complete answer. More widespread back education, with changes in life-style and changes in the ergonomic environment of the workplace and at home, will also be required. The importance of regular movement/exercise in maintaining good nutrition of joint cartilages and in healing damaged tissues should be emphasized.

Clinical studies that correlate diagnosis with physical treatment need to be energetically pursued, and should enable more accurate prescription. Such studies need to concentrate, at least in part, on the recurrence rates of back pain in relation to treatment and on the relationship between back education, body awareness, and self-help (self-treatment) with episodic low-back pain.

REFERENCES

1. Nachemson AL: The lumbar spine: An orthopaedic challenge. Spine 1:1, 59, 1976
2. Kelsey J, White AA: Epidemiology and impact of low back pain. Spine 5:2, 133, 1980
3. Glover JR: Occupational health research and problems of back pain. Trans Soc Occup Med 21:2, 1970
4. Troup D: The biology of back pain. New Scientist 2 Jan., 17, 1975
5. Twomey LT: Age changes in the human lumbar spine. PhD thesis, University of Western Australia, 1981
6. Taylor JR, Twomey LT: Innervation of lumbar intervertebral discs. NZ J Physiother 8:36, 1980
7. Giles L, Taylor J: Human zygapophyseal joint capsule and synovial fold inner-vation. Br J Rheumatol in press, 1986
8. Nachemson A: Recent advances in the treatment of low back pain. Int Orthhop 9:1, 1985
9. Taylor JR, Twomey LT: Sagittal and horizontal plane movement of the human lumbar vertebral column in cadavers and in the living. Rheumatol Rehabil 19:223, 1980
10. Twomey LT, Taylor JR: Flexion creep deformation and hysteresis in the lumbar vertebral column. Spine 7:2, 116, 1982
11. Hall H, Iceton JA: Back school: An overview with special reference to the Canadian Back Education Units. Clin Orthop 179:10, 1983
12. Berquist-Ullman M, Larson U: Acute low back pain in industry. Acta Orthop Scand suppl 170, 1977
13. McKenzie R: The Lumbar Spine. Spinal Publications, Waikanae, New Zealand, 1980
14. Kopp JR, Alexander AH, Turocy RH et al: The use of lumbar extension in the

evaluation and treatment of patients with acute herniated nucleus pulposis. A preliminary report. Clin Orthop 202:211, 1986

15. Hall DM: The Ageing of Connective Tissue. Academic Press, London, 1976
16. Salter RB, Simmonds DF, Malcolm BW et al: Effects of continuous passive motion on the healing of articular cartilage defects. J Bone Joint Surg 57A:4, 570, 1975
17. Mooney V, Ferguson AB: The influence of immobilisation and motion on the formation of fibrocartilage in the repair granuloma after joint resection in the rabbit. J Bone Joint Surg 48A:6, 1145, 1966
18. Rubak JM, Poussa M, Ritsila V: Effects of joint motion on the repair of articular cartilage with free periosteal grafts. Acta Orthop Scand 53:187, 1982
19. Frank C, Akeson WH, Woo SL-Y et al: Physiology and therapeutic value of passive joint motion. Clin Orthop 185:113, 1984
20. Salter RB, Simmonds DF, Malcolm BW et al: The biological effect of continuous passive motion in the healing of full thickness defects in articular cartilage. J Bone Joint Surg 62A:1232, 1980
21. Frank C, Amiel D, Woo SL-Y et al: Normal ligament properties and ligament healing. Clin Orthop 196:15, 1985
22. Woo SL-Y, Gelberman RH, Cobb NG et al: The importance of controlled passive mobilisation of flexor tendon healing. Acta Orthop Scand 52:615, 1981
23. Tanner JM: Foetus Into Man. Open Books, London, 1978
24. Walker J: Exercise & ageing. NZ J Physiother 14:1, 8, 1986
25. Shephard RJ: Management of exercise in the elderly. Can J Appl Sport Sci 9:3, 109, 1984
26. Twomey LT, Taylor JR: Old age and physical capacity. Aust J Physiotherapy 30:4, 115, 1984
27. Gracovetsky S, Farfan H, Helleur C: The abdominal mechanism. Spine 10:4, 317, 1985
28. Pardini A: Exercise, vitality and aging. Aging 344:19, 1984
29. Twomey LT, Taylor J, Furniss B: Age changes in the bone density and structure of the lumbar vertebral column. J Anat 136:1, 15, 1983
30. Twomey LT, Taylor JR: Age changes in the lumbar articular triad. Aust J Physiotherapy 31:3, 106, 1984
31. Smith EL, Reddan W, Smith PE: Physical activity and calcium modalities for bone mineral increase in aged women. Med Sci Sports Exerc 13:60, 1981
32. Aloia JF, Cohn SH, Ostuni JA et al: Prevention of involutional bone loss by exercise. J Clin Endocrinol Metab 43:992, 1978
33. Dixon AStJ: Non hormonal treatment of osteoporosis. Br Med J 286:999, 1983
34. Spencer H, Kramer L, Lesniak M et al: Calcium requirements in humans. Clin Orthop 184:270, 1984
35. Haldeman S: Spinal manipulative therapy: A status report. Clin Orthop 179:62, 1983
36. Tyrrell AR, Reilly T, Troup JDG: Circadian variation in stature and the effects of spinal loading. Spine 10:2, 161, 1985
37. Larsson U, Choler U, Lindstrom A et al: Auto-traction for treatment of lumbago-sciatica. Acta Orthop Scand 51:791, 1980
38. Saunders HD: use of spinal traction in the treatment of neck and back conditions. Clin Orthop 179:31, 1983
39. Kennedy B: Dynamic back care. Blake & Hargreaves Pty, Sydney, 1985
40. Paris SV: Spinal manipulative therapy. Clin Orthop 179:55, 1983
41. Deyo RA: Conservative therapy for low back pain. JAMA 250:8, 1057, 1983

42. Zusman M: Reappraisal of a proposed neurological mechanism for the relief of joint pain with passive movements. Physiother Pract 1:2, 64, 1986
43. Farrell JP, Twomey LT: Acute low back pain: Comparison of two conservative treatment approaches. Med J Aust 1:160, 1982
44. Rasmussen GG: Manipulation in low back pain: A randomised clinical trial. Manuelle Med 1:8, 1977
45. Evans DP, Burke MS, Lloyd KN et al: Lumbar spinal manipulation on trial Part I—Clinical assessment. Rheumatol Rehabil 17:46, 1978
46. Nachemson A: Lumbar intradiscal pressure. Acta Orthop Scand suppl 43, 1960

Index

Page numbers followed by *f* denote figures; those followed by *t* denote tables.

Muscles (*Continued*)
   hip flexor evaluation of, 266–267,
     267f
   imbalance of muscle action and,
     159, 257–260, 258t
   impairment of muscle function and,
     256–257
   layer syndrome, 262f, 263
   movement patterns evaluation of,
     269–272
   muscle length evaluation of, 266–
     269, 267–270f
   pelvic crossed syndrome, 260–263,
     261f
   piriformis evaluation of, 269, 270f
   quadratus lumborum evaluation of,
     267–268, 268f, 269f
   as reaction to pain, 254, 255f
   as source of pain, 159, 254–255
   standing posture evaluation of, 264–
     266
   treatment approach for, 272–276,
     273f
   trunk curl up evaluation of, 271–272
   examination of. *See* Examination of
     muscles
Myotomes, 28

Nerve(s), spinal, 6–8, 8f
Nerve roots
   adherence of, 230, 248
   anatomy of, 7, 8f, 86–89, 86f, 87f
Nerve root pain
   from irritation and compression, 93–
     95, 202
   manipulative therapy for, 211–215
     chronic pain, 213–215, 215f
     severe pain, 211–213
Neural tube formation
   abnormal, 26–27
   normal, 19–20, 21f
Notochord
   development of, 19–20, 21f
   vertebral anomalies due to, 26–29
Nucleus pulposus
   aging effects on, 39
   anatomy of, 4f, 14
     anomalies in, 28–29
     postnatal, 14, 35–36
     prenatal, 21, 22f, 24f, 26–28

   extrusion of, 7
   function of, 14
   height adjustments due to, 15
   vascularity of, 15
Nutrition, 306

Obesity, 306
Osteoporosis
   bone strength and, 308–309
   incidence of, 79
   prevention of, 79
   symptoms of, 79
   of zygopophyseal joints, 44, 46, 47

Pain, back. *See* Back pain
Passive movement treatment
   Maitland concept of, 141–142
   manipulative. *See* Manipulative
     therapy
   mobilization in, 160, 206–207, 311
Pelvic crossed syndrome, 260–263, 261f
Physical examination. *See* Examination
     procedures
Piriformis, 269, 270f
Postural syndrome
   manipulative therapy for, 222–223
   McKenzie approach to
     diagnosis, 230–231
     treatment, 247
   mechanical therapies for, 162–163, 171
Posture
   aging effects on, 57–58, 57f
   definition of, 51
   erect, prolonged maintenance of, 57
   examination of, 178
     McKenzie approach, 239–240
     in muscle dysfunction evaluation,
      264–266
   joint positions and, 52, 52f
   leg-length inequality and, 58–59
   line of gravity and, 52, 52f
   lordosis and, 52–53
   lumbar curve analysis of, 54–55, 54f
   muscle action in, 53–54, 53f, 123
   for prevention of back pain, 306–307
   sagittal pelvic tilt and, 53–54
   sexual dimorphism in, 55–56, 56f, 57f
   variations in, 56–58
   in vertebral body growth and
     development, 35–36